A Comprehensive Guide to Degenerative Spine Disorders

Vineet Kumar • Prakhar Mishra
Editors

A Comprehensive Guide to Degenerative Spine Disorders

Springer

Editors
Vineet Kumar
Department of Orthopedic Surgery
Dr. Ram Manohar Lohia Institute of Medical Sciences
Lucknow, Uttar Pradesh, India

Prakhar Mishra
Department of Orthopaedic Surgery
Dr. Ram Manohar Lohia Institute of Medical Sciences
Lucknow, Uttar Pradesh, India

ISBN 978-981-96-9090-9 ISBN 978-981-96-9091-6 (eBook)
https://doi.org/10.1007/978-981-96-9091-6

This Springer imprint is published by the registered company Springer Nature Singapore Pte Ltd.
The registered company address is: 152 Beach Road, #21-01/04 Gateway East, Singapore 189721, Singapore

Foreword

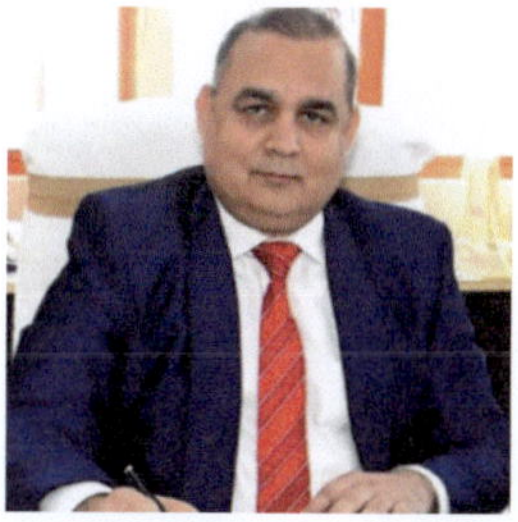

The field of spinal disorders has witnessed remarkable advancements in recent years, yet degenerative spine diseases remain a significant challenge for both patients and healthcare professionals. With an ageing population and a rising prevalence of lifestyle-related spinal conditions, the need for a comprehensive, evidence-based resource on degenerative spine disorders has never been greater. *A Comprehensive Guide to Degenerative Spine Disorders* is a timely and invaluable contribution to the field, offering a detailed exploration of the anatomy, pathophysiology, diagnostic techniques, and evolving treatment modalities for these complex conditions.

I am immensely pleased to introduce this book, edited by Dr. Vineet Kumar, Head of the Department of Orthopaedics at Dr Ram Manohar Lohia Institute of Medical Sciences, Lucknow, and Dr. Prakhar Mishra, Senior Resident, Department of Orthopaedics. Dr. Kumar and his team of esteemed contributors have meticulously compiled a wealth of knowledge, blending fundamental principles with the latest advancements in spinal care. Each chapter is crafted with precision, covering a wide array of topics, from the biomechanics of the spine and the degenerative cascade to non-surgical and surgical treatment approaches. By integrating scientific rigour with clinical relevance, this book ensures that readers gain a holistic understanding of degenerative spine disorders, enabling them to make informed decisions in clinical and personal contexts.

I extend my heartfelt congratulations to Dr. Vineet Kumar and his team for this commendable effort. I am confident that *A Comprehensive Guide to Degenerative*

Spine Disorders will serve as a cornerstone in spinal health, guiding practitioners and patients in navigating these conditions' complexities. I highly recommend this book to all those interested in studying and managing degenerative spine diseases, as it will undoubtedly contribute to enhanced patient care and improved treatment outcomes.

Director, Dr Ram Manohar Lohia Institute of Medical Sciences C. M. Singh
Lucknow, Uttar Pradesh, India

Preface

The human spine, a remarkable structure that provides support, flexibility, and protection to the central nervous system, is also vulnerable to a range of degenerative conditions that can significantly impact an individual's quality of life. As life expectancy increases and sedentary lifestyles become prevalent, degenerative spine disorders emerge as a significant healthcare concern, affecting millions worldwide. These disorders, ranging from degenerative disc disease and spondylolisthesis to facet joint arthritis and spinal stenosis, often lead to persistent pain, mobility issues, and functional limitations. Given the complexity of these conditions and the myriad of treatment options available, there is a pressing need for a comprehensive, accessible resource that addresses the full spectrum of degenerative spine disorders. *A Comprehensive Guide to Degenerative Spine Disorders* is designed to fulfil this need by offering an in-depth exploration of spinal anatomy, the pathophysiology of degeneration, diagnostic approaches, and surgical and non-surgical treatment modalities.

This book aims to bridge the gap between medical expertise and patient education, equipping healthcare providers with evidence-based knowledge while empowering individuals affected by spinal disorders to make informed decisions about their care. Each chapter systematically unpacks essential aspects of spinal health—beginning with the intricate anatomy of the spine, followed by discussions on various degenerative conditions, diagnostic methodologies, and the latest advancements in pain management and surgical interventions. By integrating clinical expertise with a patient-centred approach, this guide aspires to be an indispensable resource for spine specialists, general practitioners, physiotherapists, and patients. Whether you are a healthcare professional seeking to refine your understanding of spinal disorders or an individual striving to regain control over your spinal health, this book provides a roadmap to clarity, comprehension, and effective management.

With an emphasis on both fundamental principles and cutting-edge developments, *A Comprehensive Guide to Degenerative Spine Disorders* is a valuable companion for navigating the challenges of spinal degeneration, fostering a deeper understanding of these conditions, and ultimately contributing to improved patient outcomes and overall well-being.

Lucknow, Uttar Pradesh, India — Vineet Kumar
Lucknow, Uttar Pradesh, India — Prakhar Mishra

About the Book

The book functions as a guidebook, offering valuable insights into the symptoms associated with degenerative spine disorders, the various diagnostic methods available, and a wide array of treatment options. By presenting this information in an accessible manner, the book empowers medical professionals and laypeople to navigate the complexities of these prevalent and often debilitating spine diseases. It delves deep into the core of each disorder, dissecting the underlying causes, unravelling the complexities, and presenting a holistic understanding that goes beyond the surface.

In essence, this comprehensive guide is a vital resource for anyone involved in spinal health. Medical professionals will find it a valuable reference, providing in-depth knowledge and insights to enhance their understanding and treatment strategies. Simultaneously, individuals grappling with degenerative spine disorders will discover a roadmap to comprehend, manage, and navigate the challenges posed by these conditions, ultimately fostering a sense of empowerment on their journey towards spinal health.

Contents

About the Editors

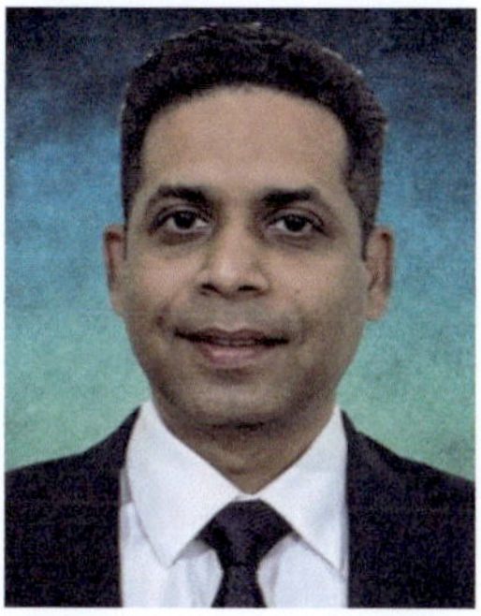

Vineet Kumar (MBBS, MS Orthopaedics) completed his postgraduate studies at King George's Medical College in Lucknow, India. Currently serving as a consultant orthopaedic surgeon and Head of the Department of Orthopaedics at Dr. Ram Manohar Lohia Institute of Medical Sciences in Lucknow, India, he specializes in Spine Surgery. He has contributed significantly to the field, with numerous original research papers published in esteemed international and national journals, alongside delivering scientific presentations at various conferences. He is the recipient of the esteemed B.N. Sinha gold medal K.G.M.U, named after the father of Indian Orthopaedics, and has been honoured with multiple fellowships from organizations such as the Indian Orthopaedic Association, Asia Pacific Orthopaedic Association, and various state orthopaedic associations.

Recognized for his outstanding work, he has received several awards for the best papers and posters at both national and international conferences. A dedicated academic, he is a life member of several national and international academic bodies and has actively participated in research under the Indian Council of Medical Research (ICMR). Additionally, he has authored numerous chapters and books aimed at the training of medical students.

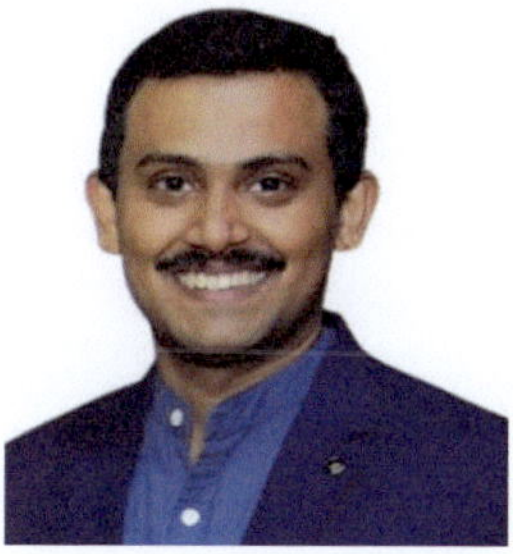

Prakhar Mishra (MBBS, MS orthopaedics, DNB) post-graduated from King George's Medical College, Lucknow, India. He served as a Senior Resident in the Department of Orthopaedics at Dr. Ram Manohar Lohia Institute of Medical Sciences, Lucknow. He is also the recipient of the B.N. Sinha gold medal K.G.M.U. Presently he is working as an Assistant Professor at Department of orthopaedics, Naraina Medical College, Panki, Kanpur.

Introduction to Degenerative Spine Disorders

1

Vineet Kumar and Prakhar Mishra

1.1 Overview

Low back pain is a common and ancient ailment, with its history stretching back thousands of years. The Edwin Smith Papyrus, an ancient Egyptian medical text, is one of the earliest documents that describe spinal disorders (1500 BCE) [1]. It details injuries to the spine and mentions treatments for back pain, such as massage and physical manipulation. Hippocrates, often called the "Father of Medicine", wrote extensively about various ailments, including back pain (c. 460–370 BCE). He advocated for treatments like spinal traction and the use of poultices.

During the Middle Ages, medical knowledge was largely influenced by religious and superstitious beliefs. Treatments for back pain often involved herbal remedies, bloodletting, and prayer. The Renaissance saw a revival of medical knowledge from ancient texts. Anatomists like Andreas Vesalius published detailed works on human anatomy, which helped improve the understanding of the spine and musculoskeletal system.

The Industrial Revolution of the eighteenth and nineteenth centuries led to an increase in manual labour, which in turn led to more cases of back pain. Medical practitioners began to take a more scientific approach to understanding and treating the condition. It was also during this period that Orthopaedics as a medical speciality began to develop, focusing on correcting deformities in bones and muscles. Treatments for back pain included bracing, traction, and rudimentary physical therapy [2].

In the twentieth century, the invention of X-rays, CT scans, and MRI revolutionized the diagnosis of back pain, allowing for better identification of underlying

V. Kumar (✉) · P. Mishra
Dr. Ram Manohar Lohia Institute of Medical Sciences, Lucknow, India

V. Kumar, P. Mishra (eds.), *A Comprehensive Guide to Degenerative Spine Disorders*, https://doi.org/10.1007/978-981-96-9091-6_1

causes such as herniated discs, spinal stenosis, and other spinal abnormalities. The twentieth century saw the rise of physical therapy as a standard treatment for back pain. Techniques such as exercise, stretching, and ergonomic training became widely adopted. Advances in surgical techniques, including minimally invasive surgery, provided new options for patients with severe back pain that did not respond to conservative treatments.

Modern treatment of back pain often involves a combination of physical therapy, medication, lifestyle changes, and in some cases, surgery. There is also a growing emphasis on preventive measures and the management of chronic pain through holistic and integrative medicine. Ongoing research continues to improve the understanding of back pain, with studies focusing on genetics, biomechanics, and the role of psychological factors in chronic pain.

The Global Burden of Disease (GBD) study identifies low back pain as a leading cause of disability worldwide, affecting approximately 9–12% of the global population at any given time and having a lifetime prevalence of around 60–70% in industrialized nations. It is the foremost cause of years lived with disability (YLDs) [3], surpassing conditions like depression and cardiovascular diseases. Low back pain prevalence increases with age and impacts both genders, with a slightly higher incidence in women. Economically, it imposes substantial costs, including direct healthcare expenses and indirect costs from lost productivity and absenteeism, highlighting the need for effective prevention, management, and policy measures to mitigate its global impact.

Degenerative spine disorders represent a spectrum of conditions resulting from the wear-and-tear or age-related deterioration of the spine's anatomical components. These disorders commonly affect the intervertebral discs, facet joints, vertebrae, ligaments, and spinal cord. The prevalence of degenerative spine disorders increases with age, making them a significant health concern in ageing populations.

1.2 Anatomy of the Spine

Vertebral Column

The vertebral column, or spine, is a complex structure composed of 33 vertebrae, segmented into five regions: cervical, thoracic, lumbar, sacral, and coccygeal. These vertebrae are separated by intervertebral discs and are supported by muscles, ligaments, and tendons, providing both stability and flexibility to the body.

- *Intervertebral Discs*

The intervertebral discs (Fig. 1.1) play several critical roles in the spine, contributing to its overall function, flexibility, and stability. Here are the primary functions of intervertebral discs:

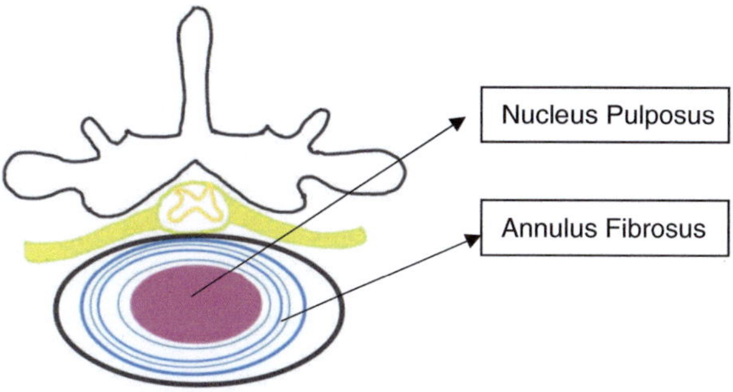

Fig. 1.1 Anatomy of disc and its relation to nerve roots

1. *Shock Absorption*
   Intervertebral discs act as cushions between the vertebrae, absorbing and dissipating the mechanical loads and shocks that the spine experiences during activities such as walking, running, and lifting. This function helps protect the vertebrae and other spinal structures from damage.
2. *Load Distribution*
   The discs help evenly distribute the weight and stresses exerted on the spine. By dispersing the forces, they prevent any single vertebra from bearing too much pressure, which helps maintain the structural integrity of the spine and reduces the risk of injury.
3. *Spinal Flexibility*
   Intervertebral discs contribute to the flexibility and mobility of the spine, allowing for a wide range of movements, including bending, twisting, and flexing. This is due to the unique structure of the disc, which consists of a gel-like nucleus pulposus surrounded by a tough, fibrous annulus fibrosus.
4. *Height and Spacing*
   The discs maintain the proper spacing between the vertebrae, which is essential for the overall height of the spine and the maintenance of spinal curves. This spacing also allows for the exit of spinal nerves from the spinal column through the intervertebral foramina without compression.
5. *Stabilization*
   By maintaining the alignment of the vertebrae, intervertebral discs contribute to the overall stability of the spine. They help keep the vertebrae in place during movement, which is crucial for both structural integrity and the protection of the spinal cord and nerves.
6. *Facilitating Movement*
   The discs allow for slight movement between the vertebrae, enabling the spine to bend and twist while maintaining its structural integrity. The nucleus pulposus permits a degree of movement by shifting within the annulus fibrosus in response to motion and load.

7. *Providing a Hydraulic Cushion*
   The nucleus pulposus, the gel-like core of the intervertebral disc, has a very high water content, typically ranging from 70% to 90% in healthy, young individuals. This water content is essential for its function as a shock absorber and for maintaining disc height and flexibility. In addition to this, the nucleus contains a large amount of proteoglycans, particularly aggrecan, which attract and retain water due to their hydrophilic nature. This allows the nucleus to swell and maintain its turgidity and ability to distribute loads evenly. This property allows the disc to adapt to varying pressures and maintain its height and function under different conditions.
8. *Supporting Posture*:
   Intervertebral discs play a role in maintaining proper posture by supporting the natural curves of the spine. They help sustain the spine's alignment and curvature, which is essential for efficient weight distribution and minimizing strain on the muscles and ligaments.

- *Facet Joints*

Facet joints are located between the pedicle and lamina of the same vertebra, forming articular pillars that stabilize the vertebral column (Fig. 1.2). The vertebral motion segment consists of two adjacent vertebrae, an intervertebral disc, and two facet joints. The posterior part guides spinal movement, with motion determined by facet orientation. Thoracic facets are coronally oriented, limiting extension but allowing rotation, while lumbar facets are sagittal oblique, restricting rotation. The posterior ligamentous complex (PLC), vital for stability, includes the supraspinous and interspinous ligaments, facet capsules, and ligamentum flavum

- *Ligaments and Muscles*

Ligaments play a crucial role in supporting the spine by connecting bones, maintaining stability, and allowing for controlled movement. Key ligaments include the anterior longitudinal ligament (ALL) and the posterior longitudinal ligament (PLL),

Fig. 1.2 Orientation of facet joints

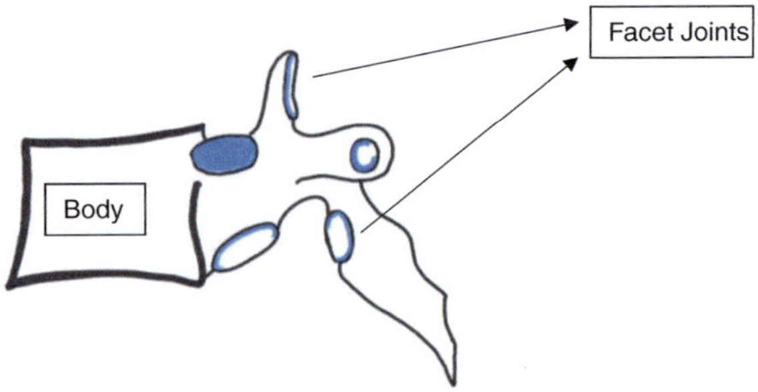

which run along the front and back of the vertebral bodies, respectively, preventing excessive extension and flexion.

The ligamentum flavum, located between the laminae of adjacent vertebrae, helps preserve the normal curvature of the spine and assists in returning it to an upright position after flexion. The interspinous and supraspinous ligaments connect the spinous processes, contributing to the spine's resistance to shear and rotational forces. Additionally, the capsular ligaments surrounding the facet joints stabilize these articulations while permitting necessary movement. Collectively, these ligaments work in harmony to ensure the spine's structural integrity, flexibility, and protection against injury.

1.3 Pathophysiology of Degenerative Spine Disorders

The pathophysiology of degenerative spine disorders involves a complex interplay of mechanical, biochemical, and genetic factors leading to the progressive deterioration of spinal structures. Key components affected include intervertebral discs, facet joints, vertebrae, ligaments, and the spinal cord. Here's an overview of the main pathological mechanisms:

1. *Intervertebral Disc Degeneration*

The intervertebral disc consists of three layers: the fibrous annulus (with outer and inner parts), the central pulpous nucleus, and the terminal plates. This avascular structure is composed of fibrous tissue and cartilage. Microscopically, it contains sparse fibroblast-like cells within an extracellular matrix, which constitutes most of the disc's structure. Both the cells and the matrix are essential for the normal function of the intervertebral disc.

Various factors, such as mechanical, traumatic, genetic, and nutritional influences, significantly contribute to the degenerative process. The fibres in the fibrous annulus become disorganized, and the network of elastin and collagen fibres gradually deteriorates. Cells in the nucleus undergo apoptosis and necrosis, while also exhibiting excessive proliferation. These degenerative changes are common, with up to 50% of cells in an adult intervertebral disc being necrotic.

The primary factor in disc degeneration is the loss of proteoglycans, which degrade into smaller fragments and are lost from the disc tissue. Degenerated discs contain less water, reducing their ability to sustain pressure, leading to bulging and height loss. Proteoglycan loss also impairs the movement of other molecules in and out of the disc matrix. Serum proteins and cytokines infiltrate the matrix, affecting cells and accelerating degeneration.

Pain during the degenerative process arises from a combination of structural and mechanical deformation and the activity of inflammatory mediators. Spinal nerve roots are often involved in the degenerative cascade, causing chronic pain due to compression and the ingrowth of neural endings into the degenerated disc, which are activated by the constant release of inflammatory mediators.

2. *Facet Joint Osteoarthritis*

Lumbar facet joints were first linked to low back and lower extremity pain in 1911, introducing the concept of "facetogenic back pain", now widely recognized but debated. These joints are formed by the articulation of the inferior and superior articular processes of adjacent vertebrae, with their orientation shifting from sagittal at L3 to coronal at S1. This transition helps limit rotation and resist flexion forces.

Each facet joint is innervated by the medial branches of nerves from its level and the one above, which also innervate nearby muscles and ligaments. Facet joints are vital for load transmission, stabilizing flexion/extension, and limiting axial rotation, but are prone to degeneration, often linked to disc disease, especially at L4/L5 and L5/S1.

Factors like disc dehydration, ageing, obesity, poor posture, and prior surgeries accelerate degeneration. This leads to inflammation and pain from overstressed joints and nociceptive nerve stimulation. Trauma and fusion surgery can also worsen facet joint pain.

3. *Spinal Stenosis*

Stenosis refers to the narrowing of a passage or canal. Spinal stenosis involves a progressive, irreversible narrowing of the spinal canal. Patients often experience neurogenic claudication, or limping, after walking due to nerve function disruption. While radicular symptoms can occur, claudication is key in diagnosing spinal canal stenosis (SCS) through:

(a) Claudication limiting leg function
(b) Clinical signs of chronic nerve root compression
(c) Imaging showing stenosis
(d) No vascular impairment in the lower extremities

Neurogenic claudication typically manifests as calf discomfort (pain, numbness, paraesthesia, weakness, tiredness, heaviness), worsened by walking and standing, and relieved only after resting in a flexed lumbar spine position [4].

The most common causes of stenosis are acquired, often resulting from degenerative changes in the central spinal canal, including disc bulging or herniation, osteophyte formation, and thickening of the ligamentum flavum.

At least 50% of patients with SCS eventually require surgery. While conservative measures can provide temporary relief, the degenerative process is relentless, and the spinal canal may continue to narrow. Surgical options include simple canal decompression, wider decompression with facet joint removal, and stabilization procedures for slipped levels, all of which have shown good results.

4. *Spondylolisthesis*

Spondylolisthesis can be classified into several types, with degenerative spondylolisthesis being the most common in adults. It occurs due to the degeneration of intervertebral discs and facet joints, leading to instability and vertebral slippage (Fig. 1.3). This degeneration is influenced by various factors, including ageing, genetics, and biomechanical stress.

The condition leads to mechanical instability, nerve compression, and inflammation, contributing to a spectrum of symptoms, including chronic low back pain, radiculopathy, and neurogenic claudication. A comprehensive approach to diagnosis and management, incorporating conservative treatments, interventional procedures, and surgical interventions, is essential to alleviate pain and improve the quality of life for individuals affected by this debilitating condition. Understanding the complex interplay of factors in spondylolisthesis-related low back pain can guide effective therapeutic strategies and enhance patient outcomes.

5. *Degenerative Scoliosis*

Degenerative scoliosis, also known as adult-onset scoliosis, is a condition characterized by a lateral curvature of the spine that develops due to degenerative changes in the spinal discs and facet joints. This condition is distinct from idiopathic scoliosis, which typically manifests during adolescence. Degenerative scoliosis primarily affects individuals over the age of 50 and is associated with progressive

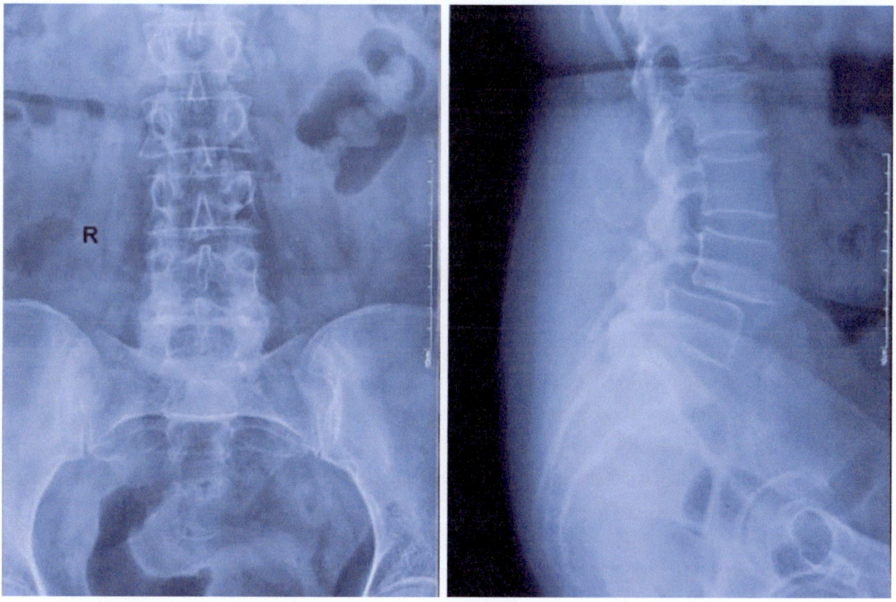

Fig. 1.3 Spondylolisthesis L4-L5

spinal degeneration, which can lead to significant morbidity, including chronic low back pain. Understanding the pathophysiology, clinical presentation, diagnostic evaluation, and treatment options for degenerative scoliosis is crucial for managing this complex condition.

The pathogenesis of degenerative scoliosis is multifactorial, involving a combination of degenerative changes in the intervertebral discs, facet joint arthropathy, and asymmetric loading of the spinal column. The intervertebral discs, composed of the nucleus pulposus and annulus fibrosus, lose hydration and elasticity with age. This disc degeneration leads to a loss of disc height and subsequent vertebral instability.

The facet joints, which are synovial joints that connect adjacent vertebrae, also undergo degenerative changes, including cartilage erosion, osteophyte formation, and subchondral sclerosis. These changes contribute to facet joint hypertrophy and ligamentous laxity, further destabilizing the spine. As the spine degenerates asymmetrically, it can develop a lateral curvature, resulting in scoliosis.

6. *Biochemical and Genetic Factors*

1. *Intervertebral Disc Degeneration*
   - The intervertebral discs are pivotal in maintaining spinal flexibility and absorbing mechanical loads. Genetic variations can affect the integrity and function of these discs. Key genes implicated in disc degeneration include:
     - *COL9A2 and COL9A3*: These genes encode collagen proteins that are essential for the structural integrity of the intervertebral discs. Mutations in these genes can lead to weakened disc structures and increased susceptibility to degeneration.
     - *Aggrecan Gene (ACAN)*: Aggrecan is a major component of the extracellular matrix in intervertebral discs. Variations in the ACAN gene can affect the water-binding capacity of the discs, leading to dehydration and degeneration.
2. *Facet Joint Osteoarthritis*
   - Facet joints are synovial joints that stabilize the vertebrae and facilitate movement. Genetic factors can influence the susceptibility to osteoarthritis in these joints:
     - *Genes Involved in Cartilage Metabolism*: Variations in genes related to cartilage synthesis and degradation, such as those coding for matrix metalloproteinases (MMPs) and tissue inhibitors of metalloproteinases (TIMPs), can contribute to the development of facet joint osteoarthritis.
3. *Spinal Structural Variations*
   - Genetic predisposition can influence the overall structure of the spine, leading to variations that may predispose individuals to LBP:
     - *Congenital Abnormalities*: Genetic mutations can result in congenital spinal abnormalities such as scoliosis, spondylolisthesis, and transitional vertebrae, which can predispose individuals to LBP.

4. *Pain Perception and Inflammatory Response*
   - Genetic variations can affect how individuals perceive pain and respond to inflammation, which are crucial factors in the experience of LBP:
     - *Cytokine Genes*: Variations in genes encoding cytokines such as interleukin-1 (IL-1), interleukin-6 (IL-6), and tumour necrosis factor-alpha (TNF-α) can influence the inflammatory response and pain perception. Elevated levels of these cytokines are associated with increased pain sensitivity and chronic inflammation in the spine.
     - *COMT Gene*: The catechol-O-methyltransferase (COMT) gene influences the metabolism of neurotransmitters involved in pain signalling. Variations in this gene can affect pain sensitivity and the likelihood of developing chronic pain conditions, including LBP.
5. *Heritability of Low Back Pain*: Twin and family studies have provided evidence for the heritability of LBP, suggesting that genetic factors account for a significant proportion of the risk. Heritability estimates for LBP range from 30% to 70%, indicating a substantial genetic component. These studies have shown that individuals with a family history of LBP are more likely to develop the condition themselves.

1.4 Prognosis and Prevention

- *Prognosis*

The prognosis for degenerative spine disorders varies depending on the specific condition, severity, and response to treatment. While some patients experience significant relief with conservative measures, others may require surgical intervention for lasting improvement. Early diagnosis and appropriate management are key to optimizing outcomes.

- *Prevention*

Preventive strategies are essential to mitigate the progression of these degenerative changes and reduce the risk of developing chronic low back pain. Effective preventive measures encompass lifestyle modifications, physical activity, ergonomic practices, and medical interventions. This comprehensive approach can help maintain spinal health and minimize the risk of low back pain.

1. *Lifestyle Modifications*
   (a) *Weight Management*:
      - Maintaining a healthy weight is crucial in reducing the load on the spine. Excess body weight, particularly around the abdomen, increases the stress on the lower back, contributing to disc degeneration and joint wear. A balanced diet and regular physical activity are fundamental in achieving and maintaining a healthy weight.

(b) *Smoking Cessation*:
  - Smoking has been linked to increased risk of degenerative disc disease and low back pain. Nicotine restricts blood flow to the discs and accelerates degeneration. Quitting smoking can improve overall health and reduce the risk of developing spinal conditions.

(c) *Adequate Hydration*:
  - Proper hydration is vital for maintaining the health of intervertebral discs. Discs are composed largely of water, and staying hydrated helps preserve their height and elasticity, reducing the risk of degeneration.

2. *Physical Activity and Exercise*

(a) *Regular Exercise*:
  - Engaging in regular physical activity strengthens the muscles supporting the spine, improves flexibility, and enhances overall fitness. Exercises such as walking, swimming, and cycling are low-impact activities that promote spinal health without excessive strain.

(b) *Core Strengthening*:
  - Strengthening the core muscles, including the abdominal, back, and pelvic muscles, provides better support for the spine. Core exercises (Fig. 1.4), such as planks, bridges, and Pilates, help maintain proper spinal alignment and reduce the risk of injury.

(c) *Flexibility and Stretching*:
  - Maintaining flexibility through regular stretching exercises can prevent stiffness and improve the range of motion. Yoga and specific stretching routines for the back and hamstrings are beneficial in keeping the spine flexible and reducing the risk of low back pain.

(d) *Posture Training*:
  - Proper posture minimizes the strain on the spine. Training oneself to maintain a neutral spine position while sitting, standing, and lifting can

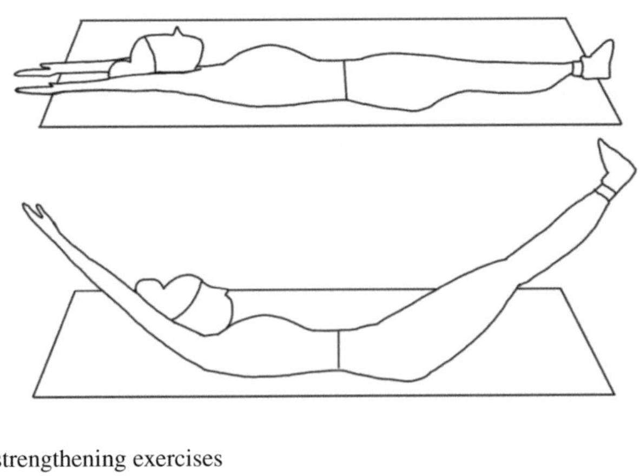

Fig. 1.4 Core strengthening exercises

prevent excessive stress on the intervertebral discs and facet joints. Ergonomic chairs and supportive cushions (Fig. 1.5) can aid in maintaining good posture.

3. *Ergonomic Practices*
   (a) *Workplace Ergonomics*:
   - Ergonomically designed workstations can prevent strain and injury. Adjusting the height of chairs and desks, using lumbar support cushions, and positioning computer screens at eye level are simple modifications that can reduce the risk of low back pain.

   (b) *Proper Lifting Techniques*:
   - Learning and practising proper lifting techniques is crucial in preventing low back injuries. Lifting with the legs rather than the back, keeping the load close to the body, and avoiding twisting motions can protect the spine from excessive strain.

   (c) *Frequent Breaks*:
   - Taking regular breaks to stand, stretch, and move around can prevent the negative effects of prolonged sitting. Implementing a routine of standing or walking for a few minutes every hour can significantly reduce the risk of developing low back pain.

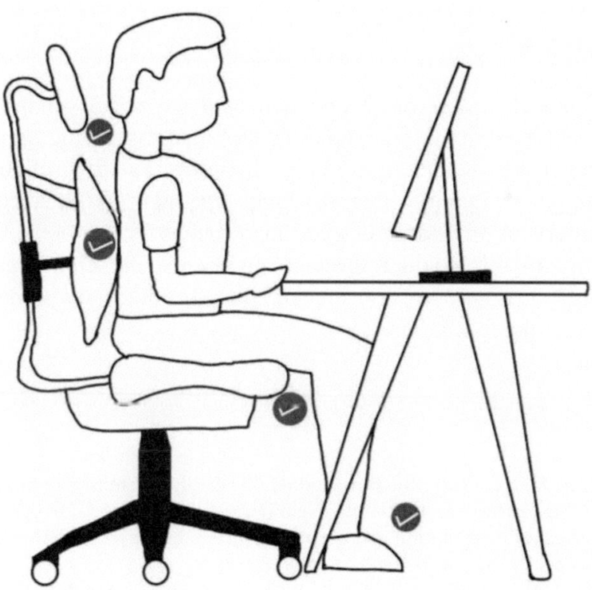

Fig. 1.5 Proper posture for deskwork

4. *Medical Interventions*
   (a) *Regular Check-ups*:
      - Regular medical check-ups can help identify early signs of spinal degeneration. Early detection allows for timely intervention and management to prevent the progression of degenerative changes.
   (b) *Physical Therapy*:
      - Physical therapists can provide personalized exercise programmes and manual therapy techniques to strengthen the spine and improve mobility. Physical therapy is particularly beneficial for individuals at risk of developing low back pain or those experiencing early symptoms.
5. *Educational Programmes*
   (a) *Health Education*:
      - Educational programmes that teach individuals about spine health, risk factors for degenerative conditions, and preventive measures can empower them to take proactive steps in maintaining spinal health.
   (b) *Workplace Training*:
      - Implementing training programmes in workplaces to educate employees on ergonomic practices, proper lifting techniques, and the importance of regular breaks can reduce the incidence of work-related low back pain.

1.5 Conclusion

Degenerative spine disorders are a prevalent and impactful group of conditions, particularly in older adults. Understanding the anatomy of the spine, the pathophysiological mechanisms underlying these disorders, and their clinical manifestations is essential for effective diagnosis and treatment. With a combination of conservative, interventional, and surgical approaches, many patients can achieve significant symptom relief and improved quality of life. Ongoing research and advances in medical technology continue to enhance our ability to manage and prevent these debilitating conditions.

References

1. Van Middendorp JJ, Sanchez GM, Burridge AL. The Edwin Smith papyrus: a clinical reappraisal of the oldest known document on spinal injuries. Eur Spine J. 2010;19:1815–23.
2. Evans DP. Backache: its evolution and conservative treatment: its evolution and conservative treatment. Springer Science & Business Media; 2012.
3. Wu A, March L, Zheng X, Huang J, Wang X, Zhao J, Blyth FM, Smith E, Buchbinder R, Hoy D. Global low back pain prevalence and years lived with disability from 1990 to 2017: estimates from the global burden of disease study 2017. Ann Transl Med. 2020;8(6):299.
4. Wilson CB, Ehni G, Grollmus J. Neurogenic intermittent claudication: chapter 5. Neurosurgery. 1971;18:62–85.

Anatomy of the Spine: Foundation for Understanding Degeneration

2

Ajay Bharti

2.1 Introduction

The spine, also known as the vertebral column, is a crucial structure in the human body, serving as the central support system for skeletal and neuromuscular functions. Structurally composed of 33 vertebrae arranged into five primary regions—cervical, thoracic, lumbar, sacral, and coccygeal (Fig. 2.1)—the spine provides an intricate combination of strength, flexibility, and protection for the spinal cord, which is essential for neural communication between the brain and the rest of the body [1]. The architecture of the spine, with its stacked vertebrae and cushioning intervertebral discs, allows for both stability and mobility, supporting the body's weight, enabling various movements, and absorbing mechanical stress during activities like walking, running, and lifting [2] (Fig. 2.2).

Over time, however, this critical structure undergoes inevitable wear and tear, which can lead to degenerative changes. Spinal degeneration, a process often accelerated by age, lifestyle factors, and mechanical stress, can cause conditions such as degenerative disc disease, spinal stenosis, and spondylosis. These conditions are among the leading causes of chronic back and neck pain, which are significant contributors to disability worldwide [3]. Degenerative changes in the spine can compromise its function, resulting in pain, limited movement, and neurological symptoms due to the compression of nerves within the spinal canal. These symptoms can impact a person's daily activities, quality of life, and ability to work, creating a substantial economic and healthcare burden [4].

Understanding the anatomy of the spine is essential for medical professionals and researchers to effectively diagnose, treat, and prevent degenerative spinal conditions. Anatomical knowledge provides a foundation for identifying structural changes, localizing sources of pain, and designing targeted interventions to restore

A. Bharti (✉)
All India Institute of Medical Sciences (AIIMS), Gorakhpur, India

V. Kumar, P. Mishra (eds.), *A Comprehensive Guide to Degenerative Spine Disorders*, https://doi.org/10.1007/978-981-96-9091-6_2

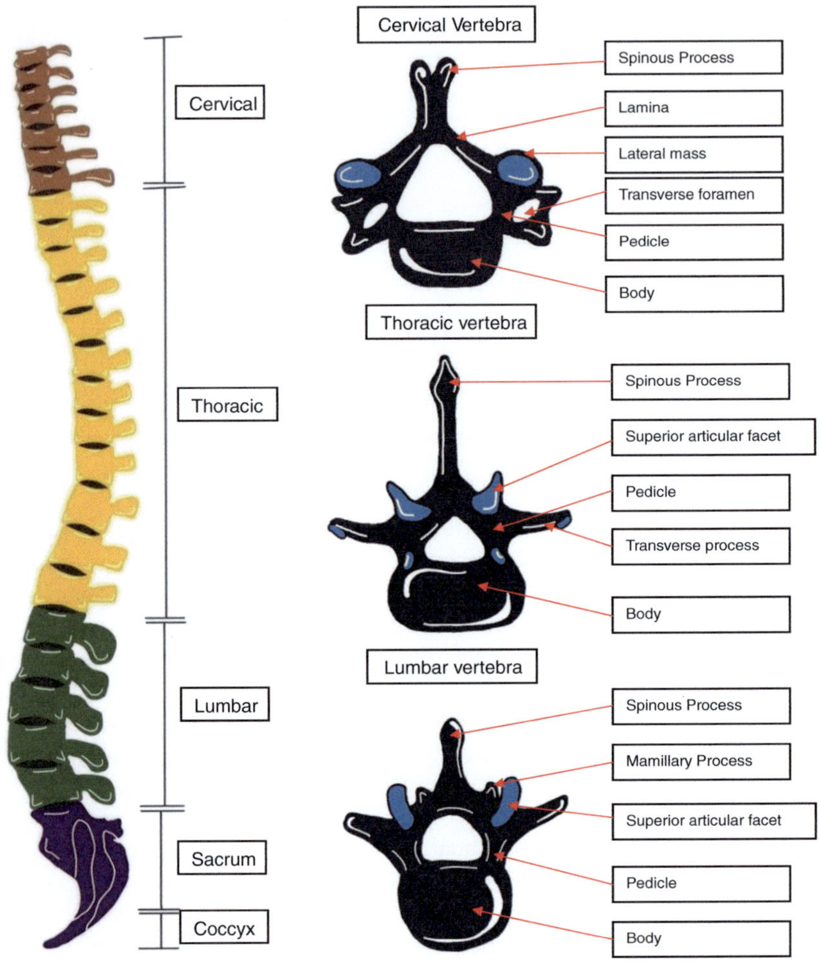

Fig. 2.1 Anatomy of the spine

function or alleviate symptoms [5]. For example, recognizing the unique roles and vulnerabilities of different spinal regions—such as the high mobility of the cervical spine and the load-bearing responsibilities of the lumbar spine—helps clinicians understand why certain areas are more prone to degeneration than others [6]. Table 2.1 depicts an overview of spinal regions and their functions.

In addition, the study of spinal anatomy illuminates the biomechanical interactions between vertebrae, discs, and ligaments that allow for flexibility and stability. Each segment of the spine is tailored to serve specific functions, and these functions affect the ways in which degenerative changes manifest clinically. For instance, degeneration in the cervical spine, due to its role in supporting the head and facilitating a wide range of motion, can lead to neck pain, stiffness, and nerve

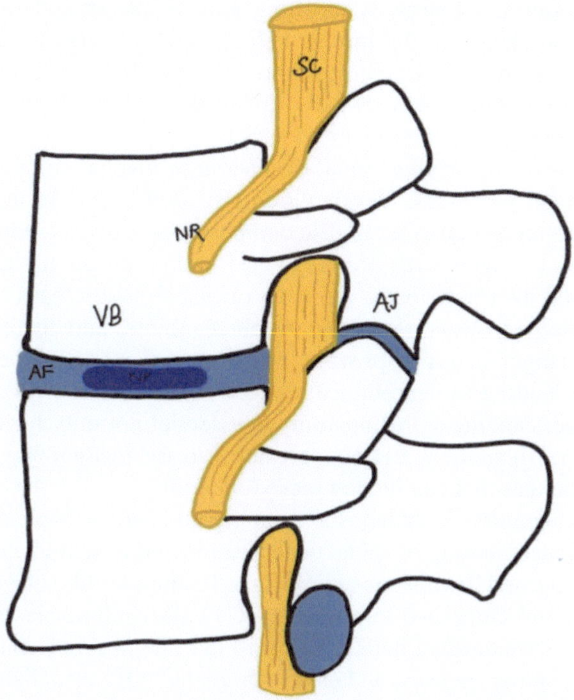

Fig. 2.2 Schematic view of a spinal segment and the intervertebral disc. The figure shows the organization of the disc with the nucleus pulposus (NP) surrounded by the lamellae of the annulus fibrosus (AF) and separated from the vertebral bodies (VB). The figure also shows the relationship between the intervertebral disc and the spinal cord (SC), the nerve root (NR), and the apophyseal joints (AJ)

Table 2.1 Overview of spinal regions and their functions

Spinal region	Vertebrae count	Key functions	Unique features
Cervical spine	7 (C1–C7)	Supports the head, allows for mobility	High flexibility; atlas (C1) and axis (C2) specialized for rotation
Thoracic spine	12 (T1–T12)	Protects thoracic organs, adds stability	Articulates with ribs, limited mobility due to rib cage
Lumbar spine	5 (L1–L5)	Bears most body weight, enabling flexion and extension	Large, robust vertebrae for load-bearing
Sacral spine	5 (fused, S1–S5)	Supports pelvis, transfers load to legs	Fused structure, articulates with pelvis at sacroiliac joints
Coccygeal spine	3–5 (fused)	Minor support, attachment for muscles	Small and triangular, prone to injury rather than degeneration

impingement, often presenting as radiating pain in the shoulders and arms [7]. Meanwhile, degeneration in the lumbar spine, which endures greater mechanical stress from supporting body weight, commonly results in lower back pain and conditions like sciatica, where pain radiates down the legs [8]. Table 2.2 enumerates anatomical differences across spinal regions.

The mechanisms underlying spinal degeneration involve complex biochemical and biomechanical processes. Degeneration typically begins in the intervertebral discs, where age-related changes in disc composition—such as reduced water content and altered collagen structure (Fig. 2.3)—compromise the disc's ability to absorb shock and distribute loads. This loss of disc function leads to further structural deterioration in the surrounding vertebrae, joints, and ligaments [9]. Such degenerative changes can also provoke inflammatory responses, exacerbate pain and potentially leading to neurological deficits if nerve structures are compressed [10]. Thus, understanding spinal anatomy is essential not only for comprehending the mechanics of movement and support but also for recognizing the cascade of degenerative changes that can disrupt these functions.

Recent advancements in diagnostic imaging and biomechanical research have enhanced our understanding of spinal degeneration and have informed the development of preventive and therapeutic approaches. Techniques like magnetic resonance imaging (MRI) and computed tomography (CT) allow clinicians to visualize soft tissue and bone structures in detail, aiding in the diagnosis of conditions such as herniated discs, spinal stenosis, and osteoarthritis [11]. By visualizing the anatomical structures and pathological changes, imaging helps tailor treatments to individual patients' conditions, which may range from conservative management with physical therapy and lifestyle modifications to surgical interventions like discectomy or spinal fusion [12].

Table 2.2 Anatomical differences across spinal regions

Feature	Cervical spine	Thoracic spine	Lumbar spine	Sacral spine	Coccygeal spine
Vertebral body shape	Small, oval-shaped	Heart-shaped	Large, kidney-shaped	Fused into triangular sacrum	Small, fused vertebrae
Movement	High flexibility	Limited rotation, some flexion	Flexion and extension	Minimal movement	Minimal movement
Facet joint orientation	Horizontal (facilitates rotation)	Vertical (limits lateral movement)	Vertical (limits rotation)	Fused	Fused
Unique features	Atlas and axis specialized for head rotation	Articulates with ribs	Thick intervertebral discs for shock absorption	Provides stability for pelvis	Attachment site for pelvic muscles

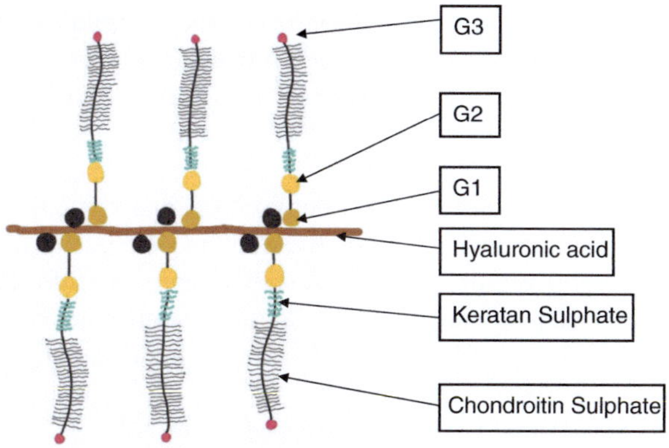

Fig. 2.3 Proteoglycan aggregates entrapped in a collagen fibre network. The proteoglycan aggregates are depicted as a central hyaluronan molecule substituted with aggrecan molecules possessing a central core protein and sulphated glycosaminoglycan side chains. Compressive loading of the spine forces some water from the disc effectively increasing the aggrecan concentration and its swelling potential, and resisting further compression. On removal of the compressive load, disc height is restored as water is drawn back into the tissue to restore the original equilibrium conditions. Any parameter that decreases proteoglycan concentration or weakens the collagen network will be detrimental to disc function

2.2 Overview of Spinal Anatomy

The spine is divided into five distinct regions: cervical, thoracic, lumbar, sacral, and coccygeal. Each region has unique anatomical features that allow it to fulfil specific roles, from supporting the skull to distributing body weight and maintaining structural stability [3].

2.2.1 Cervical Spine

The cervical spine is the uppermost section of the spinal column, comprising seven vertebrae designated C1 through C7. This segment is unique in its function and structure, providing both flexibility and support to the head. As the most mobile part of the spine, the cervical spine allows for a wide range of head movements, including rotation, flexion, extension, and lateral bending. Its role in supporting the head's weight while enabling such dynamic motion makes it particularly susceptible to mechanical stresses and age-related degeneration [1, 2].

Unique Structure of C1 and C2: The Atlas and Axis

The first two cervical vertebrae, C1 and C2, also known as the atlas and axis, are anatomically distinct and specialized for head movement. The atlas (C1) is a ring-shaped vertebra that lacks a body and spinous process, differentiating it from other vertebrae. It forms the atlanto-occipital joint with the occipital condyles at the base of the skull, allowing for the "yes" nodding motion of the head [3]. The axis (C2) has a distinctive bony projection called the odontoid process, or dens, which fits into the atlas and forms the atlanto-axial joint. This joint allows for significant rotational movement, enabling the head to turn from side to side, as in a "no" motion [4].

The atlas and axis are stabilized by a network of ligaments, including the transverse ligament of the atlas, which holds the dens in place, and the alar ligaments, which restrict excessive rotation. While these ligaments provide stability, the flexibility of the atlanto-occipital and atlanto-axial joints contributes to the high mobility and increased vulnerability of this region to trauma and degeneration [5].

Functional and Structural Characteristics of C3 to C7

The remaining cervical vertebrae (C3–C7) exhibit a more typical vertebral structure but are uniquely adapted for mobility and load distribution. Each vertebra has a relatively small body compared to thoracic and lumbar vertebrae, as it only needs to support the weight of the head. These vertebrae have bifid (split) spinous processes, which serve as attachment points for the muscles and ligaments involved in head and neck movement. Additionally, the transverse processes of C3–C7 contain openings called transverse foramina, which house the vertebral arteries that supply blood to the brain. This anatomical feature is unique to the cervical spine and highlights its importance in supporting both structural and vascular functions [6].

The facet joints, also known as zygapophyseal joints, between adjacent vertebrae in the cervical spine are oriented in a way that allows for multidirectional movement. However, this orientation can also contribute to joint degeneration as the facet joints are subjected to repetitive stress during head and neck movements. The intervertebral discs between C3 and C7 provide cushioning and absorb shock, but as they age, they tend to lose water content and elasticity, leading to decreased disc height and increased stress on the facet joints and vertebrae [7].

Age-Related Degeneration and Cervical Spondylosis

The cervical spine is particularly prone to degenerative changes, especially in the lower segments (C5–C7), which bear more mechanical stress due to their load-bearing role and frequent movement [13]. Cervical spondylosis, a common degenerative condition affecting the cervical spine, is characterized by age-related changes in the intervertebral discs, facet joints, and vertebral bodies. Degeneration typically begins in the intervertebral discs, where dehydration and loss of disc height led to increased stress on the adjacent vertebrae and joints. This process can result in osteophyte (bone spur) formation along the vertebral bodies, facet joint hypertrophy, and ligament thickening, contributing to narrowing of the spinal canal and foramina [9].

The narrowing of the spinal canal and foramina can compress the spinal cord and nerve roots, leading to symptoms such as neck pain, radiculopathy (nerve pain radiating into the arms), and even myelopathy (spinal cord dysfunction). Myelopathy is often characterized by weakness, numbness, and difficulty with coordination in the arms and legs. Studies have shown that cervical spondylosis affects a significant portion of the adult population, with prevalence increasing with age. It is estimated that over 85% of individuals over 60 years old show some degree of cervical spondylosis on imaging, even if they are asymptomatic [14].

Common Degenerative Conditions in the Cervical Spine

Degenerative disc disease (DDD) is a hallmark of cervical spine ageing. The intervertebral discs undergo biochemical changes, such as reduced proteoglycan content and collagen breakdown, which diminish their ability to retain water and absorb shock. This loss of disc function can lead to disc bulging or herniation, particularly in the lower cervical segments (C5–C7). A herniated disc can compress nearby nerve roots, resulting in pain, numbness, and tingling that radiates down the arm, a condition known as cervical radiculopathy [15].

Another degenerative condition that affects the cervical spine is facet joint arthritis, which often co-occurs with disc degeneration. As disc height decreases, the facet joints bear more load, leading to cartilage breakdown and joint inflammation. This degeneration can cause neck pain, stiffness, and reduced range of motion. Hypertrophy of the facet joints can further narrow the spinal canal and contribute to cervical spinal stenosis, a condition where the spinal canal becomes constricted, leading to myelopathy [12].

Implications of Cervical Spine Degeneration

The high mobility and structural complexity of the cervical spine make it vulnerable to degenerative conditions that can impact daily function and quality of life. Degenerative changes in the cervical spine can affect posture, balance, and movement, and can also compromise the vertebral artery, leading to vascular symptoms in severe cases. Additionally, cervical spine degeneration is associated with significant healthcare costs and disability, as it can lead to chronic pain and limited functionality. Understanding the anatomical and mechanical factors that predispose the cervical spine to degeneration is essential for developing targeted preventive and therapeutic strategies to mitigate these effects [16] (Fig. 2.4) [13].

2.2.2 Thoracic Spine

The thoracic spine, which consists of twelve vertebrae labelled T1 through T12, forms the central section of the spinal column. Unlike the cervical and lumbar regions, which prioritize mobility to allow for head and torso movement, the thoracic spine is more structurally oriented towards stability. This is largely due to its direct connection with the rib cage, which creates a protective enclosure around vital organs such as the heart and lungs. Each thoracic vertebra articulates with a pair of ribs, and these rib attachments, along with associated ligaments and muscles, restrict movement in the thoracic spine, making it the least mobile of all spinal regions [1, 2].

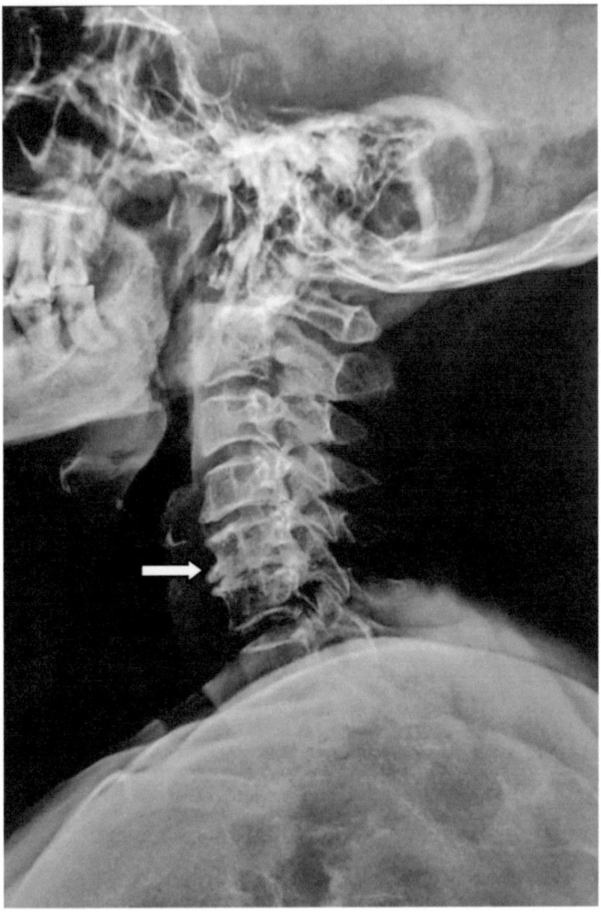

Fig. 2.4 Lateral X-ray of the cervical spine demonstrating severe spondylosis at the levels of C5/C6 with the loss of height of the disc space and osteophyte formation

Structural and Functional Characteristics of the Thoracic Vertebrae

The thoracic vertebrae are distinct from those in the cervical and lumbar regions in terms of shape, size, and functional adaptations. Thoracic vertebrae generally have larger, heart-shaped bodies to support the weight of the upper body and provide a base for the rib cage. The transverse processes of the thoracic vertebrae are longer than in other spinal regions and serve as articulation points for the ribs via costal facets. These costal facets on the sides of the vertebral bodies and the transverse processes enable the thoracic spine to support the rib cage and protect internal organs [17].

The facet joints in the thoracic spine are oriented in a way that favours flexion and extension, with some rotational capability but limited lateral bending. This orientation, combined with the rib attachments, prevents excessive movement and adds stability, which is beneficial for protecting the spinal cord and organs from traumatic forces. The restricted range of motion reduces the mechanical load on thoracic intervertebral discs and facet joints, contributing to a lower incidence of degenerative conditions compared to the cervical and lumbar regions [18].

Reduced Mobility and Degenerative Changes

The relative immobility of the thoracic spine compared to the cervical and lumbar regions means that it is less exposed to the stresses and wear that often lead to degeneration. This reduced mobility, along with the structural support provided by the rib cage, helps protect the thoracic intervertebral discs, facet joints, and vertebrae from excessive mechanical load. As a result, degenerative disc disease (DDD) and osteoarthritis are less common in the thoracic spine than in other spinal regions [18].

However, when degeneration does occur in the thoracic spine, it can lead to conditions that significantly affect posture and function. For example, degenerative changes in the vertebrae and discs can contribute to kyphosis, an exaggerated forward curvature of the thoracic spine. Kyphosis can be particularly problematic in elderly individuals, as it affects posture, reduces lung capacity, and can lead to chronic pain [19].

Common Conditions in the Thoracic Spine

Although degenerative diseases are less frequent in the thoracic spine, specific conditions can still affect this region, especially in older adults. Two of the most common thoracic spinal conditions are kyphosis and vertebral compression fractures. Table 2.3 enlists common conditions in spinal regions.

Table 2.3 Common conditions in spinal regions

Condition	Affected spinal region	Description	Symptoms	Common treatments
Cervical spondylosis	Cervical	Age-related degeneration of discs and joints	Neck pain, radiating arm pain	Physical therapy, medication, surgery
Kyphosis	Thoracic	Abnormal forward curvature of the thoracic spine	Rounded back, stiffness, pain	Bracing, physical therapy, surgery
Disc herniation	Lumbar	Protrusion of disc material compressing nerve roots	Lower back pain, leg pain (sciatica)	Medication, physical therapy, surgery
Sacralization	Sacral	Fusion of L5 with sacrum, altering lumbar mechanics	Lower back pain	Physical therapy, ergonomic modifications
Coccydynia	Coccygeal	Pain and inflammation in the coccyx	Pain when sitting, localized tenderness	Pain relief, physical therapy, coccygectomy (rare)

1. *Kyphosis*
   Kyphosis is a spinal deformity characterized by an abnormal forward curvature of the thoracic spine. This condition can arise from multiple causes, including age-related degenerative changes, osteoporosis, and compression fractures. In elderly populations, kyphosis is often associated with osteoporosis, where decreased bone density weakens vertebrae, making them more susceptible to compressive forces. As vertebral bodies lose height and shape, the spine's natural curvature increases, resulting in a rounded back or "humpback" appearance [19].

Degenerative kyphosis typically occurs as intervertebral discs lose height and elasticity, causing the vertebrae to shift forward. This shift in alignment places stress on the posterior elements of the spine, which can lead to further degenerative changes in the ligaments and facet joints. In severe cases, kyphosis can lead to pain, limited mobility, respiratory issues, and difficulties with balance and gait [8]. Thoracic kyphosis can be diagnosed through physical examination and imaging, such as X-rays, which reveal changes in vertebral alignment and height (Fig. 2.5).

2. *Vertebral Compression Fractures*
   Vertebral compression fractures are among the most common thoracic spine injuries, particularly in older adults with osteoporosis. Compression fractures occur when the vertebral body collapses under pressure, often due to weakened bone structure. These fractures are most common in the thoracic spine, where

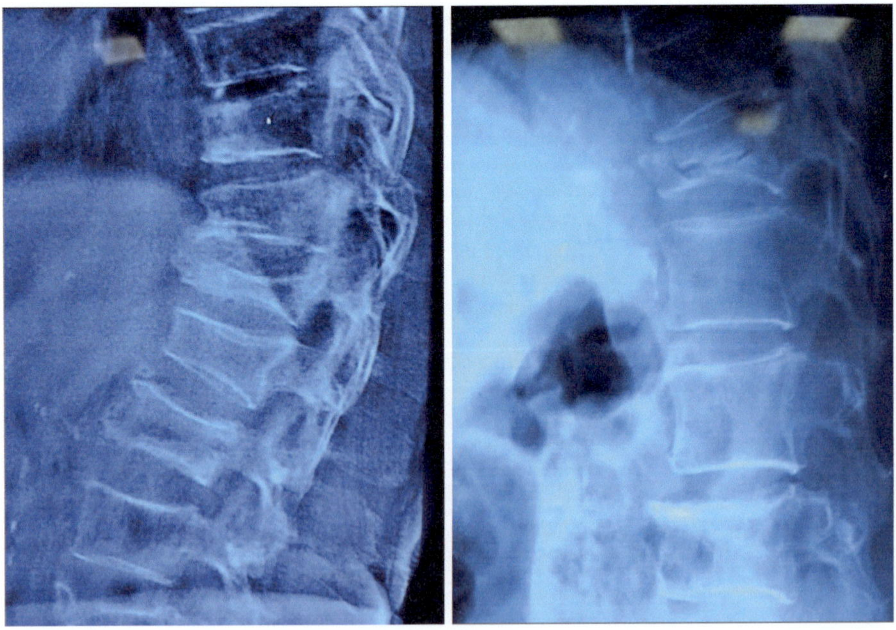

Fig. 2.5 Osteoporotic compression fractures in thoracic vertebra

the vertebrae bear significant loads from the upper body and are less flexible than those in the cervical and lumbar regions. Vertebral compression fractures can cause sudden, sharp pain that worsens with movement and may lead to a gradual loss of height and increased kyphotic curvature if untreated [19].

Compression fractures are often asymptomatic initially, especially in individuals with advanced osteoporosis. However, if multiple fractures accumulate over time, they can result in chronic pain, deformity, and impaired pulmonary function due to the altered thoracic cage shape. Treatment for compression fractures includes pain management, physical therapy, and in severe cases, procedures like vertebroplasty or kyphoplasty, where bone cement is injected into the fractured vertebra to restore height and stability [19].

Clinical Implications of Thoracic Spine Degeneration
Degenerative changes in the thoracic spine, though less common than in other spinal regions, can have significant clinical implications. Kyphosis and compression fractures, in particular, can severely impact quality of life in elderly individuals, particularly concerning in older adults, as diminished respiratory function can contribute to other health complications and exacerbate comorbidities.

Degeneration in the thoracic spine can also impact the upper and lower regions of the spine. For example, kyphotic deformities can lead to compensatory hyperextension in the cervical and lumbar spine, which may accelerate degenerative changes in those regions. This compensatory mechanism often leads to a "forward head" posture and increased lordosis in the lumbar spine, potentially contributing to pain and dysfunction in the cervical and lumbar regions [20].

In summary, the thoracic spine's unique structural characteristics, including its connection to the rib cage, contribute to its relative resistance to degenerative changes. While conditions like kyphosis and vertebral compression fractures can impact the thoracic spine, their prevalence is generally lower than in the cervical and lumbar regions. Understanding the anatomy and mechanics of the thoracic spine is essential for diagnosing and managing these conditions, particularly in ageing populations where bone health and spinal stability are critical.

2.2.3 Lumbar Spine

The lumbar spine, located in the lower back, consists of five vertebrae (L1–L5) that play a critical role in supporting the body's weight and enabling movements such as bending, twisting, and lifting. This region is distinct from the cervical and thoracic spine in both structure and function, as the lumbar vertebrae are the largest and most robust, designed to endure the considerable forces imposed by body weight and physical activity. The lumbar spine's primary functions include weight-bearing, flexibility, and providing stability for the lower body. However, due to the high mechanical loads it sustains, the lumbar region is especially vulnerable to degenerative conditions, which are a major source of lower back pain and disability [5, 21].

Structural and Functional Characteristics of Lumbar Vertebrae

The lumbar vertebrae are structurally unique, with larger and thicker vertebral bodies compared to the cervical and thoracic vertebrae. These vertebral bodies provide a wide base to distribute the load from the upper body, while their large surface area minimizes the risk of fractures under heavy loads. The transverse processes in the lumbar region are also more prominent, serving as attachment points for muscles and ligaments that stabilize and mobilize the spine [22]. Additionally, the spinous processes are shorter and project directly backwards, a feature that accommodates the demands of extension and flexion without restricting movement as much as in the thoracic spine.

The lumbar facet joints, located on the posterior side of the vertebrae, are oriented in a nearly vertical plane. This orientation allows for significant flexion and extension while restricting excessive rotation, which helps protect the intervertebral discs and ligaments from rotational stress. Each lumbar vertebra is separated by an intervertebral disc, which acts as a shock absorber and provides cushioning between vertebrae. The intervertebral discs in the lumbar spine are the thickest of all spinal regions, reflecting their essential role in load-bearing and impact absorption [2].

High Mechanical Loads and Susceptibility to Degeneration

The lumbar spine endures considerable mechanical loads, particularly during activities like lifting, twisting, and bending. These forces create compressive, tensile, and shear stresses on the vertebrae, discs, and facet joints, increasing the risk of degenerative changes over time. As people age, the intervertebral discs undergo biochemical changes, such as reduced water content and collagen degradation, which impair their elasticity and shock-absorbing capacity. This degeneration often leads to a loss of disc height, which in turn alters the load distribution across the vertebrae and facet joints, accelerating wear and tear in the lumbar region [5].

Degenerative conditions in the lumbar spine commonly include degenerative disc disease (DDD), disc herniation, and lumbar spinal stenosis [2]. Degenerative disc disease occurs when the intervertebral discs lose their ability to cushion and distribute loads effectively, causing chronic pain and stiffness. The loss of disc height can lead to instability, prompting the body to form osteophytes (bone spurs) as a compensatory mechanism (Fig. 2.6). Although these osteophytes can provide some stability, they may also narrow the spinal canal or foramen, contributing to nerve impingement and pain [12].

Common Degenerative Conditions in the Lumbar Spine

1. *Lumbar Disc Herniation*
   Disc herniation is a 3common condition in the lumbar spine, particularly at the lower segments (L4-L5 and L5-S1), which endure the most stress during movement and load-bearing. A herniated disc occurs when the nucleus pulposus, the gel-like centre of the disc, protrudes through a tear in the annulus fibrosus, the tough outer layer (Fig. 2.7) [6]. This protrusion can compress nearby nerve roots, leading to symptoms such as lower back pain, numbness, and radiating pain down the legs, a condition known as sciatica [7, 23].

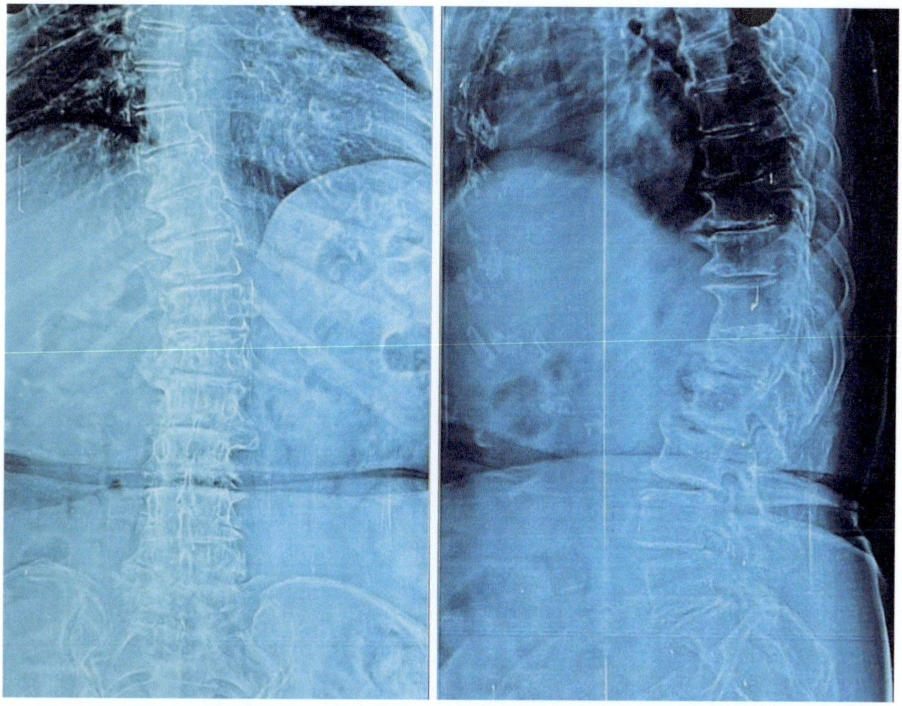

Fig. 2.6 Radiograph of an elderly female dorso-lumbar spine. The radiograph depicts how severe disc narrowing can be associated with vertebral osteophytes, sclerosis of the vertebral endplates, and selective loss of horizontal trabeculae from the vertebral body

Sciatica is one of the hallmark symptoms of lumbar disc herniation and is characterized by sharp or burning pain that travels along the sciatic nerve pathway from the lower back down to the buttocks, thighs, and lower legs. The pain is often exacerbated by movements such as bending or sitting and can significantly affect mobility and quality of life [8]. Risk factors for lumbar disc herniation include age, physical activity levels, and occupations that involve heavy lifting or prolonged sitting.

2. *Lumbar Spinal Stenosis*

   Lumbar spinal stenosis is another common degenerative condition, typically affecting older adults. This condition occurs when the spinal canal narrows due to a combination of disc degeneration, ligamentous thickening, and bone spur formation. The narrowing of the canal can compress the spinal cord or nerve roots, causing pain, numbness, and weakness in the lower extremities [9]. In severe cases, lumbar stenosis can lead to neurogenic claudication, a symptom where pain and weakness in the legs are exacerbated by walking or standing and relieved by sitting or bending forward.

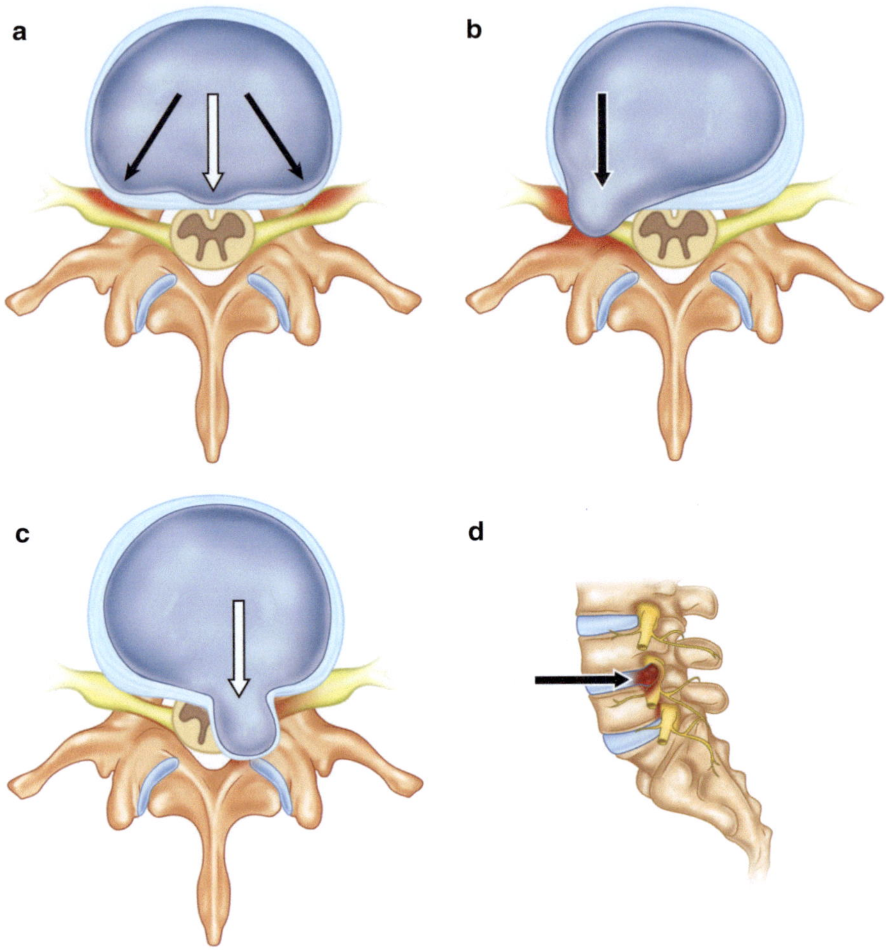

Fig. 2.7 Disc degenerative changes on MRI. (**a**) Bulging disc on axial T2-weighted MRI. (**b**) Right-central disc protrusion demonstrated on axial T2-weighted MRI. (**c**) Subarticular disc extrusion (note that the herniated material is hyperintense, a favourable prognostic sign) observed on T2-weighted MRI. (**d**) Sagittal T2-weighted MRI shows migrated herniation with preserved continuity with the disc

Lumbar spinal stenosis is often progressive, with symptoms gradually worsening over time. Patients with lumbar stenosis frequently report difficulties with activities that require prolonged standing or walking, which can impact daily life and limit physical activity. Treatment options for lumbar stenosis include conservative measures such as physical therapy and anti-inflammatory medications, with surgical decompression considered for severe cases where conservative treatment fails to alleviate symptoms [10, 24].

3. *Facet Joint Arthritis*
   Facet joint arthritis, or facet arthropathy, is common in the lumbar spine due to the increased stress placed on these joints as the intervertebral discs degenerate. As disc height decreases, the facet joints bear more of the load, which can lead to cartilage degradation and inflammation. Facet joint arthritis can cause localized lower back pain, particularly with extension and rotation movements. This condition can also contribute to spinal stenosis if hypertrophic (enlarged) facet joints encroach on the spinal canal or neural foramen, compressing nerve roots [11] (Figs. 2.8, 2.9, and 2.10).

Clinical Implications of Lumbar Spine Degeneration

Lumbar spine degeneration is one of the leading causes of lower back pain, a prevalent and often disabling condition affecting millions of people globally. Lower back pain resulting from lumbar degeneration can range from intermittent, mild discomfort to chronic, severe pain that impacts physical activity, sleep, and mental health. Studies estimate that up to 80% of individuals experience lower back pain at some point in their lives, with lumbar degeneration being a primary contributor, especially in older populations [12].

The symptoms of lumbar degeneration, such as radiating pain, numbness, and weakness in the lower extremities, can significantly affect mobility and independence. Chronic lower back pain can also lead to a cycle of physical inactivity, muscle weakness, and further deterioration of spinal health, creating additional burdens on healthcare systems and economies. Effective management of lumbar spine degeneration is essential to minimize pain, maintain function, and prevent disability in affected individuals [25]. Table 2.4 compares degenerative potential by spinal region.

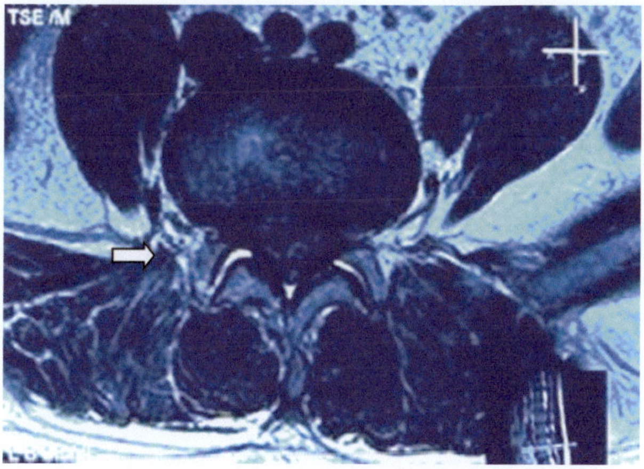

Fig. 2.8 Facet joint degenerative changes. Ligamentum flavum thickening, facet hypertrophy and coronal orientation of facet joints

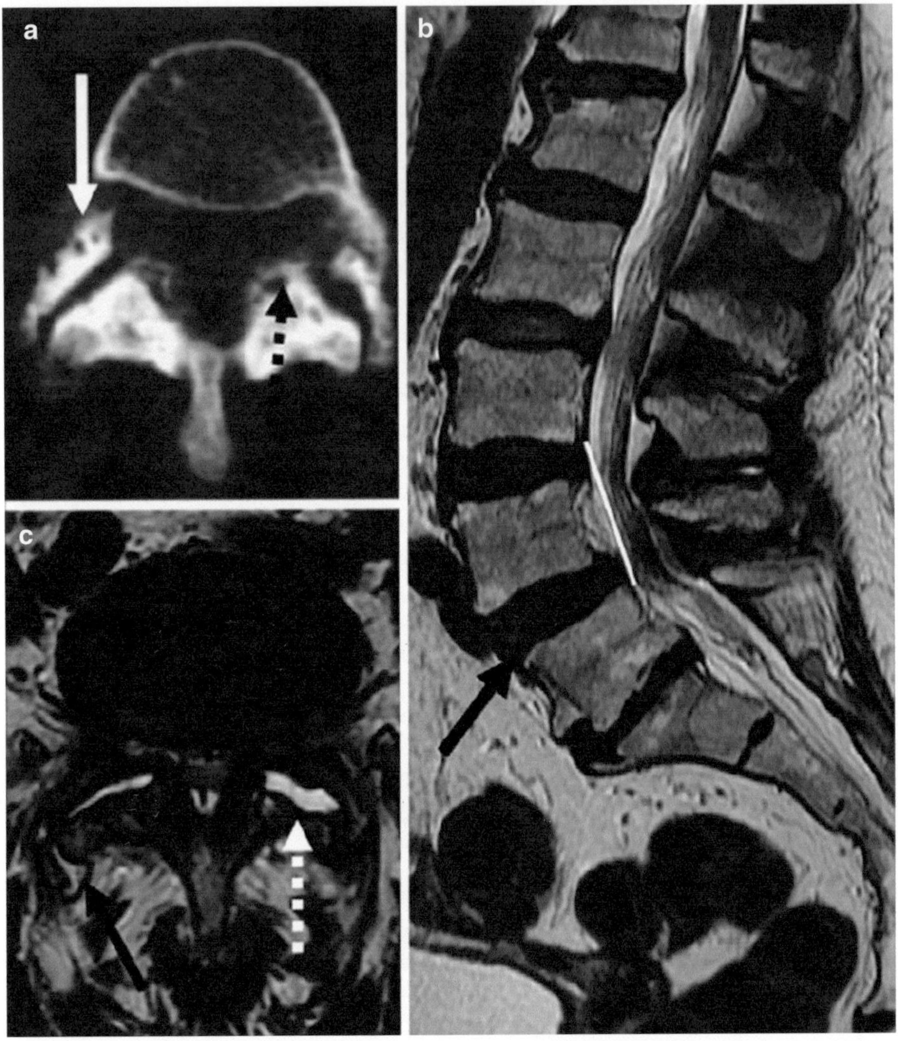

Fig. 2.9 Facet joints osteoarthritis. (**a**) On CT subchondral sclerosis, geodes and widening of the joint rim (white arrow) are demonstrated. Calcification of the ligamentum flavum is also evident (dotted black arrow). (**b**) On MRI, bone abnormalities are less clear but the examination is more accurate for visualization of ligament thickening and articular space widening. Lateral stenosis is well demonstrated. Note the right posterior synovial cyst (black arrow). (**c**) Sagittal Fast Spin-Echo T2-weighted sequence shows L4 low-grade spondylolisthesis. Note also anterior osteophytes in L5-S1

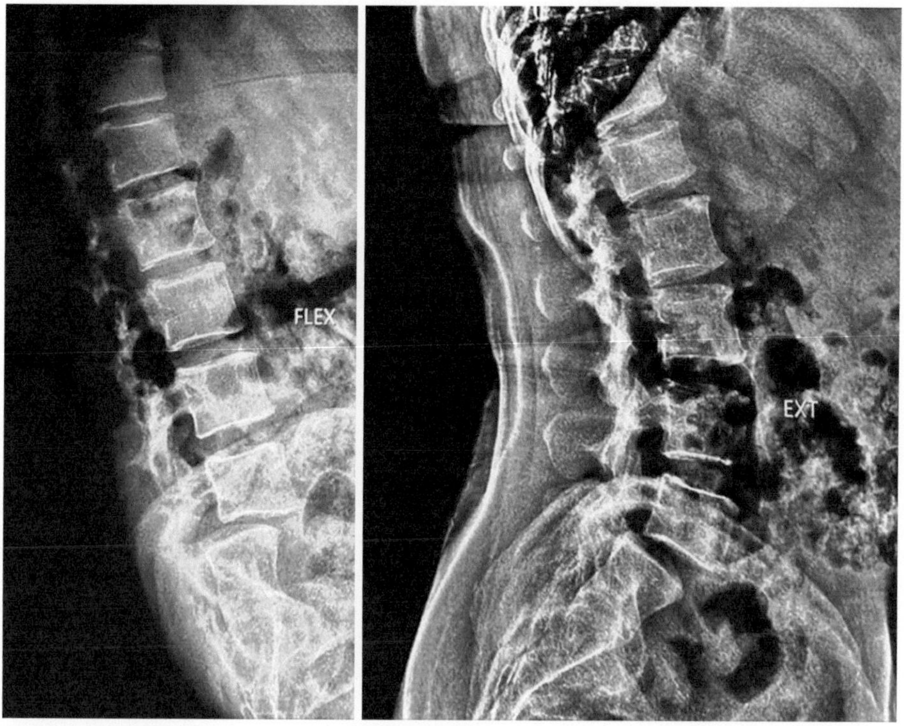

Fig. 2.10 Degenerative spondylolisthesis. Dynamic radiographs. Note the increase of vertebral slippages during flexion

Prevention and Management of Lumbar Spine Degeneration

Prevention of lumbar degeneration focuses on minimizing risk factors and promoting a healthy lifestyle that supports spinal health. Core-strengthening exercises, regular physical activity, weight management, and proper ergonomics in lifting and posture are critical for reducing the risk of lumbar spine degeneration. Smoking cessation and maintaining adequate hydration are also important, as they contribute to disc health and help prevent early degeneration [26].

Management of lumbar degeneration often starts with conservative measures such as physical therapy, anti-inflammatory medications, and lifestyle modifications. Physical therapy focuses on strengthening core and back muscles to support the lumbar spine, which can help reduce pain and improve stability. For individuals with severe symptoms unresponsive to conservative treatments, surgical options such as laminectomy, discectomy, or spinal fusion may be considered. These procedures aim to relieve pressure on nerve roots, stabilize the spine, and restore function, but they are generally reserved for cases where nonsurgical treatments have proven ineffective [26].

Table 2.4 Comparison of degenerative potential by spinal region

Spinal region	Degenerative risk	Common degenerative conditions	Typical symptoms
Cervical spine	High	Cervical spondylosis, disc herniation	Neck pain, arm pain, numbness
Thoracic spine	Moderate to low	Kyphosis, compression fractures	Mid-back pain, rounded posture
Lumbar spine	High	Degenerative disc disease, spinal stenosis, facet joint arthritis	Lower back pain, leg pain (sciatica)
Sacral spine	Low	Sacralization, sacroiliac joint dysfunction	Lower back pain, pelvic instability
Coccygeal spine	Very low	Coccydynia	Tailbone pain, worsens with sitting

2.2.4 Sacral and Coccygeal Spine

The sacral and coccygeal regions are located at the base of the spine and play a vital role in supporting the pelvis, distributing body weight, and providing structural stability for the lower body. Although not as mobile as the other regions of the spine, these sections are essential for maintaining an upright posture, supporting movements such as sitting, and serving as points of attachment for various muscles and ligaments involved in movement and balance [27].

The Sacrum

The sacrum is a triangular-shaped bone (Fig. 2.11) formed by the fusion of five sacral vertebrae (S1–S5) during late adolescence to early adulthood. Unlike the cervical, thoracic, and lumbar regions, the sacral vertebrae are fused into a single, solid structure, which provides stability and supports the upper body's weight as it is transferred to the pelvic girdle and lower limbs. This fusion results in a strong and rigid bone that can withstand significant forces without the risk of the degenerative processes commonly observed in the more mobile regions of the spine [28].

Anatomically, the sacrum connects the spine to the iliac bones of the pelvis at the sacroiliac joints. These joints bear substantial load and are key to maintaining stability during weight-bearing activities like walking, running, and sitting. The sacrum's broad, concave shape fits securely between the iliac bones, creating a stable base for the spine. The sacral promontory, the uppermost part of the sacrum, articulates with the fifth lumbar vertebra (L5), forming the lumbosacral junction. This junction is critical for transferring loads from the upper body to the sacrum and pelvis, which helps maintain balance and proper posture [28].

The sacral canal, a continuation of the vertebral canal, houses the sacral nerves, which exit through foramina on either side of the sacrum to innervate the lower body, including the pelvis, legs, and feet. Damage or degeneration within the sacral region can compress these nerves, potentially leading to conditions such as sacral radiculopathy, although this is relatively rare given the sacrum's fused structure

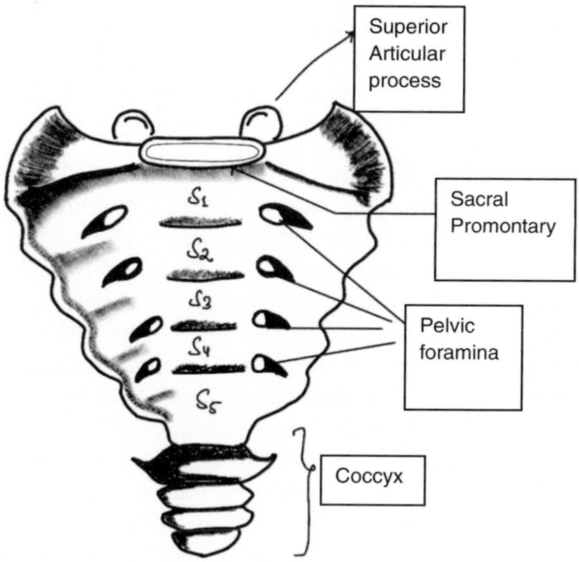

Fig. 2.11 Anterior view of sacrum and coccyx

[27]. Unlike the more mobile regions of the spine, the sacrum's stability makes it less prone to degenerative changes, although trauma or congenital abnormalities can affect its function.

The Coccyx

The coccyx, commonly referred to as the tailbone, is a small, triangular bone at the very base of the spinal column, directly below the sacrum. It typically comprises three to five small, partially fused vertebrae. While the coccyx has minimal weight-bearing function, it serves as an attachment point for several muscles, tendons, and ligaments, including those involved in pelvic floor support, sitting balance, and the movements of the hip joint [5].

The coccyx is relatively immobile compared to other regions of the spine, but it can move slightly when pressure is applied, such as during sitting. This minor movement is enabled by the fibrocartilaginous joint between the coccyx and the sacrum, as well as the ligaments connecting the coccyx to the sacrum. Unlike the other spinal regions, the coccyx does not experience significant degenerative changes because of its limited mobility. However, it is more susceptible to injury, particularly from falls or prolonged pressure during activities like cycling or extended sitting on hard surfaces. Injuries to the coccyx can result in a condition known as coccydynia, characterized by localized pain and tenderness that may be aggravated by sitting or certain movements [7].

Clinical Conditions of the Sacral and Coccygeal Spine

While the sacral and coccygeal spine are not prone to degeneration in the way that other spinal regions are, they are vulnerable to specific injuries and conditions that can cause significant discomfort and functional limitations (Table 2.5).

1. *Sacralization and Lumbosacral Transitional Vertebrae (LSTV)*
   Sacralization is a congenital condition where the fifth lumbar vertebra (L5) is partially or completely fused to the sacrum. This results in an anatomical variation known as a lumbosacral transitional vertebra (LSTV). Sacralization can alter the mechanics of the lumbosacral junction, potentially leading to lower back pain or altered load distribution on the lumbar spine. Individuals with sacralization may be at increased risk of developing degenerative changes in the lumbar region due to the altered biomechanics at the lumbosacral junction [29].
2. *Coccydynia*
   Coccydynia, or tailbone pain, is a condition characterized by inflammation and pain in the coccyx. It is commonly caused by trauma, such as a fall that directly impacts the tailbone, or repetitive strain from activities that place prolonged pressure on the coccyx, such as cycling or extended sitting. In some cases, coccydynia can also arise from childbirth, where the coccyx can be strained or even fractured during labour. Treatment typically involves pain management, ergonomic adjustments, and, in severe cases, interventions like corticosteroid injections or surgical removal of the coccyx (coccygectomy) [30].
3. *Sacral Fractures*
   Sacral fractures, although uncommon, can occur due to high-impact trauma, such as falls or car accidents, or as a result of weakened bone from conditions like osteoporosis. Sacral fractures are often stable due to the fused nature of the

Table 2.5 Conditions affecting sacral and coccygeal spine

Condition	Description	Causes	Symptoms	Treatment options
Sacralization	Fusion of L5 with sacrum, forming a lumbosacral transitional vertebra	Congenital condition	Lower back pain, altered mobility	Physical therapy, ergonomic adjustments
Sacroiliac joint dysfunction	Dysfunction in the sacroiliac joint between sacrum and pelvis	Trauma, arthritis, pregnancy	Lower back/ buttock pain, leg pain	Physical therapy, joint injections
Coccydynia	Pain and inflammation in the coccyx, often after trauma	Falls, prolonged sitting, childbirth	Pain in tailbone, worse with sitting	Pain management, injections, coccygectomy (rare)
Sacral fractures	Fracture in the sacrum, often stable due to fusion	Trauma, osteoporosis	Lower back pain, difficulty walking	Pain management, physical therapy, surgery (if severe)

sacral vertebrae, but they can cause significant pain and impair mobility. In cases of severe or displaced fractures, surgical fixation may be required to stabilize the sacrum and promote healing [31] (Figs. 2.12, 2.13, and 2.14) [31].

4. *Sacroiliac Joint Dysfunction*
   While not a direct pathology of the sacral vertebrae, sacroiliac joint dysfunction is a condition that affects the joints connecting the sacrum to the pelvis. Dysfunction in these joints can lead to pain in the lower back, buttocks, and legs. Sacroiliac joint pain is often exacerbated by activities that place asymmetrical stress on the pelvis, such as climbing stairs, prolonged standing, or shifting weight from one leg to the other. Treatment options include physical therapy, pain relief medications, and, in some cases, sacroiliac joint injections for inflammation relief [32].

Functional Significance and Stability of the Sacral and Coccygeal Spine
The sacral and coccygeal spine's main functions are to provide structural stability to the pelvis, enable effective weight distribution, and serve as anchor points for ligaments and muscles that aid in movement and support of the lower body. The sacrum's fusion and integration with the pelvis make it a strong and stable structure, minimizing the risk of degenerative changes and ensuring that it can withstand the forces exerted during weight-bearing activities. Additionally, the coccyx's role, though limited, is vital for sitting stability and pelvic floor function, which are essential for postural support and balance [33].

Unlike other spinal regions, the sacral and coccygeal spine experience limited mobility, which contributes to their resilience against degeneration. Their susceptibility to injury, however, underscores the importance of understanding the role of biomechanics, anatomy, and preventive care, particularly for those engaged in activities that place stress on the tailbone or pelvic region.

In summary, the sacral and coccygeal spine are specialized structures that provide foundational support for the pelvis and lower body. While they are less prone to degenerative changes, they are vulnerable to specific injuries and congenital variations that can lead to pain and functional impairment. Recognizing the unique structural characteristics and potential conditions associated with these regions is

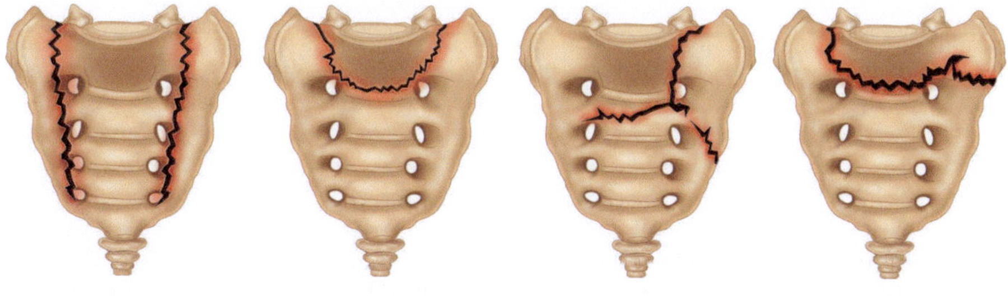

Fig. 2.12 Four combined sacral fracture types: (**a**) H-shaped; (**b**) U-shaped; (**c**) Lambda-shaped (λ); (**d**) T-shaped

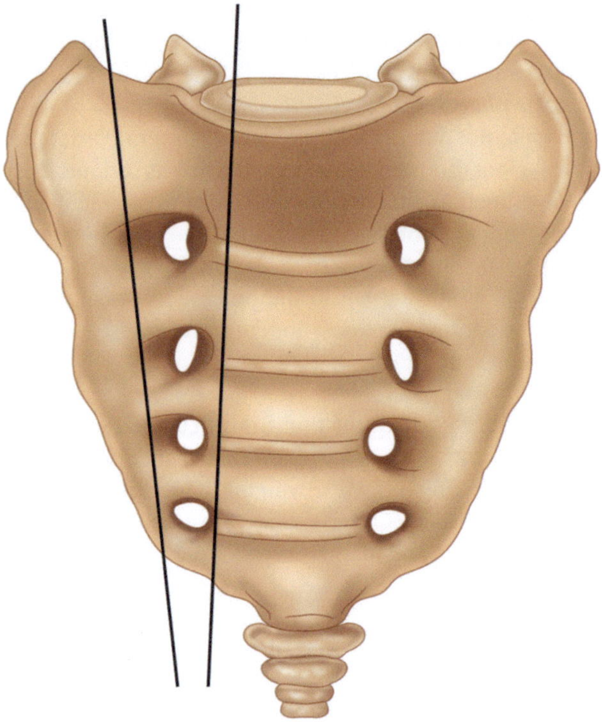

Fig. 2.13 Denis classification: Zone I fracture involves the sacral ala lateral to the foramina; zone II fracture at the level of the foramina; and zone III fracture affects the sacral canal medial to the neural foramina

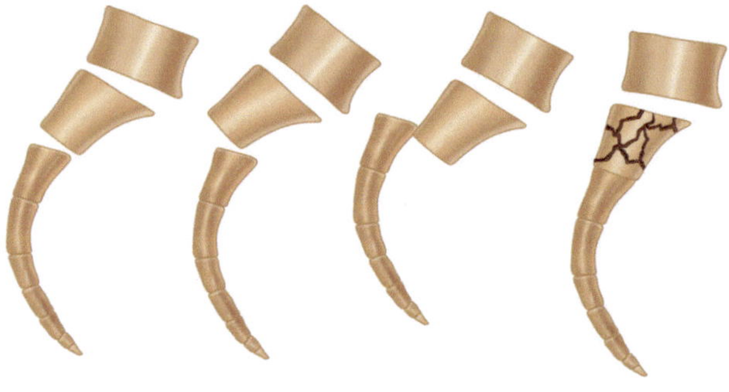

Fig. 2.14 Roy-Camille classification: Type I fractures show kyphotic angulation only; type II fractures demonstrate both kyphosis and retrolisthesis; type III fractures have complete anterior listhesis; and type IV fractures characterized by severe comminution of the S1 body

essential for managing lower spinal health and ensuring effective treatment for related disorders.

2.3 Conclusion

The anatomy of the spine provides a critical framework for understanding the progression of degenerative spinal conditions. Degeneration in the spine is a multifactorial process influenced by ageing, biomechanics, and lifestyle factors. An in-depth understanding of spinal anatomy and biomechanics is essential for recognizing degenerative patterns, predicting clinical manifestations, and applying targeted interventions. Through a combination of lifestyle changes, conservative therapies, and, when necessary, surgical intervention, the impact of spinal degeneration on quality of life can be minimized. Continuing research on the molecular and cellular underpinnings of spinal degeneration holds promise for innovative therapeutic approaches that may prevent or even reverse degenerative changes in the future. (Hand drawn Images Courtesy: Dr. Prakhar Mishra, Senior Resident, Dr. Ram Manohar Lohia Institute of Medical Sciences, Lucknow, India.)

References

1. Bogduk N. Biomechanics of the cervical spine. In: Physical therapy of the cervical and thoracic spine. Churchill Livingstone; 2002. p. 26–44.
2. Adams MA, Roughley PJ. What is intervertebral disc degeneration, and what causes it? Spine. 2006;31(18):2151–61. https://doi.org/10.1097/01.brs.0000231761.73859.2c.
3. Hoy D, March L, Brooks P, Blyth F, Woolf A, Bain C, Williams G, Smith E, Vos T, Barendregt J, Murray C. The global burden of low back pain: estimates from the global burden of disease 2010 study. Ann Rheum Dis. 2014;73(6):968–74.
4. Katz JN. Lumbar disc disorders and low-back pain: socioeconomic factors and consequences. JbJs. 2006;88(suppl_2):21–4.
5. Dagenais S, Caro J, Haldeman S. A systematic review of low back pain cost of illness studies in the United States and internationally. Spine J. 2008;8(1):8–20.
6. Gallucci M, Limbucci N, Paonessa A, Splendiani A. Degenerative disease of the spine. Neuroimaging Clin N Am. 2007;17(1):87–103. https://doi.org/10.1016/j.nic.2007.01.002.
7. Frymoyer JW. Lumbar disk disease: epidemiology. Instr Course Lect. 1992;41:217–23.
8. Goode AP, Carey TS, Jordan JM. Low back pain and lumbar spine osteoarthritis: how are they related? Curr Rheumatol Rep. 2013;15:1–8.
9. Urban JP, Roberts S. Degeneration of the intervertebral disc. Arthritis Res Ther. 2003;5:1–1.
10. Le Maitre CL, Hoyland JA, Freemont AJ. Catabolic cytokine expression in degenerate and herniated human intervertebral discs: IL-1β and TNFα expression profile. Arthritis Res Ther. 2007;9:1–1.
11. Modic MT, Ross JS. Lumbar degenerative disk disease. Radiology. 2007;245(1):43–61.
12. Weinstein JN, Tosteson TD, Lurie JD, Tosteson AN, Blood E, Hanscom B, Herkowitz H, Cammisa F, Albert T, Boden SD, Hilibrand A. Surgical versus nonsurgical therapy for lumbar spinal stenosis. N Engl J Med. 2008;358(8):794–810.
13. Lee BS, Benzel EC. Cervical spine biomechanics. In: Kaiser M, Haid R, Shaffrey C, Fehlings M, editors. Degenerative cervical myelopathy and radiculopathy. Cham: Springer; 2019. https://doi.org/10.1007/978-3-319-97952-6_2.
14. Wang XR, Kwok TCY, Griffith JF, Man Yu BW, Leung JCS, Wáng YXJ. Prevalence of cervical spine degenerative changes in elderly population and its weak association with aging, neck pain, and osteoporosis. Ann Transl Med. 2019;7(18):486. https://doi.org/10.21037/atm.2019.07.80. PMID: 31700922; PMCID: PMC6803181.
15. Caridi JM, Pumberger M, Hughes AP. Cervical radiculopathy: a review. HSS J. 2011;7(3):265–72. https://doi.org/10.1007/s11420-011-9218-z. Epub 2011 Sep 9. PMID: 23024624; PMCID: PMC3192889.
16. Jaumard NV, Welch WC, Winkelstein BA. Spinal facet joint biomechanics and mechanotransduction in normal, injury and degenerative conditions. J Biomech Eng. 2011;133(7):071010. https://doi.org/10.1115/1.4004493. PMID: 21823749; PMCID: PMC3705911.

17. Cramer GD, Darby SA. Clinical anatomy of the spine, spinal cord, and ANS. 3rd ed. St. Louis: Mosby; 2014.
18. Iorio JA, Jakoi AM, Singla A. Biomechanics of degenerative spinal disorders. Asian Spine J. 2016;10(2):377–84. https://doi.org/10.4184/asj.2016.10.2.377. Epub 2016 Apr 15. PMID: 27114783; PMCID: PMC4843079.
19. Ailon T, Shaffrey CI, Lenke LG, Harrop JS, Smith JS. Progressive Spinal Kyphosis in the aging population. Neurosurgery. 2015;77:S164–72. https://doi.org/10.1227/NEU.0000000000000944.
20. Joshi S, Balthillaya G, Neelapala YVR. Thoracic posture and mobility in mechanical neck pain population: a review of the literature. Asian Spine J. 2019;13(5):849–60. https://doi.org/10.31616/asj.2018.0302. PMID: 31154701; PMCID: PMC6773982.
21. Bogduk N, Mercer S. Biomechanics of the lumbar spine. Clin Biomech. 2000;15(9):633–48.
22. Waxenbaum JA, Reddy V, Williams C, et al. Anatomy, back, lumbar vertebrae [Updated 2023 Jul 30]. In: StatPearls [Internet]. Treasure Island: StatPearls Publishing; 2024. Available from: https://www.ncbi.nlm.nih.gov/books/NBK459278/.
23. Pal GP, Routal RV. Transmission of weight through the lower thoracic and lumbar regions of the vertebral column in man. J Anat. 1987;152:93–105. PMID: 3654379; PMCID: PMC1261749.
24. Wu L, Munakomi S, Cruz R. Lumbar spinal stenosis [Updated 2024 Jan 30]. In: StatPearls [Internet]. Treasure Island: StatPearls Publishing; 2024. Available from: https://www.ncbi.nlm.nih.gov/books/NBK531493/.
25. Donnally CJ III, DiPompeo CM, Varacallo M. Vertebral compression fractures [Updated 2023 Aug 4]. In: StatPearls [Internet]. Treasure Island: StatPearls Publishing; 2024. Available from: https://www.ncbi.nlm.nih.gov/books/NBK448171/.
26. Rainville J, Nguyen R, Suri P. Effective conservative treatment for chronic low back pain. Semin Spine Surg. 2009;21(4):257–63. https://doi.org/10.1053/j.semss.2009.08.009. PMID: 20161564; PMCID: PMC2805825.
27. Sattar MH, Guthrie ST. Anatomy, back, sacral vertebrae [Updated 2023 Jul 30]. In: StatPearls [Internet]. Treasure Island: StatPearls Publishing; 2024. Available from: https://www.ncbi.nlm.nih.gov/books/NBK551653/.
28. Panjabi MM, White AA 3rd. Basic biomechanics of the spine. Neurosurgery. 1980;7(1):76–93. https://doi.org/10.1227/00006123-198007000-00014.
29. Pal GP. Weight transmission through the sacrum in man. J Anat. 1989;162:9–17. PMID: 2808126; PMCID: PMC1256432.
30. Garg B, Ahuja K. Coccydynia-A comprehensive review on etiology, radiological features and management options. J Clin Orthop Trauma. 2021;12(1):123–9. https://doi.org/10.1016/j.jcot.2020.09.025. Epub 2020 Sep 24. Erratum in: J Clin Orthop Trauma. 2021;21:101561. https://doi.org/10.1016/j.jcot.2021.101561. PMID: 33716437; PMCID: PMC7920198.
31. Santolini E, Kanakaris NK, Giannoudis PV. Sacral fractures: issues, challenges, solutions. EFORT Open Rev. 2020;5(5):299–311. https://doi.org/10.1302/2058-5241.5.190064. PMID: 32509335; PMCID: PMC7265089.
32. Raj MA, Ampat G, Varacallo M. Sacroiliac joint pain [Updated 2023 Aug 14]. In: StatPearls [Internet]. Treasure Island: StatPearls Publishing; 2024. Available from: https://www.ncbi.nlm.nih.gov/books/NBK470299/.
33. Mostafa E, Varacallo M. Anatomy, back, coccygeal vertebrae [Updated 2023 Jun 5]. In: StatPearls [Internet]. Treasure Island: StatPearls Publishing; 2024. Available from: https://www.ncbi.nlm.nih.gov/books/NBK549870/.

Common Types of Degenerative Spinal Disorders: An Overview

3

Vishal Kumar and Manoj Kumar

3.1 Introduction

Degenerative spinal conditions involve a Degeneration of normal spinal structure and normal functioning in the spine. As the word Degenerative suggests, the cause of these changes is age-related wear and tear. The changes are not due to trauma, infections, or some other reason. Degenerative disorders of spine are a major cause of morbidity in the aging population. The condition is common in older adults. After the age of 40, most people experience some spinal degeneration [1]. Prevalence of low back ache is rising due to the obesity epidemic and increased life expectancy [2]. Low back pain is also a leading cause of lost workdays, impacting the economy. These disorders are characterised by progressive deterioration of structural and functional integrity of the spine which leads to pain, disability, and reduced quality of life.

According to a 2018 meta-analysis by Vijay M. Ravindra et al., 266 million people (3.63% of the global population) have lower back pain (LBP) and lumbar degenerative spinal disease (DSD) annually. Low- and middle-income countries had four times as many instances as high-income countries based on population sizes. Spondylolisthesis was seen in 39 million people (0.53%), spinal stenosis in 103 million people (1.41%), and symptomatic disc degeneration in 403 million people (5.5%) per year [3].

The two neighbouring vertebral bodies and the intervertebral disc, which together make up the functional spinal unit, are prone to degeneration. A tri-joint complex is made up of the disc and two zygapophyseal joints that are located on the same level. Humans experience both macro- and micro-traumas as they age, and these changes cause the biomechanical forces acting on the lumbar spine to shift and redistribute unevenly [4].

V. Kumar · M. Kumar (✉)
Department of Orthopaedics, PGIMER, Chandigarh, India

V. Kumar, P. Mishra (eds.), *A Comprehensive Guide to Degenerative Spine Disorders*, https://doi.org/10.1007/978-981-96-9091-6_3

Degenerative changes in the spine can affect every structure of the spine, i.e., discs, bone and cartilages, ligaments, etc. In this chapter, discussion is mainly focused on the overview of the most common types of degenerative spinal disorders, including their pathophysiology, clinical presentation, diagnostic approach, and management strategies [5].

The differential diagnosis for back pain varies by spinal region. In the cervical spine, potential causes include rheumatic diseases (like rheumatoid arthritis and ankylosing spondylitis), trauma, regional conditions (such as myofascial pain and osteomyelitis), bone disorders (like osteoporosis and metastatic tumours), and neurological issues (like meningitis and cerebral palsy). In the thoracolumbar region, low back pain is most often mechanical, with lumbar strain or sprain being the leading cause. Other possible causes include degenerative conditions, herniated discs, spinal stenosis, neoplasms, infections, and visceral diseases like renal or pelvic organ issues [6].

3.2 Pathophysiology of Degenerative Spinal Disorders

The spine is a complex structure composed of vertebral segments, each consisting of a vertebral body, articulations with nearby vertebrae, and connections to ribs in the thoracic region (Fig. 3.1). The sacrum consists of fused vertebrae and contributes to the pelvic ring. Ligaments and muscles link these segments, enabling movements such as rotation, flexion, extension, and tilting. The intervertebral disc plays a crucial role in facilitating these movements while maintaining stability. Composed of a tough annulus fibrosus and a hydrated nucleus pulposus, the disc withstands significant mechanical load and distributes pressure across the vertebral body.

The spine endures various forces, including compression, tensile, shear, bending, and torsion. In the presence of disease, adjacent segments may bear increased load, leading to pain and dysfunction across the vertebral column. Age-related degeneration and osteoporosis further complicate spinal integrity, potentially resulting in

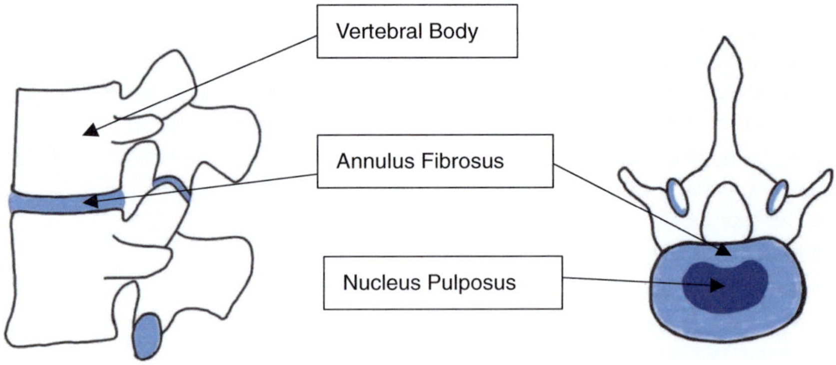

Fig. 3.1 Anatomy of intervertebral disc space

catastrophic collapse, such as insufficiency fractures. Ligaments provide both stability and flexibility, particularly in the sacroiliac region, which is susceptible to inflammatory joint diseases. Understanding the spine as a dynamic, mechanically active system is crucial in diagnosing and treating spinal disorders, as traditional static imaging often fails to capture functional abnormalities that underlie patient symptoms [7].

The intervertebral disc, a key structure in our spine, is made up of two main parts: the nucleus pulposus and the annulus fibrosus. The nucleus, filled with water, helps absorb the pressures we put on our spine, whether we are sitting or standing. Surrounding it is the annulus, which is tougher and contains layers of collagen that keep the nucleus in place.

Both the nucleus and annulus lack their own blood supply, so they depend on nearby blood vessels for nutrients. Similar to cartilage in our joints, the disc is maintained by cells that produce collagen and proteoglycans, crucial for keeping the disc strong and functional. These processes are supported by growth factors, which help repair and maintain the disc.

However, when the balance between building and breaking down this matrix is disrupted, often due to inflammation or a drop in pH, the disc can start to degrade. This delicate balance is essential for keeping our discs and our spine healthy [8].

Degenerative spine disease is driven by a mix of genetic, lifestyle, and mechanical factors, with inflammation playing a key role. Factors like aging, obesity, smoking, and mechanical stress, especially in the lower back, contribute to disc degeneration. Inflammation exacerbates this process, with elevated levels of cytokines like IL-1 and TNF-alpha found in degenerated discs. These inflammatory molecules, along with enzymes, break down the disc's matrix, leading to loss of hydration and structural integrity [9].

As the disc deteriorates, it loses height and becomes less effective at cushioning the spine. This can result in increased stress on surrounding structures like facet joints and muscles, as well as nerve compression, all of which can cause pain. Reduced blood flow and nutrient supply to the disc further worsen the condition by promoting cell death and inflammation, making the disc less capable of repairing itself and resisting further damage. Degeneration usually starts in the nucleus pulposus and progresses to the disc, annulus fibrosus, endplates, and bone marrow of the neighbouring vertebral bodies in advanced stages (Fig. 3.2). In addition, degeneration may affect structures farther away, resulting in facet joint osteoarthritis, spinal canal stenosis, and ligamentum flavum hypertrophy. Nitrogen gas can build up inside the disc as disc degeneration continues; this is referred to as the vacuum phenomenon. This process, which manifests as a signal void on T1- and T2-weighted MRI imaging, is quick, posture-dependent, and frequently associated with segmental instability. Vacuum phenomena are linked to fluid collection within the disc. In advanced degeneration, the disc may calcify, particularly in the annulus fibrosus, most commonly occurring in the lower thoracic spine.

Annular tears or fissures occur when fibres of the annulus fibrosus are avulsed, often during excessive spinal loading. These fissures can be circumferential, peripheral rim, or radial, and may cause pain. Fluid tracking through these fissures causes

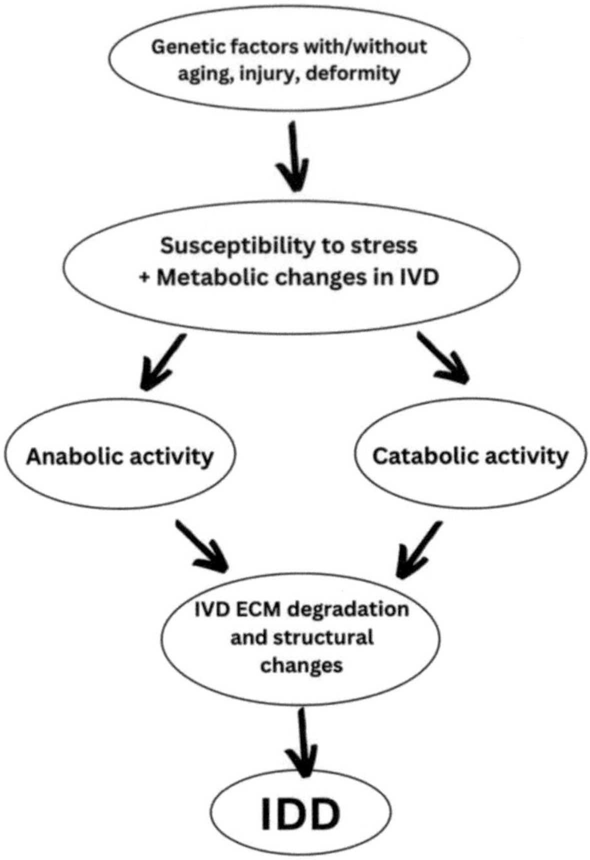

Fig. 3.2 Pathophysiology of intervertebral disc degeneration

high signal intensity on T2-weighted MRI. Disc material displacement beyond the intervertebral disc space can lead to bulging or herniation, which may occur centrally, paracentrally, foraminally, or extraforaminally, and can migrate superiorly or inferiorly within the spine.

3.3 Risk Factors for Degenerative Spinal Disorder

Rate and degree of degeneration can be affected by multiple factors. Factors which increase the risk of developing degenerative spine disease are mentioned below:

Age: Age can be considered as most consistent physiological reason behind disc degeneration. As the age of individual increases concentration of cells in the annulus decreases. The quality and rate of synthesis of proteoglycans also decreases meanwhile collagen content in the nucleus starts to increase and type

II collagen gets replaced by type I which is more vulnerable for calcification. And hence nucleus progressively becomes more dry and solid leading to degeneration of the disc [10].

Genetic Factors: Studies have suggested familial aggregation and genetics influences in DDD, though the effect size of identified genes is generally modest. Siblings of patient with disc degeneration were found to have more chances of disk degeneration than the general population [11]. Various Genes Linked to DDD are summarised below:

- *Vitamin D Receptor (VDR)*:
  - VDR gene polymorphisms, particularly TaqI and FokI, are linked to disc degeneration.
  - The TaqI polymorphism is associated with reduced MRI signals of discs in multiple ethnic groups, with the Tt genotype linked to more severe disc degeneration.
  - The FokI polymorphism impacts the efficiency of vitamin D signalling and is associated with varying transcriptional activities in different protein forms [12].
- *Collagen IX (COL9A2 and COL9A3)*:
  - COL9A2 and COL9A3 genes, coding for collagen IX in the disc matrix, are associated with DDD.
  - The Trp2 allele (COL9A2) and Trp3 allele (COL9A3) have shown significant associations with DDD, with varying prevalence across ethnic populations.
  - These mutations are linked to structural changes in the disc, contributing to disc degeneration and related conditions like sciatica.
- *Aggrecan (AGC1)*:
  - AGC1 gene, responsible for maintaining disc hydration, has VNTR polymorphisms linked to DDD.
  - The variability in VNTR length affects the structural integrity of the disc, with certain lengths associated with early onset of DDD [13].
- *Collagen I (COL1A1)*: The Sp1 polymorphism in COL1A1, which affects bone mineral density, is linked to an increased risk of disc degeneration, though further research is needed for confirmation.
- *Matrix Metalloproteinase 3 (MMP3)*: The 5A/6A polymorphism in the MMP3 gene regulates its expression, with the 5A allele associated with increased disc degeneration in older populations.
- *Interleukin-1 (IL-1) Gene Cluster*: Particularly IL-1β, linked to disc bulging and symptomatic pain in DDD.

Environmental and Lifestyle Related Risk Factors Environmental factors play a big role in how and when degenerative disc disease (DDD) might develop. Here is how various factors can contribute:

- *Physical Activity*: Regularly lifting heavy objects or performing repetitive motions, especially if done with poor form, can speed up disc wear. Jobs or activities that involve frequent bending or twisting put extra stress on your discs. Not being active enough can weaken the muscles that support your spine, making it more prone to disc problems.
- *Posture*: Sitting for long periods in a poor posture or slouching can place extra pressure on your discs, leading to problems over time.
- *Obesity*: Carrying excess weight puts extra strain on your spine, which can contribute to faster disc degeneration due to increased pressure and inflammation.
- *Smoking*: Smoking reduces blood flow to the discs, making it harder for them to get the nutrients they need and speeding up degeneration.
- *Trauma and Injury*: Sudden injuries, like falls or accidents, can damage your discs and lead to quicker degeneration.
- Metabolic disorders like diabetes mellitus and alkaptonuria, oxidative stress, and low-grade infections can also increase the risk of DDD.

Making changes like improving your posture, staying active, maintaining a healthy weight, and avoiding smoking can help lower the risk of developing DDD.

3.4 Common Types of Degenerative Spinal Disorders

Common degenerative conditions of spine can be broadly subdivided into undermentioned subheadings

- Degenerative Disc Disease (DDD)
- Spinal Osteoarthritis (Spondylosis)
- Spinal Stenosis
- Spondylolisthesis
- Cervical Myelopathy

3.4.1 Degenerative Disc Disease (DDD)

Back pain and neck pain are major public health problems and are strongly associated with degeneration of intervertebral disk. DDD is a result of several factors acting individually or collectively. Disk degeneration in symptomatic patients is also associated with sciatica and disk herniation or prolapse.

The intervertebral disc has two key parts: the nucleus pulposus and the annulus fibrosus. The nucleus pulposus is the disc's inner core, rich in water, making it ideal for cushioning the spine under pressure. Surrounding it is the annulus fibrosus, a tougher, collagen-rich layer that acts as a protective barrier. The outer fibres of the disc, known as Sharpey's fibres, anchor it securely to the vertebrae. Unlike most tissues, the nucleus and annulus do not have their own blood supply. Instead, they rely on nearby blood vessels to supply nutrients and remove waste.

Biochemically, the disc is similar to joint cartilage. Cells in the nucleus produce type II collagen and proteoglycans, which help the disc absorb shocks. In the annulus, different cells generate type I and II collagen, adding to its strength. Proteoglycans and collagen work together to maintain the disc's structure. The balance between building and breaking down the disc's matrix is tightly regulated by growth factors and enzymes, with macrophages playing a crucial role by promoting breakdown and triggering inflammation when needed. The vertebral endplates, which separate the disc from the vertebrae, have a similar makeup, allowing them to effectively transfer nutrients between the bone and the disc.

As the intervertebral disc degenerates, it loses height and cushioning ability, increasing stress on surrounding structures like facet joints, muscles, and nerves, leading to pain. Reduced blood flow and nutrient supply exacerbate the condition by promoting cell death and inflammation, hindering the disc's ability to repair itself. The degenerative process begins in the nucleus pulposus and spreads to the annulus fibrosus, endplates, and adjacent vertebral bodies. In advanced stages, this can lead to facet joint osteoarthritis, ligamentum flavum hypertrophy, and spinal canal stenosis, further contributing to spinal instability and pain. Disc material displacement beyond the intervertebral disc space can lead to bulging or herniation, which may occur centrally, paracentrally, foraminally, or extraforaminally, and can migrate superiorly or inferiorly within the spine (Fig. 3.3).

Herniated discs can be classified into three subtypes based on morphology and imaging (Figs. 3.4 and 3.5):

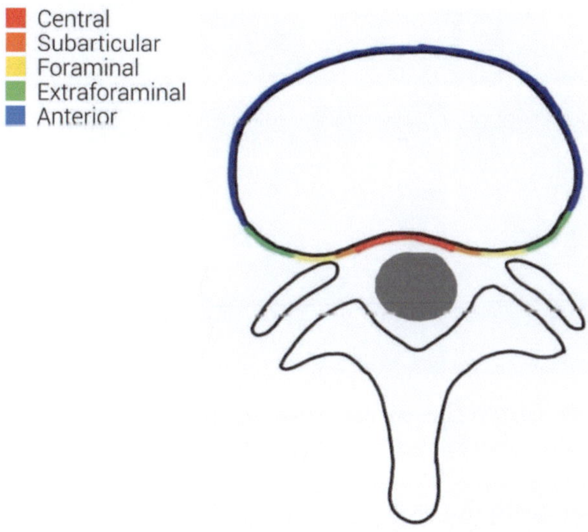

Fig. 3.3 Axial localisation of disc prolapses

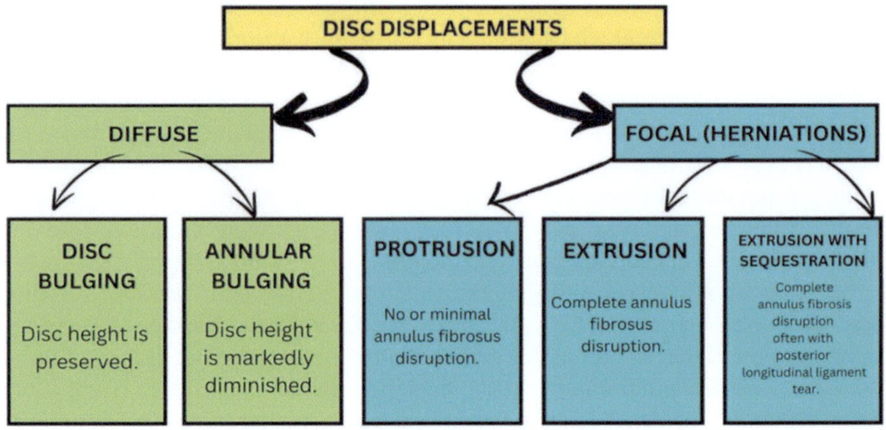

Fig. 3.4 Classification of disc displacement

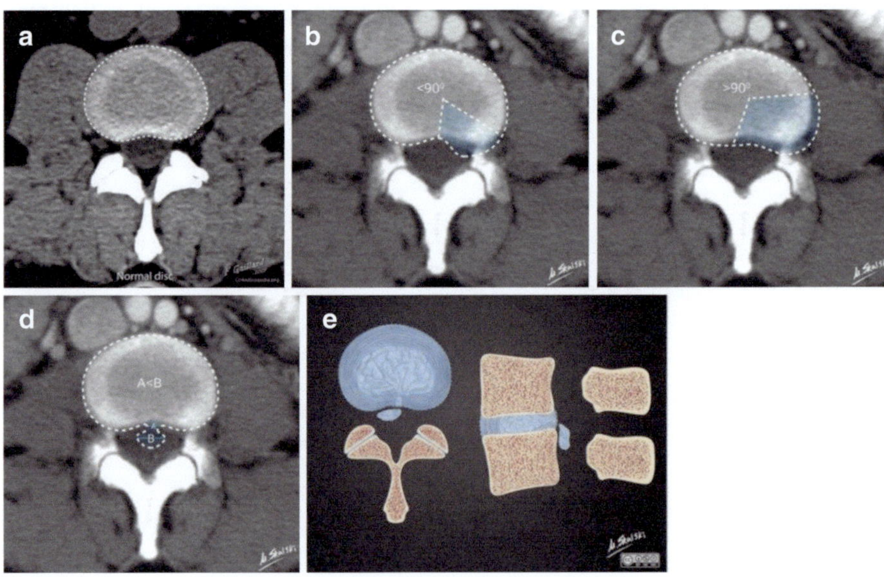

Fig. 3.5 (**a**) Normal disc, (**b**) Disc protrusion, (**c**) Disc bulge, (**d**) Disc extrusion, and (**e**) Disc sequestration

- Protrusion: Localised displacement of disc material where the distance between the displaced portion's edges is less than the base. The annulus fibrosus is minimally disrupted, and the posterior longitudinal ligament remains intact.
- Extrusion: Disc material extends beyond the disc space, with full-thickness disruption of the annulus fibrosus but usually with an intact posterior longitudinal ligament. The extrusion may cause neurological symptoms due to ligament tension.

- Sequestration: Extruded disc material loses continuity with the original disc, potentially causing severe pain and neurological symptoms, especially if it migrates within the spinal canal.

In a healthy spine, the intervertebral disc appears hyper-intense on T2-weighted MRI sequences. However, aging alters the signal within the disc space, often accompanied by changes in the vertebral endplates known as Modic changes (Fig. 3.6) [14]:

- *Modic type I*: Shows linear oedema signals along the endplates, hypo-intense on T1 and hyper-intense on T2 sequences.
- *Modic type II*: Characterised by linear fat signals, hyper-intense on both T1 and T2 sequences.
- *Modic type III*: Displays linear sclerotic signals that are hypo-intense on both T1 and T2 sequences.

3.4.1.1 Cervical Disc Degeneration

Degenerative disc disease of the cervical spine primarily affects the aging population, equally in men and women, with patients often presenting with pain and, occasionally, neurological symptoms. The cervical spine (C1–C7) provides significant range of motion, with the intervertebral discs (IVDs) playing a key role in stability and mobility. Over time, the IVDs lose water content and proteoglycans, leading to a more fibrotic nucleus pulposus (NP) and potential disc herniations or spinal stenosis.

Cervical disc degeneration is a normal part of aging that begins as early as the second decade of life. As intervertebral discs (IVDs) lose water content, they become less flexible, leading to disc height reduction, collapse, and potential spondylotic changes such as facet hypertrophy. The degeneration of the nucleus pulposus (NP) increases the load on the annulus fibrosus (AF), causing it to tear, weaken, and bulge, which further contributes to disc height loss.

Several factors can predispose individuals to cervical degenerative disc disease, including environmental influences, genetics, and chronic neck flexion due to the use of electronic devices. Increased flexion significantly raises the stress on cervical discs, accelerating degeneration. Other potential risk factors like smoking,

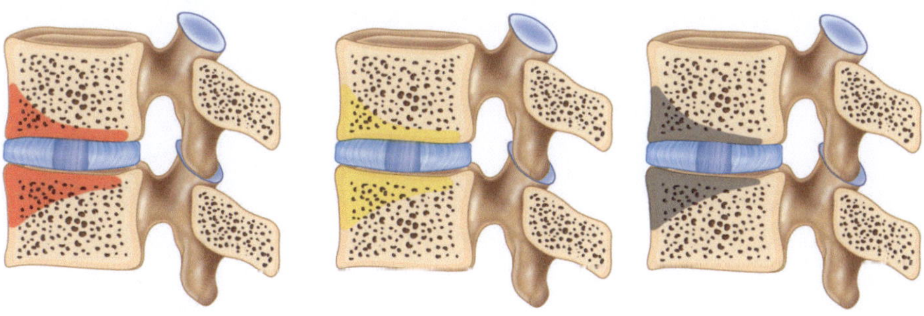

Fig. 3.6 Modic changes in vertebral end plates

occupation, and sports have been studied, but evidence regarding their impact on cervical degeneration remains inconclusive. Notably, studies have found no strong link between smoking or sports like weightlifting and increased risk of cervical spine degeneration.

A careful history and physical examination are essential to diagnose cervical disc disease and differentiate it from more serious conditions. Key history components include constitutional symptoms, oncologic history, trauma, and a detailed pain history. Neurologic symptoms such as weakness, sensory loss, and gait disturbances should also be thoroughly assessed. The physical exam should start with vitals and include a comprehensive neurologic evaluation, cervical spine range of motion, and provocative tests like Spurling and Lhermitte's signs (Fig. 3.7).

Patients often present with axial neck pain, movement difficulties, and potentially radicular symptoms. Commonly affected nerve roots are C6 and C7, leading to pain, muscle weakness, and reflex changes. Cervical spondylotic myelopathy, a more severe condition, can cause stiffness, numbness, fine motor impairment, and in advanced cases, bladder and bowel dysfunction.

- Cervical disc herniations commonly occur at C6–C7, leading to C7 nerve root compression. This results in neck pain radiating to the lateral forearm, palm, and middle finger, with potential triceps weakness and a depressed triceps reflex.
- C5 root compression causes neck pain radiating to the shoulder and periscapular area, with possible weakness in shoulder abduction, external rotation, and elbow flexion, along with diminished biceps and brachioradialis reflexes.

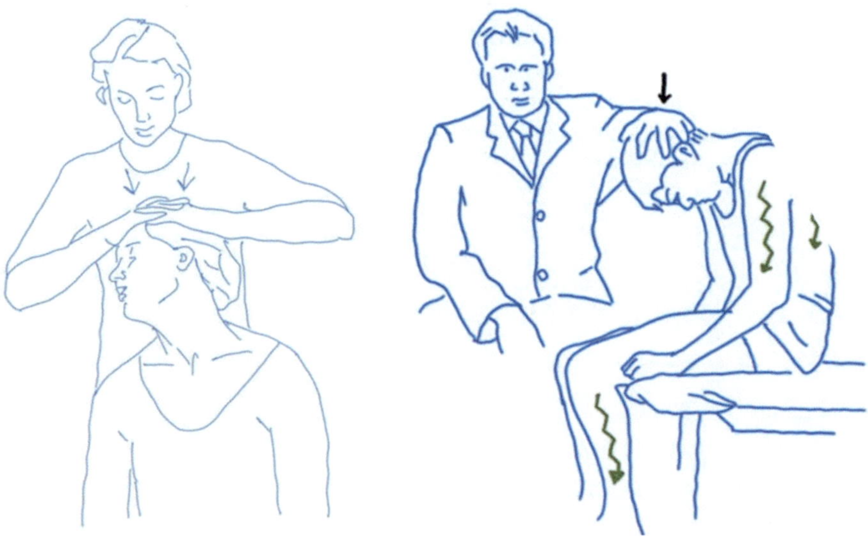

Fig. 3.7 Spurling and Lhermitte's sign

- C6 nerve involvement leads to pain radiating from the neck to the thumb and index finger, with weakness in elbow flexion and wrist extension.
- C8 and T1 root compressions cause pain radiating to the medial forearm, with C8 affecting thumb extension and T1 leading to weakness in the first dorsal interosseous muscle.

Differential diagnoses for cervical disc degeneration are mentioned below:

- Brachial plexus pathology
- Carpal/cubital tunnel syndrome
- Peripheral neuropathy or neuritis
- Complex regional pain syndrome
- Demyelinating disorder
- Malignancy (Pancoast tumour for neuropathic symptoms)
- Cervical spondylosis
- Cervical sprain and strain
- Fibromyalgia
- Shoulder pathology/rotator cuff injury
- Thoracic outlet syndrome
- Infections

Treatment for cervical disc disease focuses on reducing pain, improving function, and preventing recurrence. Initial management is nonoperative, involving rest, activity modification, medications, physical therapy, and various injections. Non-steroidal anti-inflammatory drugs (NSAIDs), steroids, and muscle relaxants provide symptom relief. Physical therapy includes passive modalities like heat, cryotherapy, and massage, as well as active exercises for muscle strengthening and range of motion. Cervical collars and traction may be used, though their efficacy is debated.

If nonoperative measures fail, surgery may be necessary, particularly in cases of severe pain, neurological deficits, or myelopathy. Surgical options include decompression with or without fusion, often performed via an anterior approach (e.g., ACDF). This approach is preferred for patients with normal to kyphotic alignment and may involve the removal of multiple discs with fusion. Posterior approaches, such as laminectomy or laminoplasty, are used for patients with multi-level compression or neutral/lordotic alignment. Cervical disc arthroplasty is an emerging alternative to fusion but is typically reserved for herniated discs rather than degenerative disc disease. Surgical outcomes are generally positive, but complications like recurrent symptoms, graft issues, and postoperative kyphosis can occur. A combined anterior-posterior approach may be necessary for complex cases [15].

3.4.1.2 Lumbar Disc Degeneration

Particularly lumbar disk degeneration occurs at the L4–L5 or L5–S1 levels, which impinge the L4, L5, or S1 nerve roots. Disc degeneration is closely linked to ageing, with men typically experiencing this degeneration earlier than women.

Although environmental factors like smoking and occupational hazards were once considered primary causes, recent research emphasises genetic factors as the most significant predictors of disc degeneration, with environmental influences playing a minor role.

When evaluating a patient who may have spinal problems, the history should concentrate on the duration of the pain, any radiation to the legs, and potential triggers, such as previous trauma. Surgical results for radiating pain, particularly to the lower extremities and buttocks, are generally more predictable than for non-specific lower back pain, which is typically the result of strained muscles. Radiating pain is frequently associated with canal stenosis. When pain is felt during specific movements, it could be an indication of instability or a degenerative fracture.

A thorough physical exam includes gait assessment, strength and reflex testing, and evaluating neurologic function in the arms, legs, bladder, and bowels. The Straight Leg Raise (SLR) test helps diagnose canal stenosis, with positive findings indicating nerve root compression (Fig. 3.8). Additionally, clinicians should inspect the skin and note any tenderness or prior surgical scars. Documentation of these findings is crucial for ongoing evaluation. Finally, consider Waddell signs to rule out non-organic causes of low back pain, particularly when psychological factors are suspected. These include inconsistent symptoms, non-anatomic tenderness, and pain with movements like axial loading.

Standard imaging for assessing individuals with low back pain consists of lateral and anterior-posterior (AP) radiographs of the afflicted region. When a suspected acute disc herniation first presents, an MRI is not advised unless there

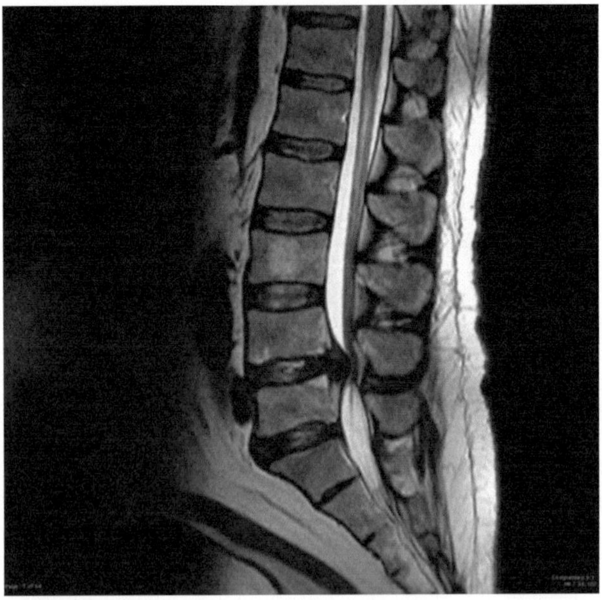

Fig. 3.8 Sagittal MRI image of prolapsed intervertebral disc at L4–L5 level

are "red flags." An MRI with a focus on T2-weighted sagittal and axial images can be acquired to detect any neurologic compression if symptoms continue following this first course of treatment. Notably, disc herniations, whether symptomatic or not, often decrease in size over time, and the presence of disc disease on MRI does not necessarily predict chronic pain or the need for surgery in the future.

Differential diagnoses for lumbar disc degeneration are mentioned below:

- Cauda equina syndrome
- Spinal cord tumour
- Muscle spasm
- Spinal infection
- Spondylolisthesis
- Spondylolysis

It is imperative to seek a timely diagnosis and explore surgical options when "red flags" are present, such as cauda equina syndrome, infection, suspected malignancy, or trauma. Nonetheless, the majority of low back pain sufferers get better without surgery. The first course of treatment usually consists of 6 weeks of physical therapy with an emphasis on core strengthening and stretching. In addition to surgery, nonsurgical therapies include NSAIDs, cognitive therapy, lifestyle modifications, and epidural injections, which may offer temporary relief [16].

Surgery is typically only recommended in cases involving neurological impairments, degenerative spondylolisthesis, or severe discomfort that substantially limits day-to-day activities. The gold standard for treating degenerative disc disease is lumbar discectomy with fusion; alternatively, lumbar total disc replacement may be a preferable option for treating single-level disc disease. Studies like the Spine Patient Outcomes Research Trial (SPORT) demonstrate that patients who have surgery frequently have better results than non-surgical patients. Surgery is a reliable treatment for radicular pain, but its efficacy in treating non-radiating lower back pain is less certain. Patients should be informed about the potential outcomes and risks before proceeding with surgery.

3.4.2 Spinal Osteoarthritis (Spondylosis)

Osteoarthritis, particularly in the spine, is a common cause of chronic low back pain, significantly affecting quality of life and leading to substantial healthcare costs. Despite the high prevalence, identifying the exact cause of pain can be challenging, as imaging results often do not correlate with symptoms.

As patient's age advances, their spines undergo degenerative changes due to alterations in load-bearing forces, starting with intervertebral disc degeneration. Normally, facet joints bear about 33% of the load, but as degeneration occurs, this increases to 70%, leading to changes like osteophyte formation and cartilage damage. These changes contribute to spinal stenosis. Additionally, the decline in synovial fluid's viscoelastic properties, along with inflammation from leukotrienes and prostaglandins, further exacerbates the condition, leading to chronic pain. Inadequate blood supply, particularly stenosis in lumbar arteries, is also linked to intervertebral disc degeneration [17].

Spine osteoarthritis is influenced by various factors, from genetics and age to lifestyle and diet. While it was once seen as simply the result of "wear and tear," we now know it is more complex. Genetics play a significant role, with certain gene mutations making some people more prone to developing osteoarthritis. As we age, our joints naturally wear down, and this, combined with factors like obesity and physical activity, can lead to the painful symptoms of osteoarthritis. Gender and ethnicity also matter—women and older men, for example, often experience more curvature in their lower back, which can increase stress on the spine and lead to degeneration. Similarly, certain ethnic groups may have differences in joint mobility, which can impact how osteoarthritis develops. Lifestyle choices, like diet and exercise, are crucial too. Being overweight can increase inflammation in the body, worsening joint damage over time. On the flip side, eating foods rich in antioxidants, like vitamins C and K, might help protect your joints from further harm. Ultimately, spine osteoarthritis is a condition shaped by a mix of who we are, how we live, and how we age. Understanding these factors can help manage and potentially reduce the impact of this condition on our lives.

Diagnosing spine osteoarthritis starts with a careful history and physical exam, but it is also crucial to rule out other serious causes of back pain, like infections or tumours. Imaging, like X-rays, is often the first step, especially if the pain has lasted more than 6 weeks without nerve symptoms. If symptoms are severe or persistent, more detailed scans like MRIs might be needed.

Treatment depends on how long the pain has been present and how severe it is. It usually begins with conservative methods, like physical therapy, exercise, and medications like NSAIDs or acetaminophen. For some, especially if the pain is disabling or neurological symptoms are worsening, more invasive options like injections or surgery might be necessary. Managing weight and maintaining a healthy diet can also help reduce symptoms, especially since obesity can worsen the condition. Personalised treatment plans are essential, particularly for older adults, to help them manage their pain and improve their quality of life.

3.4.3 Spinal Stenosis

In spinal stenosis spaces within the spine becomes narrow and causes pressure on the nerves. It usually affects the neck and lower back, resulting in pain, numbness, or weakness. While spinal stenosis becomes more common with age, not everyone will experience symptoms, and many can manage the condition through lifestyle adjustments rather than surgery. Treatment varies based on the location and type of nerve compression. Thankfully, most people recover without the need for invasive procedures, and only a small percentage develop more severe conditions like a herniated disc.

Spinal stenosis can stem from either congenital or acquired causes. Congenital factors, though less common (about 9% of cases), include conditions like achondroplasia, shortened pedicles, and spinal dysraphism. Acquired stenosis, which is more prevalent, arises from degenerative changes, trauma, iatrogenic factors, and systemic diseases. Trauma can cause acute compression of the vertebral canal, while degenerative changes such as disc herniation, ligament hypertrophy, and spondylolisthesis contribute to chronic narrowing. Surgical procedures like laminectomy or discectomy can also lead to iatrogenic stenosis. The narrowing of the spinal canal or lateral recesses often results in compression of the spinal cord, nerve tissues, and cerebrospinal fluid. Factors such as disc protrusion, epidural fat deposition, and hypertrophy of ligaments and facet joints are involved in the process. Severe cases of spinal stenosis can lead to serious complications like myelopathic syndrome or cauda equina syndrome [18].

Cervical Spine Stenosis Symptoms include neck or arm pain, radiculopathy depending on the affected disk (e.g. C6 radiculopathy from a C5–6 herniation). Common disk herniations at C6–7, C5–6, C7–T1, and C4–5 lead to specific motor and sensory deficits, including weakness, pain, and paraesthesia. Cervical spondylotic myelopathy may cause upper extremity clumsiness, gait disturbance, and lower extremity weakness (Fig. 3.9).

Lumbar Spine Stenosis Leads to neurogenic claudication, motor weakness, sensory disturbances, and pathologic reflexes. Symptoms include leg cramps, increase

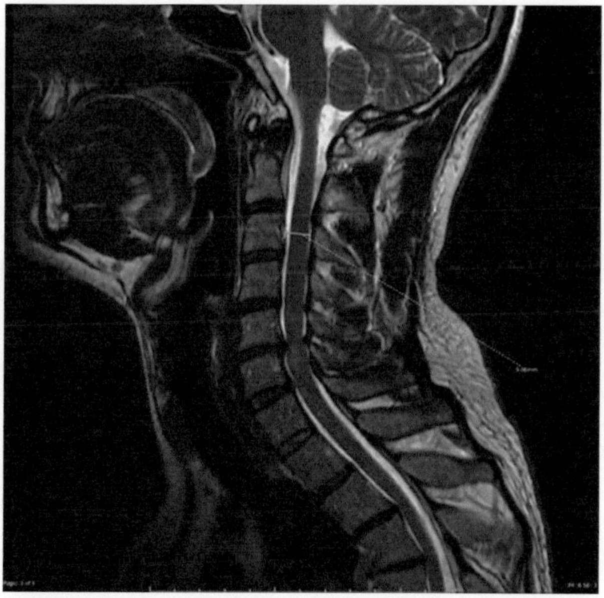

Fig. 3.9 Congenital cervical canals stenosis

in the pain while walking or standing which gets relieved while sitting or leaning forward. Common disk herniations occur at L4–5 and L5–S1, causing plantar-flexion weakness, foot drop, or numbness in specific areas (Fig. 3.10).

MRI is the gold standard for diagnosing spinal stenosis, revealing intrinsic cord abnormalities and the extent of stenosis [19]. CT helps differentiate between calcified and soft discs and detect fractures. Plain radiographs are limited but useful for assessing dynamic instability. CT myelogram is an alternative for patients with contraindications to MRI. Nerve conduction studies, somatosensory evoked potentials, and needle electromyography help in differential diagnosis.

Treatment/management options for cervical stenosis include both conservative and surgical options. Conservative management for non-myelopathy cases includes bracing, rest, and anti-inflammatory medications. In order to relieve compression and stabilise the spine, anterior or posterior decompression and fusion are surgical treatments for myelopathy. Regarding lumbar stenosis, NSAIDs and physical therapy are the first lines of treatment; for chronic pain, interventional pain management is used. Surgical options are considered for progressive myelopathy, neurologic deficits, or spinal instability, with approaches including anterior, lateral, or posterior decompression and fusion [20].

Differential diagnoses for spinal stenosis are mentioned below:

- Lumbar Compression Fracture
- Lumbar Degenerative Disk Disease
- Lumbar Spondylosis

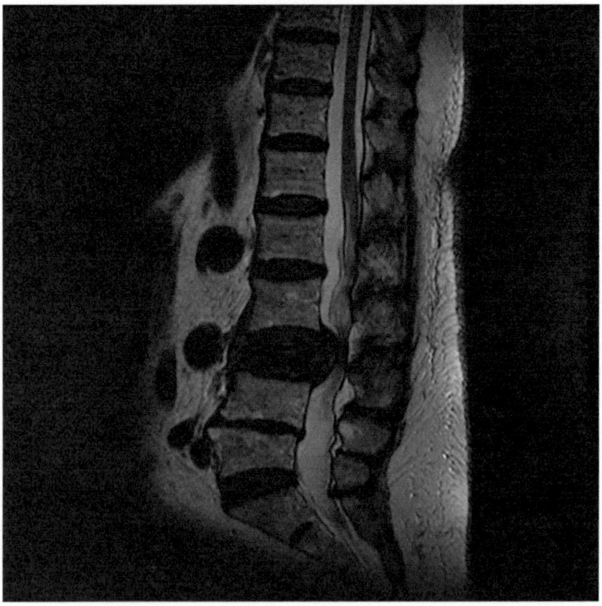

Fig. 3.10 Lumbar canal stenosis due to L5 fracture

- Lumbar Facet Arthropathy
- Rehabilitation for Osteoarthritis
- Rheumatoid Arthritis
- Spondylodiskitis
- Spondylolisthesis

3.4.4 Spondylolisthesis

Degenerative spondylolisthesis is a condition that primarily affects the lumbar spine and is rarely found in the thoracic spine. While cervical spondylolisthesis has not been studied in great depth, emerging evidence suggests it may be more prevalent than previously recognised. The underlying mechanisms for spondylolisthesis across different regions of the spine are thought to be similar. This condition typically results from severe disc degeneration, where the disc's structural integrity deteriorates over time, leading to instability and displacement of vertebrae [21].

Degenerative spondylolisthesis can be categorised into two main types: dynamic and static. Dynamic spondylolisthesis is characterised by observable instability on flexion and extension X-rays, which reveal movement between vertebrae. This type often necessitates surgical intervention, including instrumentation and fusion, to stabilise the spine and alleviate symptoms. In contrast, static spondylolisthesis does not show evidence of instability on X-rays but may still be symptomatic. The decision to use surgical instrumentation or fusion in static cases is less straightforward and depends on the patient's specific symptoms and functional impairment [22].

In addition to X-rays, MRI can reveal indirect signs of instability in the spine. These signs include facet joint fluid, interspinous fluid, synovial cysts, facet joint hypertrophy, and the vacuum phenomenon within the disc. These findings on MRI can suggest underlying instability, which might not be apparent from static X-ray images alone. Functional radiographs (flexion and extension) remain the gold standard for diagnosing degenerative instability, as they provide a dynamic view of the spinal movements that can highlight instability more clearly.

Cervical spondylolisthesis, though less frequently studied, can also be divided into two distinct types. Type I, or adjacent spondylolisthesis, occurs at the junction of a stiffer, spondylotic segment and a more mobile segment of the cervical spine. Type II, or spondylotic spondylolisthesis, develops within spondylotic segments that have undergone significant disc degeneration. Each type presents its own set of challenges for diagnosis and treatment.

In the lumbar spine, the severity of spondylolisthesis is often graded using the *Meyerding* classification system (Fig. 3.11). This method determines the degree of displacement by calculating the ratio between the superior vertebral body's overhanging segment and the neighbouring inferior vertebral body's anteroposterior length. Slippage is indicated by Grade I at 1–25% (Fig. 3.12), Grade II at 50%, Grade III at 75%, and Grade IV at 101%. Spondyloptosis, also known as Grade V spondylolisthesis, is the word used when slippage surpasses 100% (Fig. 3.13). This

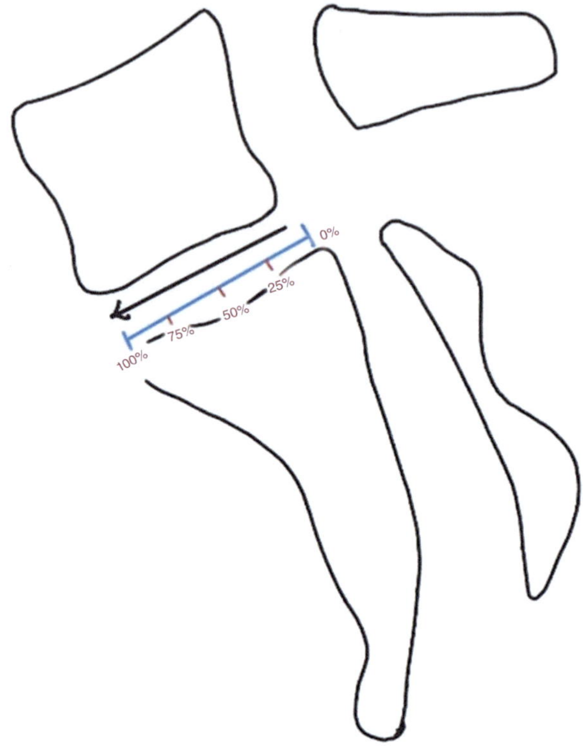

Fig. 3.11 Meyerding classification system of spondylolisthesis

classification helps in deciding the extent of the condition and planning proper treatment strategies [23].

"Isthmic spondylolisthesis" is further subdivided into three types: subtype A (stress fractures of the pars interarticularis), subtype B (elongation of pars without a clear fracture), and subtype C (acute fracture of pars). "Pathologic spondylolisthesis" has two subtypes: subtype A (due to systemic conditions) and subtype B (resulting from focal processes).

Patients with lumbar or cervical spondylolisthesis typically experience intermittent, localised pain in the lower back or neck, worsened by flexion and extension at the affected segment. This mechanical pain may be accompanied by radicular symptoms due to nerve root compression from the slippage of one vertebra on another. Pain may improve when lying supine, as this position reduces instability and pressure on the spinal canal or neural foramen. Buttock pain, leg numbness or weakness, trouble walking, and, in rare instances, loss of bladder or bowel control are some other symptoms of lumbar spondylolisthesis.

Diagnosis begins with anteroposterior and lateral plain films, along with lateral flexion-extension views to assess vertebral alignment and motion, indicating instability. In isthmic spondylolisthesis, a "*Scotty dog collar*" (Fig. 3.14) sign on imaging may indicate a pars defect. CT scans provide the highest specificity and

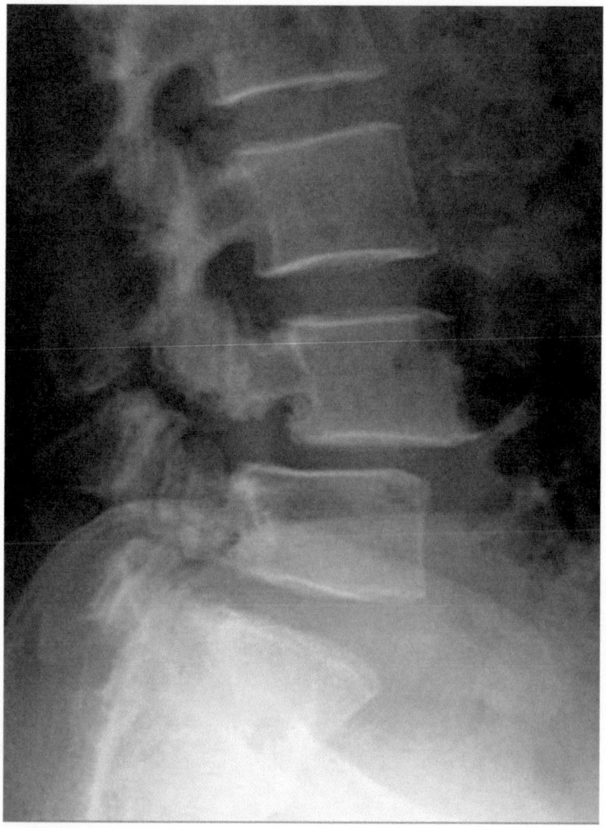

Fig. 3.12 Grade 1 spondylolisthesis

sensitivity for diagnosis, while MRI is useful for detecting associated soft tissue problems and disc abnormalities.

- Differential diagnoses for spondylolisthesis are mentioned below: Degenerative Lumbar Disc Disease
- Lumbosacral Spine Acute Bony Injuries
- Lumbosacral Discogenic Pain Syndrome
- Lumbosacral Facet Syndrome
- Lumbosacral Spondylosis
- Lumbosacral Radiculopathy

Treatment for grade I and II spondylolisthesis start with conservative measures such as NSAIDs, traction, heat, bracing, light exercise, and bed rest. However, 10–15% of younger patients with low-grade spondylolisthesis may require surgery, which can involve decompression, fusion, or inter-body fusion, especially in cases of instability.

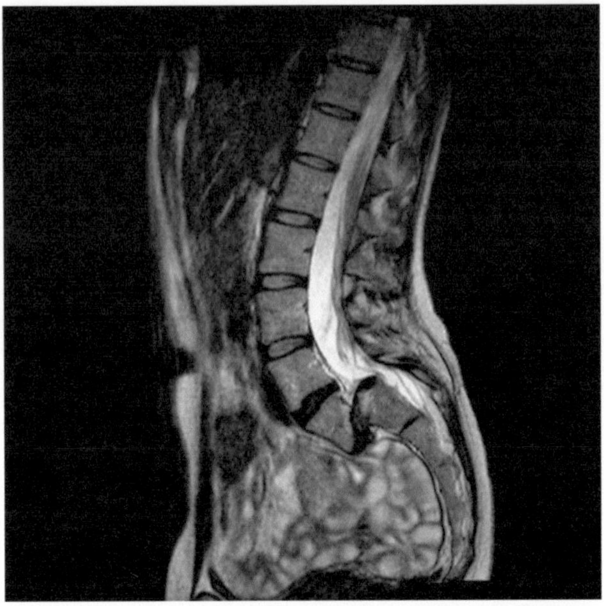

Fig. 3.13 MRI image of Grade V spondylolisthesis (spondyloptosis)

Fig. 3.14 Scotty dog collar sign

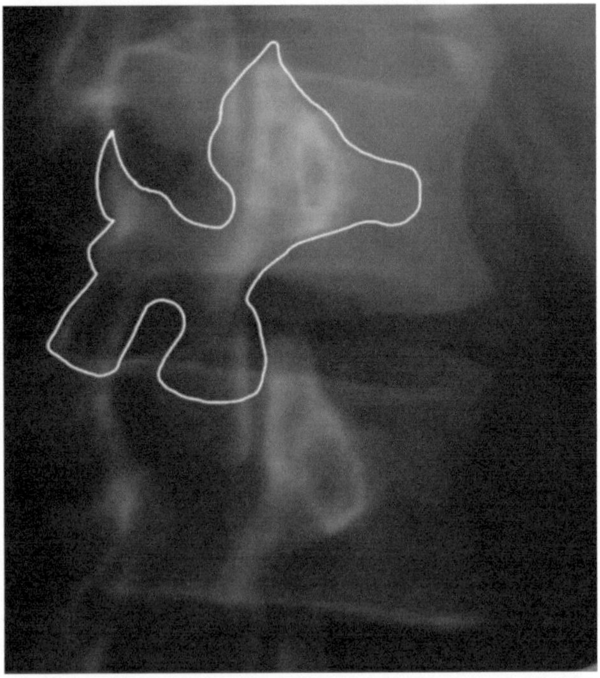

3.4.5 Cervical Myelopathy

Cervical myelopathy is a condition where the spinal cord is compressed at the cervical level, often due to congenital narrowing of the cervical canal, leading to symptoms like spasticity, hyperreflexia, hand clumsiness, and gait disturbances. It typically progresses slowly but can lead to significant paralysis without treatment. Poor prognosis is associated with long symptom duration, reduced cervical spine mobility, and female gender. Stenosis is most common at C5–C6 or C6–C7, with factors like disc herniation, ligament infolding, spondylolisthesis, and osteophyte formation contributing to the narrowing. Patients with severe canal stenosis (less than 6 mm space) are at substantial risk for developing myelopathy. Age is a strong predictor of postoperative complications and recovery.

This often causes a stiff, unsteady walk, and clumsiness in the hands, making everyday tasks like buttoning a shirt or holding small objects challenging. Some patients also feel pain or an electric shock-like sensation down their back or arms. Neck pain is common, and some experience pain radiating down their arms. If the condition progresses, it can affect bowel and bladder control, which is a sign of a more serious prognosis [24].

To diagnose this condition, history of the pain, its pattern, and any triggering fracture comes handy. A thorough physical examination to check strength, sensation, and reflexes is necessary. Surgical intervention, often involving decompression and fusion, is the primary treatment. Gait assessment is required to evaluate for balance issues or spasticity in movement. Motor reflex examination like Biceps reflex, Brachioradialis reflex, Patellar reflex, Achilles reflex, etc. need to be performed to exclude hyperreflexia. Lhermitte sign can be elicited by flexing the neck which triggers an electric shock-like sensation. Few named signs and tests which can be elicited are mentioned below:

- Hoffman Sign: Extend and quickly release the distal phalanx of the long finger to see if the patient responds with reflex flexion of the thumb and/or index finger.
- Inverted Radial Reflex: Tap the brachioradialis and watch for wrist extension and finger flexion.
- Crossed Radial Reflex: Observe for extension of both the biceps and wrist during a biceps reflex test.
- Grip Test: Assess the ability to repeatedly make a tight fist.
- Finger Escape Sign: Patient struggles to keep the ulnar digits extended and adducted.

Flexion and extension views on AP and lateral spine radiographs aid in evaluating ligamentous stability. Radiographs can be used to calculate the Torg ratio. Torg ratio compares the cervical canal's diameter to the cervical body's width on lateral radiograph. Congenital stenosis may be suggested by a ratio less than 0.8. A canal space evaluation can be performed via MRI. A less than 10 mm canal space suggests stenosis. Indicators of myelopathy include compression and alterations in signal on T1 and T2. It is important to know that up to one fifth of asymptomatic patients might show significant cervical abnormalities. MRI can also offer valuable insights for both clinicians and patients regarding potential recovery outcomes. High-intensity changes on T2-weighted images and low intensity on T1-weighted images are linked to lower recovery rates and less improvement in motor symptoms. A lower JOA recovery rate is linked to a larger ratio of T2 signal intensity between non-compressed and compressed spinal segments (C7 through T1). The presence of frequent high signal intensity on T2-weighted images is indicative of a worse recovery prognosis [25]. Central cord syndrome, Guillain-Barre syndrome, Chiari malformation, Syrinx, Multiple sclerosis, etc., can be differentials for cervical myelopathy.

Non-surgical management of cervical myelopathy includes anti-inflammatory medications, physical therapy, ultrasound treatments, and corticosteroid injections, which provide only temporary relief. For patients with progressive symptoms, surgery should be strongly considered [26]. The primary goal of surgery is to increase canal space, reducing or eliminating spinal cord compression. Early surgical intervention is generally recommended over a prolonged wait-and-see approach. Surgical options include anterior and posterior approaches. A posterior approach, such as laminectomy, is preferred for lordosis deformities and posterior canal pathology. Anterior cervical discectomy and fusion (ACDF) is performed for up to three-disc levels but may result in temporary throat discomfort and dysphagia.

3.5 Emerging Trends and Future Directions

Spinal degeneration is a major health issue, and current treatments have limitations in terms of risks and long-term effectiveness. This has led to increased scientific interest in exploring the causes and mechanisms of spinal degeneration to develop more effective therapies. Recent research is focused on finding treatments that target the root causes of spinal degeneration rather than just alleviating symptoms. Compounds such as melatonin, naringin, berberine, oestrogen, icariin, resveratrol, metformin, quercetin, vitamin D, and other growth factors could be used as potential future therapeutics [27]. Table 3.1 summarises some emerging drugs useful to prevent disc degeneration.

Additionally, cell-based therapies show promise in regenerating intervertebral discs (IVDs) or slowing their degeneration. Another area of interest is the development of artificial IVDs using biocompatible and biodegradable materials to reduce long-term complications seen with earlier implants. Continued optimisation of these strategies and their progression from preclinical testing to clinical trials could lead to significant advancements in treating spinal degeneration and improving the quality of life for millions of affected individuals in the near future [28].

An increasingly popular treatment option for intervertebral disc degeneration (IDD) is platelet-rich plasma (PRP). PRP, derived from autologous blood with a high platelet concentration, shows potential by reducing apoptosis, increasing autophagy, and stimulating cell proliferation and extracellular matrix (ECM)

Table 3.1 Summary of key compounds for treatment of intervertebral disc degeneration

Melatonin	Helps maintain structural integrity of intervertebral discs (IVDs). Promotes cell survival and enhances matrix anabolism. Accelerates damage repair in intervertebral discs. Modulates extracellular matrix (ECM) remodelling. Inhibits inflammatory pathways.
Oestrogen	Crucial in preventing disc degeneration especially in postmenopausal women. Reduces disc degeneration by inhibiting inflammatory cytokines. Lowers oxidative stress and promotes autophagy. Carries risks, including hypertension and cardiovascular issues.
Naringin	A natural flavonoid shows potential in treating intervertebral disc degeneration (IDD). Promotes nucleus pulposus (NP) cell proliferation and reduces inflammation. Regulates autophagy and oxidative stress, supporting extracellular matrix (ECM) integrity. Effects are mediated through pathways like AMP-activated protein kinase (AMPK) and PI3K/Akt. Protects NP cells from apoptosis.
Icariin	Prevents nucleus pulposus (NP) cell apoptosis. Promotes extracellular matrix (ECM) preservation. Exerts anti-inflammatory effects by inhibiting IL-1β-induced signalling pathways. Aids in recruiting stem cells to the disc region, supporting tissue regeneration.
Resveratrol	Has antioxidant properties. Supports extracellular matrix (ECM) synthesis. Enhances autophagy, promoting cellular repair and maintenance. Inhibits inflammatory responses.
Metformin	Metformin shows potential in treating intervertebral disc degeneration (IDD) by promoting autophagy. Reduces inflammation and protects against apoptosis and cellular senescence. Enhances anabolic processes, aiding tissue regeneration. Inhibits the expression of catabolic genes, slowing down degeneration.
Vitamin D	Vitamin D, recognised for its immunomodulatory properties, contributes to intervertebral disc (IVD) health. It helps slow down intervertebral disc degeneration (IDD) by reducing inflammation, oxidative stress, and cell aging. Vitamin D administration is associated with increased collagen II levels and decreased collagen X levels.

regeneration. While in vitro and in vivo studies have demonstrated these benefits, clinical studies suggest that intradiscal PRP injections can alleviate low back pain associated with disc degeneration, although they may not lead to structural or functional improvements [29].

Additionally, Artificial Intelligence (AI) is emerging as a tool to enhance the prevention, diagnosis, and treatment of IDD. Machine learning (ML) algorithms, such as decision trees and artificial neural networks, have shown promise in early disease detection and risk assessment, offering personalised insights for patient care [30].

3.6 Conclusion

Degenerative spine disease continues to be a major health issue with incomplete understanding and solutions. A broad understanding of these conditions is essential for radiologists. Imaging plays a crucial role in managing these diseases, particularly in assessing spinal stability and guiding treatment decisions, such as the use of potent anti-inflammatory medications. While MRI is typically the primary imaging tool for many spinal disorders, conventional radiographs and CT scans remain essential as first-line techniques, especially in trauma cases. In some instances, a combination of imaging modalities may be necessary to achieve an accurate and safe diagnosis. While conventional treatments, including conservative and surgical options, are widely used, regenerative therapies offer promising potential but are currently experimental. These regenerative approaches focus on two main strategies: using growth factors to boost extracellular matrix synthesis by disc cells and employing agents to inhibit cytokines that contribute to matrix degradation. A broad understanding of these conditions is essential for radiologists. Imaging plays a crucial role in managing these diseases, particularly in assessing spinal stability and guiding treatment decisions, such as the use of potent anti-inflammatory medications. While MRI is typically the primary imaging tool for many spinal disorders, conventional radiographs and CT scans remain essential as first-line techniques, especially in trauma cases. In some instances, a combination of imaging modalities may be necessary to achieve an accurate and safe diagnosis.

Image Disclaimer Images used in this chapter are for educational purposes only. They are sourced from Radiopaedia and subject to their terms of use and Indian copyright laws.

References

1. Kos N, Gradisnik L, Velnar T. A brief review of the degenerative intervertebral disc disease. Medical Archives.2019 Dec;73(6):421.
2. DeWitt D. What is spinal osteoarthritis (Facet Joint Arthritis)? https://www.arthritis-health.com/types/osteoarthritis/what-spinal-osteoarthritis-facet-joint-arthritis
3. Ravindra VM, Senglaub SS, Rattani A, Dewan MC, Härtl R, Bisson E, Park KB, Shrime MG. Degenerative lumbar spine disease: estimating global incidence and worldwide volume. Global Spine J. 2018;8(8):784–94.
4. Scarcia L, Pileggi M, Camilli A, Romi A, Bartolo A, Giubbolini F, Valente I, Garignano G, D'Argento F, Pedicelli A, Alexandre AM. Degenerative disc disease of the spine: from anatomy to pathophysiology and radiological appearance, with morphological and functional considerations. J Pers Med. 2022;12(11):1810.
5. Wilson DJ, de Abreu M. Spine degeneration and inflammation. In Hodler J (Eds.) et. al., Musculoskeletal diseases 2021-2024: diagnostic imaging. Springer; 2021. pp. 197–213.
6. Amirdelfan K, McRoberts P, Deer TR. The differential diagnosis of low back pain: a primer on the evolving paradigm. Neuromodulation. 2014;17:11–7.
7. Bogduk N. Functional anatomy of the disc and lumbar spine. In: The artificial disc. Berlin, Heidelberg: Springer Berlin Heidelberg; 2003. p. 19–32.

8. Kushchayev SV, Glushko T, Jarraya M, Schuleri KH, Preul MC, Brooks ML, Teytelboym OM. ABCs of the degenerative spine. Insights Imaging. 2018;9:253–74.
9. Manshaii F, Tawil B. Degenerative disc disease: causes, symptoms, anatomy, market trends, and emerging treatment strategies. J Appl Biotechnol Bioeng. 2023;10(4):113–8.
10. Green BN, Johnson CD, Haldeman S, Griffith E, Clay MB, Kane EJ, Castellote JM, Rajasekaran S, Smuck M, Hurwitz EL, Randhawa K. A scoping review of biopsychosocial risk factors and co-morbidities for common spinal disorders. PLoS One. 2018;13(6):e0197987.
11. Chan D, Song Y, Sham P, Cheung KM. Genetics of disc degeneration. Eur Spine J. 2006;15:317–25.
12. Fang Y, van Meurs JB, d'Alesio A, Jhamai M, Zhao H, Rivadeneira F, Hofman A, van Leeuwen JP, Jehan F, Pols HA, Uitterlinden AG. Promoter and 3′-untranslated-region haplotypes in the vitamin D receptor gene predispose to osteoporotic fracture: the Rotterdam study. Am J Hum Genet. 2005;77(5):807–23.
13. Kawaguchi Y, Osada R, Kanamori M, Ishihara H, Ohmori K, Matsui H, Kimura T. Association between an aggrecan gene polymorphism and lumbar disc degeneration. Spine. 1999;24(23):2456.
14. Zhang YH, Zhao CQ, Jiang LS, Chen XD, Dai LY. Modic changes: a systematic review of the literature. Eur Spine J. 2008;17(10):1289–99.
15. Margetis K, Dowling TJ. Cervical Degenerative Disc Disease. 2025 Aug 2. In: StatPearls [Internet]. Treasure Island (FL): StatPearls Publishing; 2025 Jan–. PMID: 32809607.
16. Donnally III CJ, Hanna A, Varacallo MA. Lumbar Degenerative Disk Disease. 2023 Aug 4. In: StatPearls [Internet]. Treasure Island (FL): StatPearls Publishing; 2025 Jan–. PMID: 28846354. Donnally III CJ, Hanna A, Varacallo M. Lumbar degenerative disk disease.
17. Laplante BL, DePalma MJ. Spine osteoarthritis. PM&R. 2012;4:S28–36.
18. Raja A, Patel P, Mesfin FB. Spinal Stenosis. 2023 Jun 12. In: StatPearls [Internet]. Treasure Island (FL): StatPearls Publishing; 2025 Jan–. PMID: 28723018.
19. Schroeder GD, Kurd MF, Vaccaro AR. Lumbar spinal stenosis: how is it classified? J Am Acad Orthop Surg. 2016;24(12):843–52. [PubMed].
20. Munakomi S, Cruz R. Lumbar Spinal Stenosis. 2024 Jan 30. In: StatPearls [Internet]. Treasure Island (FL): StatPearls Publishing; 2025 Jan–. PMID: 30285388.
21. Margetis K, Gillis CC. Spondylolisthesis. [Updated 2025 Mar 28]. In: StatPearls [Internet]. Treasure Island (FL): StatPearls Publishing; 2025 Jan.
22. Shamrock AG, Donnally III CJ, Varacallo MA. Lumbar Spondylolysis and Spondylolisthesis. 2023 Aug 7. In: StatPearls [Internet]. Treasure Island (FL): StatPearls Publishing; 2025 Jan–. PMID: 28846329.
23. Koslosky E, Gendelberg D. Classification in brief: the Meyerding classification system of spondylolisthesis. Clin Orthop Relat Res. 2020;478(5):1125–30.
24. Donnally CJ III, Hanna A, Odom CK. Cervical myelopathy. In: StatPearls [Internet]. StatPearls Publishing; 2023.
25. McCormick JR, Sama AJ, Schiller NC, Butler AJ, Donnally CJ. Cervical spondylotic myelopathy: a guide to diagnosis and management. J Am Board Fam Med. 2020;33(2):303–13.
26. Fehlings MG, Kwon BK, Tetreault LA. Guidelines for the management of degenerative cervical myelopathy and spinal cord injury: an introduction to a focus issue. Global Spine J. 2017;7(3_suppl):6S–7S.
27. Costăchescu B, Niculescu AG, Teleanu RI, Iliescu BF, Rădulescu M, Grumezescu AM, Dabija MG. Recent advances in managing spinal intervertebral discs degeneration. Int J Mol Sci. 2022;23(12):6460.
28. Loughran MJ, Hunt JA. Stem cells for disc regeneration. In: Biomaterials for spinal surgery. Woodhead Publishing; 2012. p. 536–62.
29. Everts P, Onishi K, Jayaram P, Lana JF, Mautner K. Platelet-rich plasma: new performance understandings and therapeutic considerations in 2020. Int J Mol Sci. 2020;21(20):7794.
30. Soin A, Hirschbeck M, Verdon M, Manchikanti L. A pilot study implementing a machine learning algorithm to use artificial intelligence to diagnose spinal conditions. Pain Physician. 2022;25(2):171.

Understanding Degenerative Disc Disease

4

Aditya Gupta and Vishal Kumar

4.1 Introduction

Annular fissure, disc extrusion, disc protrusion, spondylolisthesis and disc degeneration are different stages of the same pathological process. The aetiology and development of disc herniation involve multiple factors including genetics, biology, mechanics, and the environment and this is still a matter of debate. The majority of discal nutrients will enter the disc through the adjacent vertebral endplates. Discal imbibitions (hydration) are facilitated by the high proteoglycan content of the central area of the disc [1]. These proteoglycans have a strong hydrophilic tendency, which obliges water molecules into the disc, maintaining the vascular volume and supporting the role of the highly hydrophilic hydrated nucleus in the short-term regulation of diurnal and postural related changes in disc deformation. Drying of these proteoglycans, together with collagen denaturation, results in the other hallmark of disc degeneration: a desiccated and brittle nucleus (dry degeneration) [2]. This is reversible in mild to moderate cases and majority of the cases can be managed with conservative treatment options, such as rest and/or physical therapy. However, the risk factors for disc degeneration are not clearly understood, which may compromise preventive measures. An improved understanding of the risk factors related to annular fissure, disc extrusion, and lumbar intervertebral disc degeneration is important for the prevention and management of lumbar disc herniation and the design of better personalized medical treatment (Fig. 4.1).

A. Gupta (✉) · V. Kumar
PGIMER, Chandigarh, India

V. Kumar, P. Mishra (eds.), *A Comprehensive Guide to Degenerative Spine Disorders*, https://doi.org/10.1007/978-981-96-9091-6_4

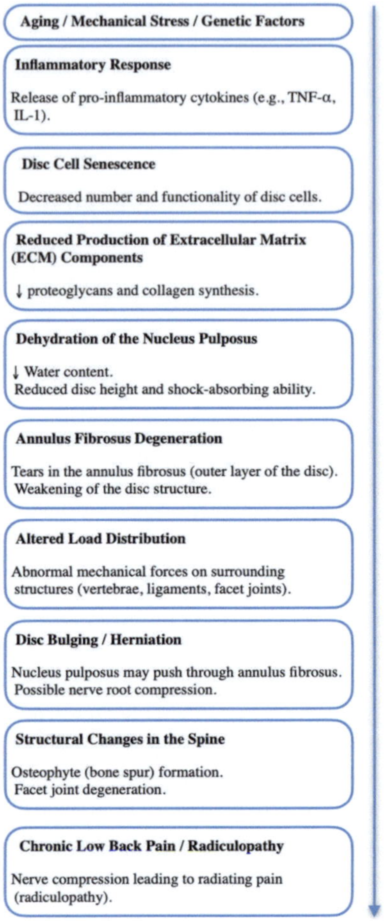

Fig. 4.1 Pathophysiology of DDD

4.2 Anatomy and Function of Intervertebral Discs

IVDs links adjacent vertebral bodies together and form 25% of spinal height. Each disc consists of two main components. (Fig. 4.2)

1. *Nucleus Pulposus*: This is the central part of the disc, composed of a gel-like substance rich in water (88%), type II collagen, and proteoglycans (mainly Aggrecans). It provides the disc with its ability to absorb shock and distribute loads. The hydrophilic matrix has a high polysaccharide content, which is responsible for height of the intervertebral disc. It contains chondrocyte-like cells responsible for producing type II collagen and proteoglycans and survive in hypoxic conditions.

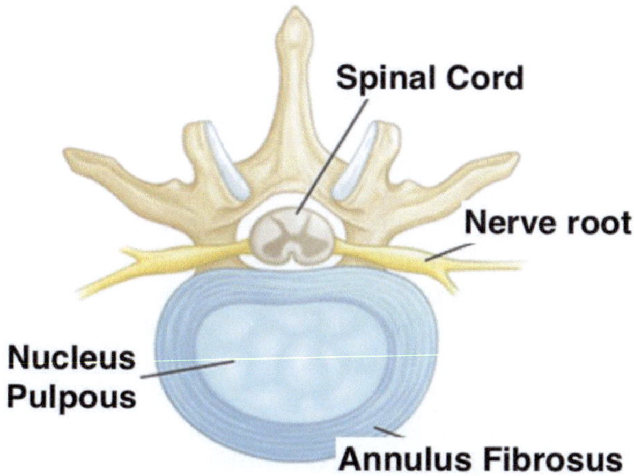

Fig. 4.2 Diagram depicting normal anatomy of disc and nucleus

2. *Annulus Fibrosus*: It is the outer structure surrounding Nucleus Pulposus. It acts as a tough, fibrous ring made up of concentric layers of collagen fibres having a high collagen/low proteoglycan ratio. The annulus fibrosus provides structural support and helps contain the nucleus pulposus. It has fibroblast-like cells, which produce Type I Collagen and proteoglycans.

The primary functions of intervertebral discs include:

- *Shock Absorption*: Discs act as cushions, absorbing the impact from daily activities such as walking, running, and lifting.
- *Load Distribution*: Discs help evenly distribute the weight and loads across the spine, reducing the stress on individual vertebrae.
- *Mobility*: Discs allow for a range of motion in the spine, including flexion, extension, and rotation.

Blood Supply The disk is an avascular structure. The structure of the endplate is a layer of cartilage and calcified cartilage, while the vertebral bony part is mainly a thin layer of trabecular bone. The transport of nutrients and waste through the endplate is an important factor that affects disc degeneration. The vertebral endplate brings nutrients to and takes waste away from the nucleus pulposus through diffusion. It not only acts as a barrier for the NP to prevent cell ingrowth from the adjacent vertebral bony structures notochordal cells but also allows cells to go through the bony tissue. The annulus is not porous enough to allow diffusion.

4.3 Aetiology and Pathophysiology of Degenerative Disc Disease

Pathological characteristics of ageing of the intervertebral disc of the lumbosacral localization are decreased height and destroyed or diluted intervertebral disc fibrous ring due to the destruction of collagen fibres of the fibrous ring of the intervertebral disc and a decrease in the water content of the core pulposus. In late stages of dystrophic changes in the fibrous structures and cartilaginous tissues, weight and gas exchange, enzymatic and biosynthetic processes are disrupted, which leads to the development of the core pulposus and the cartilaginous structures of the intervertebral disc [3].

4.3.1 Ageing and Degenerative Changes

The natural ageing process is the most significant factor contributing to DDD. As people age, the intervertebral discs undergo several changes (Table 4.1):

- *Decreased Hydration*: The nucleus pulposus loses water content, reducing its ability to absorb shock and maintain disc height.
- *Collagen Breakdown*: The collagen fibres in the annulus fibrosus weaken and become less organized, making the disc more susceptible to tears and herniation. However, there is no change in the absolute quantity of collagen.
- *Loss of Proteoglycans*: Proteoglycans, which help retain water within the disc, decrease, further contributing to dehydration and loss of disc height.

4.3.2 Other Contributing Factors

While ageing is the primary cause, other factors can accelerate or exacerbate disc degeneration:

- *Genetics*: A family history of DDD can increase an individual's risk of developing the condition.
- *Injury*: Traumatic events such as falls or car accidents can damage the discs and initiate the degenerative process.

Table 4.1 Change in IVD with ageing

Decreases with ageing	Increases with ageing
Water content	Keratin sulphate to chondroitin sulphate
Absolute viable cell number	S. lactate levels
Nutritional transport	Density of fibroblast-like cells
Proteoglycans	
pH	

- *Repetitive Stress*: Occupations or activities involving repetitive bending, lifting, or twisting can accelerate disc wear and tear.
- *Obesity*: Excess body weight increases the load on the spine, contributing to faster disc degeneration.
- *Smoking*: Nicotine impairs blood flow to the discs, reducing their ability to repair and maintain themselves.

4.3.3 Pathophysiological Changes

Degenerative disc disease is part of the natural process of growing older. During the course of the day, the intervertebral discs get compressed. This compression may cause small tears in the outer annulus fibrosus, hence known as annular tears. If the annular tears heal, the person usually is asymptomatic. If the annular tears do not heal, the internal disc material can extrude through the tears and cause pain and signs of compression [4]. This is one way a disc herniation occurs. If the disc material is pressing on a nerve, the person will feel pain radiating down the leg.

Depending on the symptomatology and prevalence of pain and lumbosacral radiculopathies after LDD (Lumbar Disc Disease), four stages of the intervertebral disc are in the focus of degeneration (Fig. 4.3).

STAGE 1 *(Disc Dehydration)*: In the early stage of DDD, the intervertebral discs lose their ability to retain water, causing dehydration. This results in a reduction in disc height and may lead to a decrease in the space between adjacent vertebrae. The annulus fibrosus may develop minor tears and cracks leading to disc instability and the potential for future damage.

STAGE 2 *(Disc Bulging)*: The nucleus pulposus pushes against the weakened annulus fibrosus, causing the disc to bulge. This puts pressure on adjacent structures causing persistent pain with radiation.

STAGE 3 *(Disc Herniation)*: In this stage, the inner nucleus pulposus extrudes through the tears in annulus fibrosus.

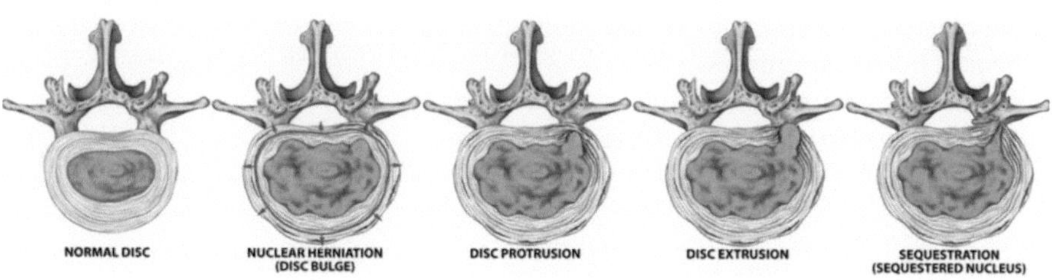

Fig. 4.3 Diagram showing different stages of degeneration

STAGE 4 *(Severe Degeneration)*: In the advanced stage of DDD, there is loss of space between the vertebrae. To compensate for the loss of disc height and instability, bony spurs grow along the edges.

- The superficial fibres of annulus are innervated by the sinuvertebral nerve. It is given off by the dorsal root ganglion. Neuropeptides released by the IVDs include substance P, calcitonin, VIP (Vasoactive Intestinal Peptide), CPON (C terminal flanking Peptide of Neuropeptide Y) [5]. Disc herniation, herniated discs, lead to increased production of neurotransmitter including:
- Osteoprotegrin (OPG)
- Interleukin-1 beta
- Receptor activator of nuclear factor-kB ligand (RANKL)
- Parathyroid hormone (PTH)

Lateral radiographs of the lumbar spine are used to make the diagnosis. Flexion and extension lateral lumbar radiographs identify the degree of instability. MRI studies are helpful for diagnosing central or foraminal stenosis.

4.4 Clinical Manifestations

- *Back Pain*: The most common symptom, which can be chronic or intermittent. The pain is often described as a deep, aching sensation and is usually relieved with rest and sitting.
- *Radicular Pain*: Pain that radiates from the spine to other areas, such as the buttocks, thighs, or legs, indicating nerve involvement. This is commonly seen in cases where the disc herniates and compresses a nerve root. It may lead to neurogenic claudication and leg pain (Table 4.2). The pain is relieved by sitting but not relieved by standing in one place (as is vascular claudication) and may be unilateral or bilateral. Cauda equina syndrome may manifest in very rare cases.
- *Stiffness and Reduced Mobility*: Loss of disc height and elasticity can lead to reduced spinal flexibility and stiffness.
- *Numbness and Tingling*: Compression of spinal nerves can cause sensory disturbances in the extremities.
- *Muscle Weakness*: In severe cases, nerve compression can lead to weakness in the muscles served by the affected nerves.

Table 4.2 Neurogenic vs vascular claudication

Feature	Neurogenic claudication	Vascular claudication
Cause	Compression of spinal nerves, often due to spinal stenosis or degenerative changes in the spine	Insufficient blood flow to leg muscles due to peripheral artery disease (PAD)
Pain	Burning, tingling, numbness, weakness, or cramping	Cramping, aching, tightness, or heaviness in the legs
Location	Lower back, buttocks, thighs, calves, feet	Calves, thighs, or buttocks (less often lower back)
Triggering factor	Walking or standing for long periods, especially when upright	Physical activity, such as walking or climbing stairs
Relief	Pain relieved by bending forward or sitting (flexing the spine)	Pain relieved by stopping activity and resting
Effect of posture	Worsens with standing or walking upright; improves with bending forward (e.g., leaning on a shopping cart)	Posture has no effect on symptoms
Walking uphill	Walking uphill or bending forward often improves symptoms	Walking uphill usually worsens symptoms
Onset	Gradual onset and varies with movement and posture	Occurs quickly after walking a certain distance
Relief time	Pain relief may take longer, not immediate with rest	Pain relief is rapid (within minutes) after stopping activity
Pulses	Pulses are usually normal and present	Weak or absent pulses in the legs or feet due to poor circulation
Skin	No associated skin changes	Skin may appear pale, cool, or show signs of poor circulation (hair loss, ulcers)
Diagnostic test	MRI or CT scan to confirm spinal stenosis or nerve compression	Ankle-brachial index (ABI) or Doppler ultrasound to assess blood flow
Treatment	Physical therapy, medications, or surgery (e.g., decompression surgery)	Lifestyle changes, medications, or surgical interventions like angioplasty or bypass

4.5 Diagnostic Evaluation

Diagnosing DDD involves a combination of patient history, physical examination, and imaging studies:

- *Patient History*: A detailed history of the patient's symptoms, including onset, duration, and factors that alleviate or exacerbate the pain, is essential.
- *Physical Examination*: The physician will assess spinal mobility, alignment, and signs of nerve compression, such as abnormal reflexes, muscle strength, and sensation.
- *Imaging Studies*:
  - *X-rays*: Useful for detecting changes in disc height, spinal alignment, and the presence of osteophytes. Recommended views are lumbar AP, lateral neutral,

lateral flexion, and lateral extension in weight bearing. The slip is evident on lateral X-ray. The flexion and extension radiographs help to exclude instability. A spine is said to be unstable if there is translation of >4 mm or 10° of angulation of motion compared to adjacent motion segment.

- *MRI (Magnetic Resonance Imaging)*: MRI is the investigation of choice to evaluate impingement of neural elements. It is indicated in persistent backache failing non operative intervention or for neurological defect and bowel bladder involvement. Provides detailed images of the discs, allowing for assessment of disc hydration, annular tears, and nerve compression. However, degenerative changes on MRI do not always correlate with the amount of back pain. Sometimes people without any back pain at all will have degenerative findings on their MRI (Fig. 4.4).
- *CT (Computed Tomography) Scans*: Can be used to evaluate bony pathology and detect disc degeneration or herniation. CT myelogram is investigation of choice where an MRI is contraindicated (e.g. pacemaker) (Fig. 4.5).

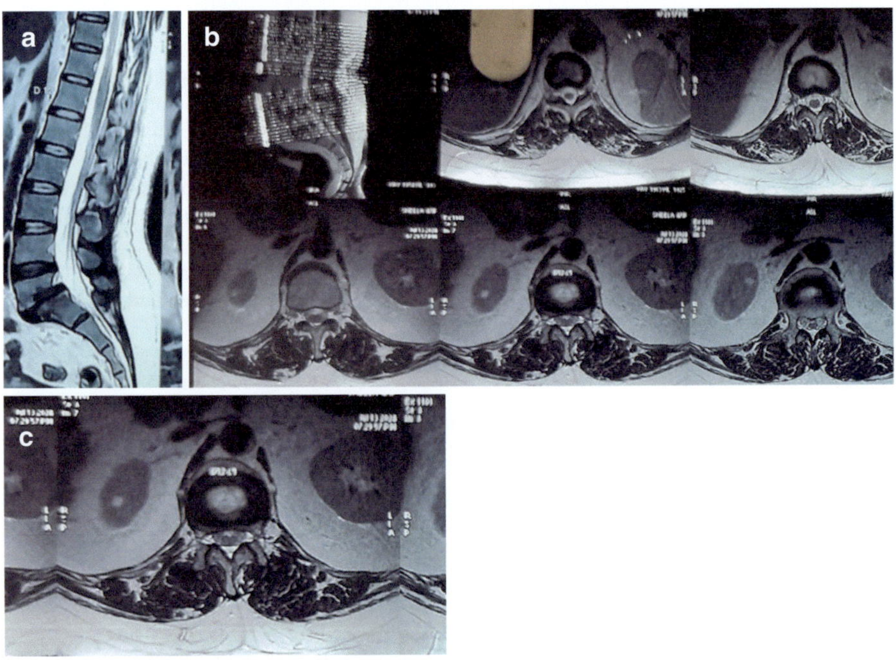

Fig. 4.4 (**a**) Sagittal cut of L/S MRI showing DDD. (**b**) Axial cut of L/S MRI showing disc protrusion. (**c**) Axial cut of L/S MRI showing disc herniation. (**d**) Axial cut of L/S MRI showing disc sequestration

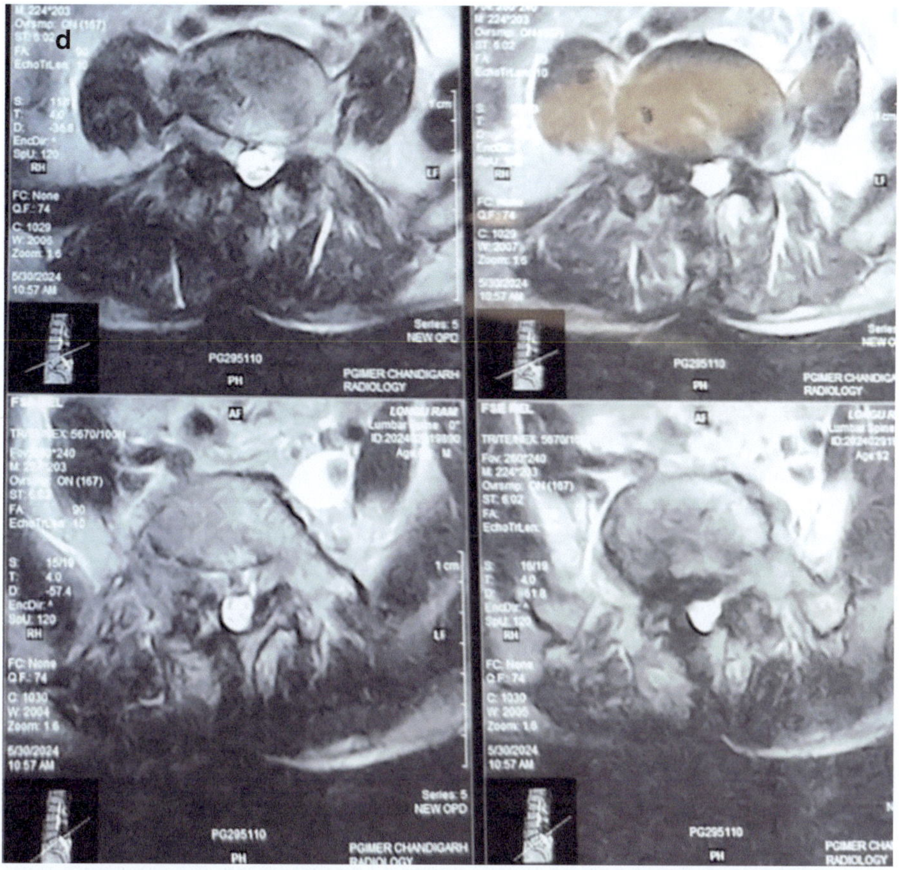

Fig. 4.4 (continued)

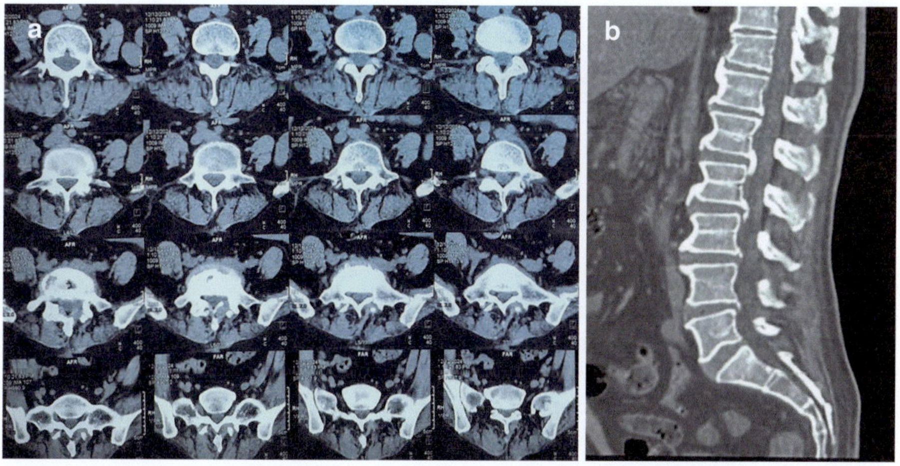

Fig. 4.5 (**a**) Axial cut of NCCT L/S Spine. (**b**) Sagittal cut of L/S MRI showing degeneration and post osteophytes

4.6 Treatment Options

4.6.1 Conservative Management

Treatment is a trial of nonoperative management with NSAIDs and physical therapy. Surgical management is indicated for progressive disabling pain that has failed nonoperative management, and/or progressive neurological deficits. Most cases of DDD can be managed with non-surgical treatments.

- *Medications*:
  - *Pain Relievers*: Most patients can be treated nonoperatively with Non-Steroidal Anti-Inflammatory Drugs (NSAIDs), activity restriction, and physiotherapy.
  - *Muscle Relaxants*: These can be prescribed to relieve muscle spasms.
  - *Corticosteroids*: Oral or injectable steroids may be used to reduce inflammation.
- *Physical Therapy*: Tailored exercises can strengthen the muscles supporting the spine, improve flexibility, and reduce pain (Fig. 4.6).
- *Lifestyle Modifications*:
  - *Weight Management*: Maintaining a healthy weight reduces the load on the spine.
  - *Ergonomic Adjustments*: Modifying workspaces and daily activities to reduce stress on the spine. General precautions include avoiding bending forward and lifting heavy weight. Cushioning should be added for prolonged sitting and desk jobs. Using a chair with proper lumbar support to maintain the natural curvature of spine and adding a small cushion or lumbar roll can help reduce pain. A good chair allows your feet to rest flat on the floor with your knees at a 90-degree angle, aligning with your hips. Standing intermittently can relieve pressure on the discs and improve circulation. Take breaks every 30 min to stand, stretch, and walk around to reduce spinal compression.
  - *Smoking Cessation*: Quitting smoking improves blood flow to the discs and enhances healing.

4.6.2 Interventional Procedures

When conservative treatments are insufficient, interventional procedures may be considered:

- *Epidural Steroid Injections*: Injections of corticosteroids into the epidural space can reduce inflammation and alleviate pain. (Fig. 4.7).
- *Facet Joint Injections*: Injections into the facet joints can help manage pain originating from these structures.
- *Radio Frequency Ablation*: This procedure uses heat to disrupt the nerves transmitting pain signals from the affected discs or facet joints.

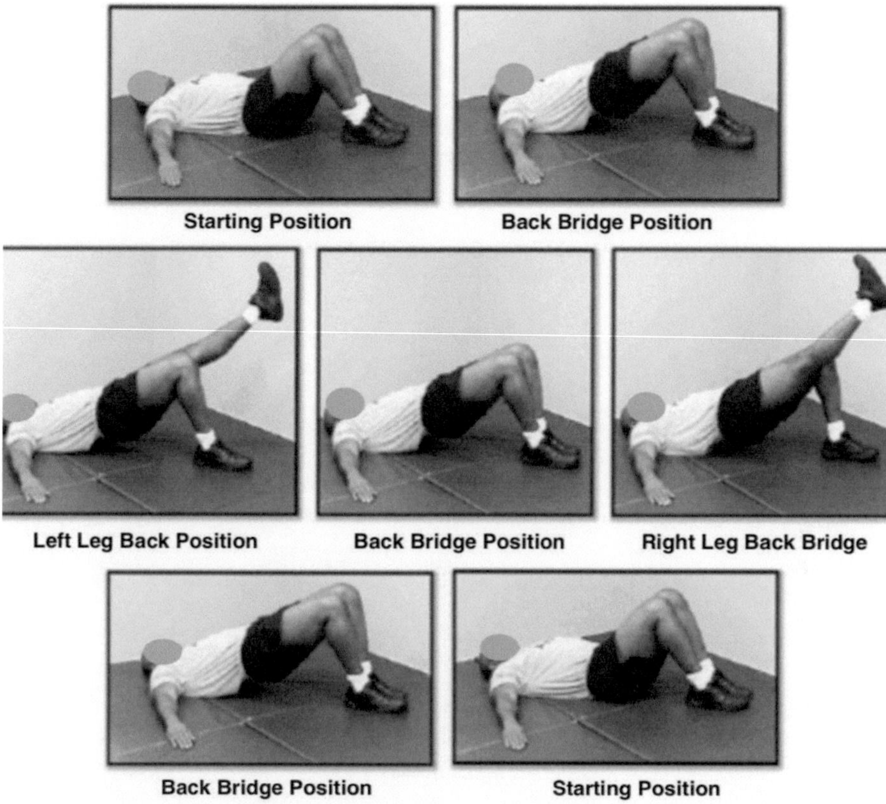

Fig. 4.6 Back and core strengthening exercises

4.6.3 Surgical Treatment

Surgery is typically reserved for severe cases of DDD that do not respond to conservative or interventional treatments. Common surgical options include:

- *Lumbar decompression*: Removal of a portion of a herniated disc that is compressing a nerve (Fig. 4.8). Indications include persistent and aggravating pain (>6 months of failed nonoperative management and epidural steroid injections), progressive neurodeficit or development of cauda equina syndrome
- *Spinal Fusion*: Joining two or more vertebrae together to stabilize the spine. This can alleviate pain but reduces spinal flexibility. There are improved fusion rates on using pedicle screws over cortical screws. The decompression is often done using a unilateral approach preserving PLC (Posterior Longitudinal Complex). Navigation and MIS (Minimal Invasive Surgery) techniques are gaining popularity nowadays, more than 80% have satisfactory outcomes. Smoking should be stopped prior to surgery since it has a poor prognosis.

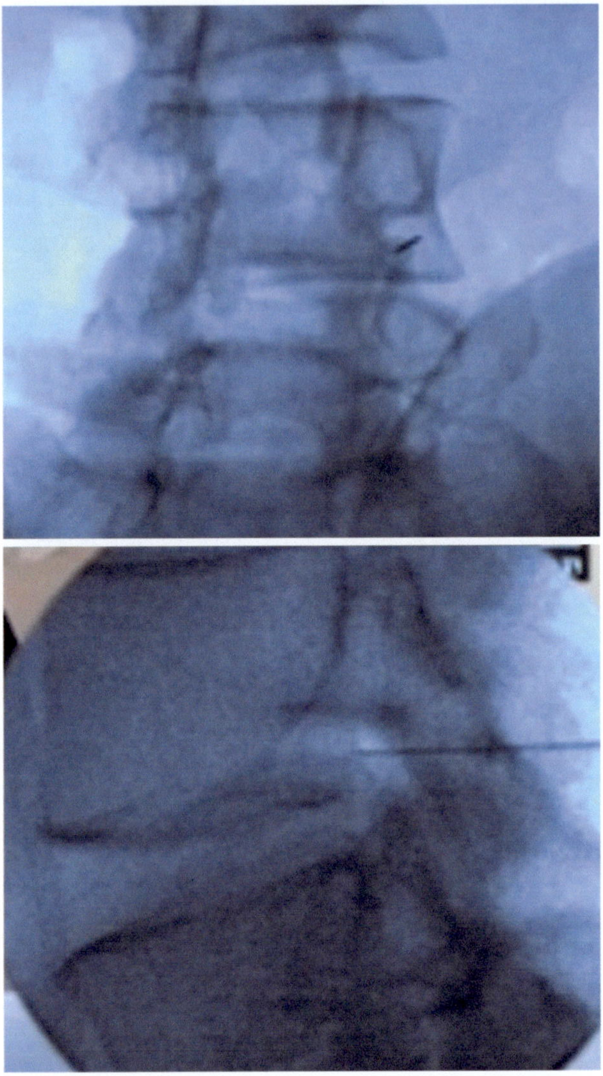

Fig. 4.7 Transforaminal nerve root block procedure

- *Artificial Disc Replacement*: The damaged disc is replaced with an artificial one to maintain spinal mobility. The preserved motion was believed to cause less Adjacent Segment Disease but results show results comparable to fusion.
- *Posterior Decompression with Posterolateral Fusion*: Laminectomy, wide decompression, and foraminotomy is done via posterior approach. TLIF/PLIF (Transforaminal Lumbar Interbody Fusion/Posterior Lumbar Interbody Fusion) is being used widely due to increase in fusion rates and decreased risk of postoperative slip progression. Reducing the slip has none to limited role in adults. Cortical bone trajectory screws are gaining popularity recently due to limited lateral exposure for obtaining screw starting points. The fusion rates and functional outcomes are similar to conventional pedicle screw fixation.

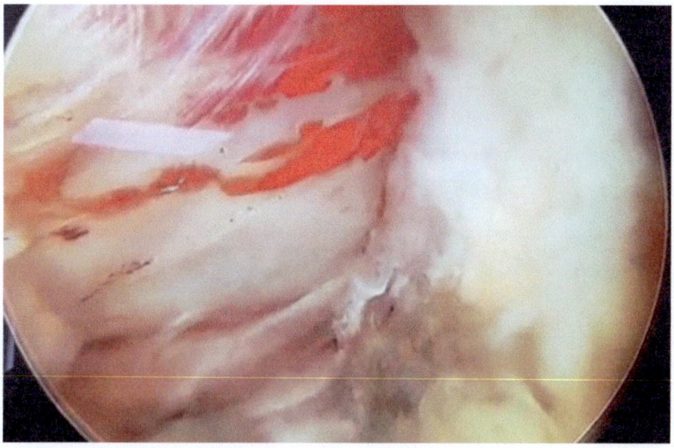

Fig. 4.8 Endoscopic discectomy showing decompressed dura

4.7 Complications

- *Pseudoarthrosis*: Seen in 5–30% of the patients. The investigation of choice is CT scan. It is more accurate than MRI for identifying failed arthrodesis.
- *Adjacent Segment Disease (2–3%)*: 20–30% cases require re-surgery at 10 years. The cause is the compensatory increase in motion due to the fused adjacent level space and soft tissue damage during surgery.
- *Surgical site infection (0.2–2%)*: Usually resolves with antibiotics and debridement. Hardware can be retained in majority of the cases.
- *Dural Tear*: Intra operative dural tear requires repair of the defect. CSF (Cerebrospinal Fluid) leakage manifests as nausea, vomiting, headaches and visual disturbances. Acetazolamide is given post operatively.
- *Neuropathy*: LFCN (Lateral Femoral Cutaneous Nerve), ulnar nerve or brachial plexopathy may be compressed due to prone positioning with incorrect position.

4.8 Prevention Strategies

4.8.1 Maintaining a Healthy Lifestyle

Adopting a healthy lifestyle can help prevent or slow the progression of DDD:

- *Regular Exercise*: Engaging in regular physical activity, including strength training, aerobic exercises, and flexibility exercises, helps maintain a healthy spine.
- *Healthy Diet*: A balanced diet rich in essential nutrients supports overall health and weight management.
- *Proper Body Mechanics*: Using proper techniques for lifting and bending can reduce the risk of injury to the spine.

- *Workplace Ergonomics*: Adjusting chairs, desks, and computer screens to maintain proper posture.
- *Supportive Footwear*: Wearing shoes that provide good support and cushioning.
- *Regular Medical Check-ups*: Regular check-ups with a healthcare provider can help detect early signs of DDD and manage risk factors effectively.

4.9 Conclusion

Degenerative Disc Disease is a common condition that affects many individuals as they age. While it can cause significant discomfort and reduce quality of life, understanding its aetiology, clinical manifestations, and treatment options can help manage the condition effectively. With appropriate interventions and lifestyle modifications, many individuals with DDD can lead active, fulfilling lives. Advances in medical research continue to improve our understanding of DDD, offering hope for more effective treatments and preventive strategies in the future.

References

1. Scarcia L, Pileggi M, Camilli A, Romi A, Bartolo A, Giubbolini F, Valente I, Garignano G, D'Argento F, Pedicelli A, et al. Degenerative disc disease of the spine: from anatomy to pathophysiology and radiological appearance, with morphological and functional considerations. J Pers Med. 2022;12(11):1810.
2. Iatridis JC, MacLean JJ, O'Brien M, Stokes IA. Measurements of proteoglycan and water content distribution in human lumbar intervertebral discs. Spine (Phila Pa 1976). 2007;32(14):1493–7.
3. Diaconu GS, Mihalache CG, Popescu G, et al. Clinical and pathological considerations in lumbar herniated disc associated with inflammatory lesions. Romanian J Morphol Embryol. 2021;62(4):951–60.
4. Dowdell J, Erwin M, Choma T, Vaccaro A, Iatridis J, Cho SK. Intervertebral disk degeneration and repair [published correction appears in neurosurgery]. Neurosurgery. 2018;83(5):1084. https://doi.org/10.1093/neuros/nyy437. Neurosurgery 2017;80(3S):S46–54.
5. Groh AMR, Fournier DE, Battié MC, Séguin CA. Innervation of the human intervertebral disc: a scoping review. Pain Med. 2021;22(6):1281–304.

Degenerative Spondylolisthesis

5

Vineet Kumar and Prakhar Mishra

5.1 Aetiology

The development of degenerative spondylolisthesis is multifactorial, with several factors contributing to its onset. Ageing is a major predisposing factor, leading to degenerative changes such as disc degeneration, pars defect (Fig. 5.1) facet joint arthritis, and ligamentum flavum hypertrophy. These age-related alterations contribute to an imbalance in the stability of the spine, allowing for the slippage of one vertebral body over another. Genetic factors [1] may also play a role in the susceptibility to degenerative spondylolisthesis, influencing the structural integrity of the spine components.

V. Kumar (✉)
Dr. Ram Manohar Lohia Institute of Medical Sciences, Lucknow, India

P. Mishra
Dr. Ram Manohar Lohia Institute of Medical Sciences, Lucknow, India

V. Kumar, P. Mishra (eds.), *A Comprehensive Guide to Degenerative Spine Disorders*, https://doi.org/10.1007/978-981-96-9091-6_5

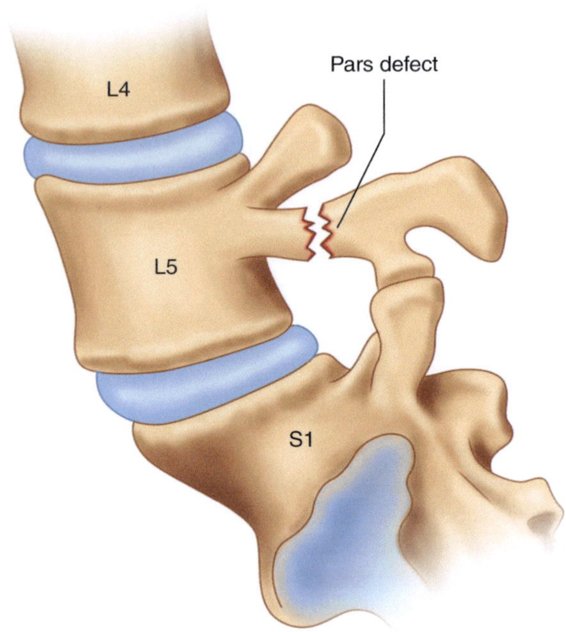

Fig. 5.1 Spondylosis showing pars interarticularis defect

5.2 Classification

The Wiltse, Newman, and Macnab classification [2] system categorizes spondylolisthesis based on aetiological factors. Developed by orthopaedic surgeons in the 1970s, this classification identifies three distinct types. Type I, or dysplastic, involves congenital abnormalities affecting the neural arch. Type II, isthmic, results from a defect in the pars interarticularis, often seen in athletes. Type III, or degenerative, occurs due to aging-related changes, affecting the posterior elements. This classification aids clinicians in tailoring treatment approaches, emphasizing the importance of understanding the underlying causes of spondylolisthesis for more precise diagnosis and effective management.

Type I	Dysplastic
Type II	Isthmic
Type III	Degenerative
Type IV	Post-traumatic
Type V	Pathologic
Type VI	Post-surgical

Degenerative spondylolisthesis can be classified based on the severity of the slippage, presence of associated symptoms, and radiographic features. The Meyerding classification [3] system categorizes spondylolisthesis into Grades I–IV, indicating the percentage of slippage relative to the width of the superior vertebral body.

Grade I	0–25% slippage
Grade II	25–50% slippage
Grade III	50–75% slippage
Grade IV	75–100% slippage
Grade V	More than 100% slippage

Additionally, the Spinal deformity Study Group (SDSG) [4] system focuses on three key traits evaluable through sagittal radiographs of the spine and pelvis: (1) the slip grade (low or high), (2) pelvic incidence (low, normal, or high), and (3) spino-pelvic balance (balanced or unbalanced). Consequently, six distinct subtypes emerge from this refined approach.

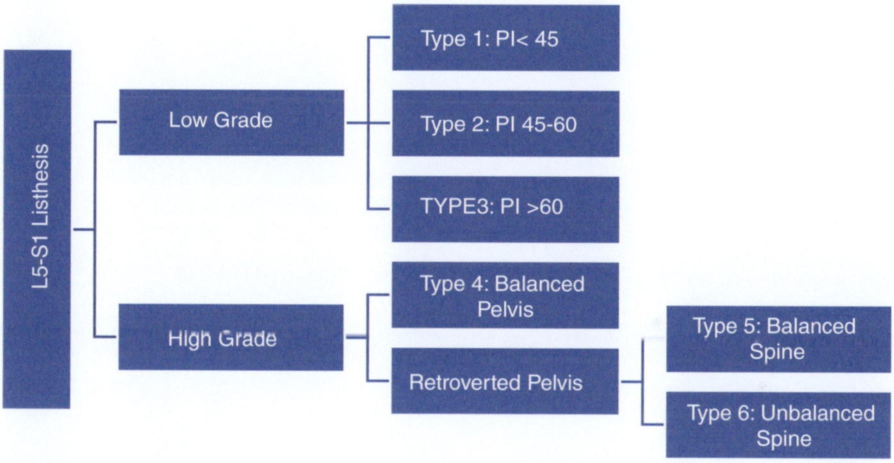

5.3 Clinical Examination

A comprehensive clinical examination is essential for diagnosing and assessing degenerative spondylolisthesis. Patients typically present with lower back pain, which may radiate into the buttocks or thighs. Neurological symptoms such as radiculopathy or claudication may also be present, depending on the degree of nerve root compression. Physical examination includes evaluating gait, assessing range of motion, and performing neurologic testing to identify any sensory or motor deficits. Understanding the clinical presentation aids in formulating an accurate diagnosis and determining the most suitable treatment approach.

5.4 Imaging

Various imaging modalities play a crucial role in the diagnosis and assessment of degenerative spondylolisthesis. Plain radiographs provide a baseline evaluation of the degree of slippage and help in classifying the condition. Advanced imaging techniques, such as magnetic resonance imaging (MRI) and computed tomography (CT), offer detailed information about the intervertebral discs, facet joints, and nerve roots. Dynamic imaging (Fig. 5.2), including flexion and extension radiographs, assists in assessing the dynamic instability of the spine. A seated lateral view and supine films suffice for patients who are not able to perform active flexion and extension postures for assessment of dynamic instability. These imaging tools collectively contribute to a comprehensive understanding of the pathology and aid in treatment planning.

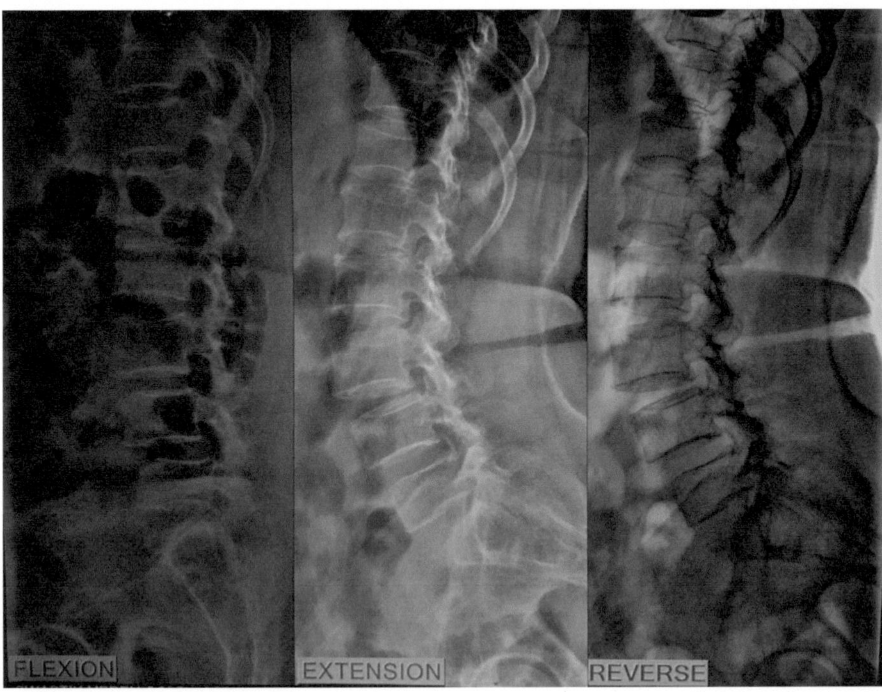

Fig. 5.2 Dynamic imaging showing flexion extension views

5.5 Conservative Treatment

For mild to moderate cases of degenerative spondylolisthesis, conservative management is typically the first line of treatment. Non-surgical interventions focus on relieving symptoms, enhancing function, and preventing further progression of the condition. Physical therapy is a key component, helping to strengthen core muscles, improve flexibility, and encourage proper body mechanics. Pain management may include the use of non-steroidal anti-inflammatory drugs (NSAIDs) and analgesics to reduce discomfort and inflammation. If the patient does not respond to oral analgesics, a trial of selective nerve root block or caudal epidural analgesia must be tried prior to resorting to surgical intervention in order to break the pain cycle and gaining patients confidence motivating him for physical therapy. Lifestyle changes, such as weight control and modifying activities, are also vital to treatment. Educating patients on correct posture and body mechanics enables them to take an active role in their care. Counselling and prognostication are important aspects of conservative management in these subgroups of patients.

5.6 Surgical Treatment

Surgical intervention becomes necessary when conservative treatments fail to provide sufficient relief or when there is progressive neurological deterioration. The selection of a surgical procedure is based on factors such as the degree of vertebral slippage, the presence of neurological symptoms, and the patient's overall health. Decompression techniques, like laminectomy and foraminotomy, are used to relieve nerve root compression, while spinal fusion, with or without instrumentation, is often performed to stabilize the affected area and prevent further slippage.

Historically, spinal fusion was the standard treatment for spondylolisthesis, a principle supported by a 1991 prospective study by Herkowitz et al. [5] published in JBJS. But is fusion necessary for every patient?

In 2016, Peter Forsth [6] and colleagues conducted a randomized controlled trial to assess the effectiveness of fusion surgery combined with decompression in patients with lumbar spinal stenosis, with or without degenerative spondylolisthesis. The study found no significant difference between the fusion and decompression-only groups in terms of average ODI scores or 6-min walk test results. However, the fusion group had longer surgeries, greater blood loss, and higher surgical costs.

In 2018, Hiroyuki [7] and colleagues evaluated long-term outcomes of three surgical approaches for degenerative spondylolisthesis: decompression alone, decompression with fusion, and decompression with stabilization. They found that both fusion and stabilization groups had increased blood loss and longer surgeries compared to the decompression-only group. Additionally, patients in the fusion group experienced longer hospital stays. Importantly, for low-grade (<30%) degenerative spondylolisthesis, the addition of instrumentation did not result in better outcomes compared to decompression alone at both 1 and 5 years post-surgery.

Even the recent literature published after 2020 [8–10] support the view that the clinical effectiveness of decompression alone was comparable to that of decompression with fusion for degenerative lumbar spondylolisthesis.

A dogmatic approach that everyone with a degenerative spondylolisthesis needs a fusion is not backed up by the literature.

So, the question is: Does the patient need fusion or we want to fuse? Or the fusion is not needed at all?

On the basis of radiologic parameters, it has been observed that both an increasing incidence over time and an increasing progression of the slip rate is seen in up to a third of the patients older than 25 years, which is important aspect for counselling patients and surgical decision making.

One may consider fusion in cases with:

(a) Instability seen on flexion extension films-

$$\text{SP}(\text{Slip percentage}) \geq 8\% \text{ or } \geq 3\text{mm}$$

(b) Sagittal alignment of facets
(c) Component of axial back pain
(d) Possible bony component of subarticular recess stenosis

Lumbar interbody fusion (LIF) is a well-established procedure for treating various spinal conditions, including degeneration, trauma, infection, and tumours. Procedure involves discectomy followed by end plate preparation and placing an implant (cage or spacer) or bone graft into the intervertebral space. Lumbar interbody fusion is performed through five main approaches:

1. Posterior lumbar interbody fusion (PLIF)
2. Transforaminal lumbar interbody fusion (TLIF or MI-TLIF)
3. Oblique lumbar interbody fusion/anterior to psoas (OLIF/ATP)
4. Anterior lumbar interbody fusion (ALIF)
5. Lateral lumbar interbody fusion (LLIF)

- *PLIF*: The PLIF (Posterior Lumbar Interbody Fusion) technique accesses the intervertebral disc through a posterior approach, with the patient positioned prone on an Andrews or Jackson table. After identifying the spinous process and laminae at the target levels (L1-S1), a laminotomy is performed medial to the facet, and the dura is retracted to access the disc space. The space and endplates are then prepared for implant or spacer insertion. However, PLIF has some drawbacks. Prolonged muscle retraction can cause paraspinal injury, delaying recovery and mobilization. Additionally, correcting coronal imbalance, restoring lordosis, and preparing endplates can be more difficult than with anterior fusion techniques.

- *TLIF*: The TLIF (Transforaminal Lumbar Interbody Fusion) approach offers several advantages, including easier access to posterior structures like the lamina, ligamentum flavum, and facet joints. Unlike PLIF, TLIF preserves key ligamentous structures, which helps maintain biomechanical stability in both the affected and adjacent segments. It provides bilateral anterior column support through a single unilateral incision. When performed using minimally invasive surgery (MIS) techniques with a mini-open incision and magnification tools, it reduces muscle injury, bleeding, and enhances recovery. However, like PLIF, TLIF can still lead to paraspinal muscle injury from prolonged retraction, and it may be challenging to correct coronal imbalance or restore lordosis.
- *ALIF*: ALIF (Anterior Lumbar Interbody Fusion) is an extremely effective technique for the management of discogenic low back pain. The front of disc is approached from anterior retroperitoneally, which enables a through discectomy and implant placement for fusion. Main advantages of this approach include a direct view of disc space from midline and wide lateral exposure of the body of vertebra, which makes discectomy easy and endplate preparation easier. The approach also allows for the use of larger implants, improving lordosis correction and restoring foraminal height. Additionally, it leads to higher fusion rates due to more extensive disc space preparation.
- *XLIF*: Extreme lateral interbody fusion (XLIF), introduced by Ozgur et al. in 2006, involves accessing the disc space through a lateral retroperitoneal and transpsoas corridor. This minimally invasive approach provides direct access to the intervertebral disc while preserving much of the surrounding tissue, making it particularly effective for correcting both sagittal and coronal deformities. XLIF is especially beneficial in cases of lumbar degenerative scoliosis with lateral listhesis, where it helps realign the spine and restore balance.

The technique allows for the placement of larger interbody devices, which aids in restoring disc height and improving segmental lordosis. Additionally, by avoiding a posterior approach, XLIF minimizes disruption to the spinal musculature, reducing postoperative pain and recovery time.

However, the XLIF, or more broadly the LLIF (Lateral Lumbar Interbody Fusion) technique, has limitations. It is less suitable for patients with severe central canal stenosis, as the lateral approach does not adequately address central compression. Similarly, cases with bony lateral recess stenosis or high-grade spondylolisthesis may not be ideal candidates, as these conditions often require direct decompression or stabilization that is difficult to achieve through a lateral approach. In such cases, posterior or other surgical techniques may be necessary to achieve optimal outcomes.

- *OLIF*: The oblique lumbar interbody fusion (OLIF), also known as the anterior to psoas (ATP) approach, was first described by Michael Mayer in 1977 and employs a minimally invasive technique to access the disc space via a path between the peritoneum and the psoas muscle. Similar to the lateral lumbar interbody fusion (LLIF), OLIF avoids posterior interventions such as laminectomy, facetectomy, or disrupting spinal or paraspinal muscles. However, unlike the lateral transpsoas approach, OLIF does not require dissection or passage through the psoas muscle, reducing the risk of nerve damage. During OLIF, the patient is positioned laterally, with either the left or right side up depending on the surgeon's preference and anatomical access to the target disc. This approach allows for easier placement of larger implants, improving lordosis correction and foraminal height restoration, while minimizing muscle trauma and postoperative recovery time. It is especially useful in cases where anterior access is needed without the complications associated with posterior surgery.

Recent advancements, such as minimally invasive surgery (MIS) and stereotactic spinal guidance, have significantly advanced the field. MIS techniques have been shown to minimize muscle damage and reduce perioperative pain, leading to faster recovery and improved quality of life. In cases of symptomatic, single-level degenerative grade-1 spondylolisthesis, MIS TLIF offers better outcomes in terms of disability, back pain, and patient satisfaction compared to posterior MIS decompression alone, and it is also associated with a lower reoperation rate.

5.7 Conclusion

Degenerative spondylolisthesis is a common spinal disorder affecting the lumbar spine, particularly in the ageing population. Understanding its aetiology, classification, clinical presentation, and appropriate imaging techniques is crucial for accurate diagnosis and effective treatment planning. Conservative measures play a vital role in managing mild to moderate cases, while surgical intervention becomes necessary in cases of severe slippage or progressive neurological compromise. Do not subject each patient of degenerative spondylolisthesis to fusion surgery. Decision to operate on degenerative listhesis should be tailor made, depending on multiple factors that have been discussed. The collaborative efforts of healthcare professionals, including orthopaedic surgeons, neurosurgeons, and physical therapists, are essential in providing comprehensive care to individuals with degenerative spondylolisthesis. Ongoing research and advancements in treatment modalities continue to shape the landscape of managing this challenging spinal condition.

References

1. Biswas A, Garg B. Decoding the genetic threads of disc degeneration. Indian Spine J. 2024;7(2):148–58.
2. Wiltse LL, Newman PH, Macnab IA. Classification of spondyloisis and spondylolisthesis. Clin Orthop Relat Res. 1976;117:23–9.
3. Koslosky E, Gendelberg D. Classification in brief: the Meyerding classification system of spondylolisthesis. Clin Orthop Relat Res. 2020;478(5):1125–30.

4. Mac-Thiong JM, Duong L, Parent S, Hresko MT, Dimar JR, Weidenbaum M, Labelle H. Reliability of the spinal deformity study group classification of lumbosacral spondylolisthesis. Spine. 2012;37(2):E95–102.
5. Herkowitz HN, Kurz LT. Degenerative lumbar spondylolisthesis with spinal stenosis. A prospective study comparing decompression with decompression and intertransverse process arthrodesis. JBJS. 1991;73(6):802–8.
6. Försth P, Ólafsson G, Carlsson T, Frost A, Borgström F, Fritzell P, Öhagen P, Michaëlsson K, Sandén B. A randomized, controlled trial of fusion surgery for lumbar spinal stenosis. N Engl J Med. 2016;374(15):1413–23.
7. Aoki Y, Takahashi H, Nakajima A, Kubota G, Watanabe A, Nakajima T, Eguchi Y, Orita S, Fukuchi H, Yanagawa N, Nakagawa K. Prevalence of lumbar spondylolysis and spondylolisthesis in patients with degenerative spinal disease. Sci Rep. 2020;10(1):6739.
8. Wei FL, Zhou CP, Gao QY, Du MR, Gao HR, Zhu KL, Li T, Qian JX, Yan XD. Decompression alone or decompression and fusion in degenerative lumbar spondylolisthesis. EClinMed. 2022;51:101559. https://doi.org/10.1016/j.eclinm.2022.101559. PMID: 35865739; PMCID: PMC9294267.
9. Kaiser R, Kantorová L, Langaufová A, et al. Decompression alone versus decompression with instrumented fusion in the treatment of lumbar degenerative spondylolisthesis: a systematic review and meta-analysis of randomised trials. J Neurol Neurosurg Psychiatry. 2023;94:657–66.
10. Kgomotso EL, Hellum C, Fagerland MW, Solberg T, Brox JI, Storheim K, Hermansen E, Franssen E, Weber C, Brisby H, Algaard KR. Decompression alone or with fusion for degenerative lumbar spondylolisthesis (Nordsten-DS): five year follow-up of a randomised, multicentre, non-inferiority trial. BMJ. 2024;386:e079771. https://doi.org/10.1136/bmj-2024-079771.

Degenerative Kyphosis and Scoliosis

6

Rakesh Kumar, Deepak Kumar Singh, Rajiv Sethi, and Neha Singh

6.1 Introduction

Kyphoscoliosis is a complex condition affecting the thoracolumbar spine, characterized by abnormal curvature in multiple planes [1]. Depending on variables like the age at which the condition first manifests and the root cause, this spinal deformity may result in a number of complications. Adult scoliosis is referred to as a coronal plane spinal deformity with a Cobbs angle exceeding 10°.

Kyphosis and lordosis are the deformity of spine in sagittal plane. Typically, Thoracic kyphosis sees a natural progression with age, reaching up to 29° in people below 40, 53° in those 60–74, and 66° in people over 75 [2]. Kyphoscoliosis can occur in the cervicothoracic area, although it most frequently affects the thoracolumbar spine. The Cobb angle is used to categorize the severity of kyphoscoliosis: moderate kyphoscoliosis falls between 25 and 100°, while severe kyphoscoliosis surpasses 100°. The degree of axial rotation, the number of involved vertebrae, the position of curvature and severity all affect how these aberrant curvatures affect

R. Kumar
Department of Neurosurgery, University of Virginia, Charlottesville, VA, USA
e-mail: Rk8nv@uvahealth.org

D. K. Singh (✉)
Department of Neurosurgery, Dr. Ram Manohar Lohia Institute of Medical Sciences, Lucknow, India

R. Sethi
Departments of Orthopaedics and Neurosurgery, Virginia Mason Medical Center, Seattle, WA, USA
e-mail: sethir@uw.edu

N. Singh
Department of Radiodiagnosis, Dr. Ram Manohar Lohia Institute of Medical Sciences, Lucknow, India

V. Kumar, P. Mishra (eds.), *A Comprehensive Guide to Degenerative Spine Disorders*, https://doi.org/10.1007/978-981-96-9091-6_6

clinical results [3]. These variables influence the function of lungs as well as the energy consumption.

A previously straight spine can develop primary degenerative scoliosis, frequently referred to as "De Novo" scoliosis, usually in middle age as a result of the rapid destruction of the facet joints and spinal discs. This process causes global spondylosis and may lead to spinal instability, which may turn up as spondylolisthesis, lateral listhesis, or vertebral rotation. Degenerative scoliosis, as a distinct entity, should be differentiated from the broader term of adult scoliosis. Degenerative scoliosis arises from the progressive degeneration of the spine's structural elements, leading to malalignment of the spinal column [4]. Adult scoliosis, on the other hand, encompasses both idiopathic and degenerative spinal deformations in a skeletally mature adult.

6.2 Epidemiology

In the adult population, scoliosis prevalence ranges considerably, from 2% to 32%, with recent studies indicating that the prevalence in elderly individuals may exceed 60%. In addition, it has been found that between 6% and 68% of people have degenerative scoliosis [4]. Degenerative scoliosis is becoming an increasingly significant healthcare concern as the population ages and quality of life along with financial considerations in the healthcare system become more important. Apart from growing cosmetic challenges, it also serves as a major source of pain and disability, impacting the overall well-being of the affected individuals.

6.3 Pathophysiology

In the lumbar spine region, the asymmetrical disc degeneration initiates a vicious cycle of degeneration, which finally lands up into degenerative adult scoliosis. This process lands up into the asymmetrical degenerative process of intervertebral discs and morphological changes in facet joints, leading to uneven loading of the functional spinal units, which turns out to be a circumferential deformity of the lumbar spine. In addition to the ongoing degeneration cycle, conditions associated with bone metabolism such as osteoporosis, particularly in post-menopausal women, where the weakened vertebrae are more susceptible to collapse, further accelerate the progression of the spinal curve [5]. The degeneration affecting the functional spinal unit, particularly facet joints, intervertebral disc, and joint capsules leads to multi-segmental instability, landing up into conditions as lumbar spondylolisthesis or rotational listhesis (Fig. 6.1).

The body creates osteophytes at the facet joints and vertebral endplates in reaction to this instability. These osteophytes, along with ligamentum flavum hypertrophy and calcification, causes narrowing of the spinal canal creating a central or lateral recesses stenosis [6]. Furthermore, foraminal stenosis carried on by the

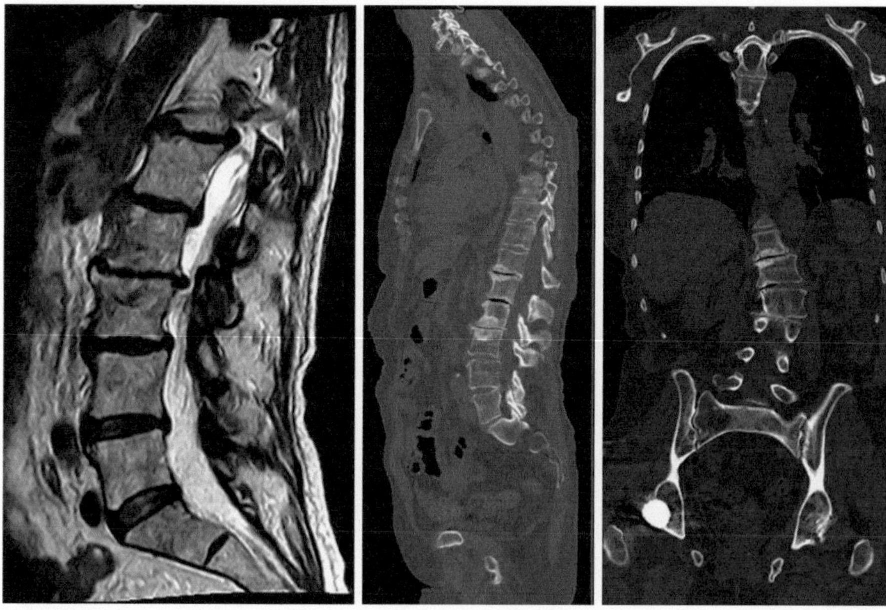

Fig. 6.1 MRI and CT spine of degenerative spine deformity patient showing multilevel degenerative changes with vacuum disc phenomena

collapse of disc height may result in neurogenic claudication or radicular pain. Degenerative scoliosis, in contrast to adolescent idiopathic scoliosis, can advance at a rate of 3° or more annually, particularly if certain conditions are present, such as a higher degree of coronal plane deformity (> 30°), apical vertebral rotation of more than 30%, a lateral subluxation of 6 mm or more, and degenerative disc disease affecting the lumbosacral spine [7]. As this condition advances, it can lead to significant disability, severely impacting daily life and reducing healthy life expectancy in elderly individuals [8].

6.4 History and Examination

6.4.1 History

Axial back pain, worries about the way one looks, or steadily declining pulmonary function are some of the main issues that elderly individuals may have when they come in for an initial assessment of kyphoscoliosis. Obtaining an entire medical history is essential, similar to paediatric situations, and it should include a check for any changes in neurological or psychosocial health. Patient's past medical history holds significant importance and needs a thorough evaluation, including any previous surgeries or therapies, a family history of spinal abnormalities, and the development of symptoms. It is also substantial to evaluate how the illness affects the patient's everyday activities and quality of life, as well as any associated symptoms such as leg pain, numbness, or weakness, which may indicate neurological involvement.

6.4.2 Examination

The patient's entire height, gross anatomy, and symmetry should be carefully evaluated at the commencement of the physical examination. The patient's spinal alignment, flexibility, and ease of movement needs to be assessed with great diligence. Assessing the patient's posture and gait might reveal important information about how severe the deformity is. Hyperextension of the vertebrae during the exam can help rule out conditions like Scheuermann disease. A comprehensive examination of the skin is also required to spot any indications of dimpling, hyperpigmentation, hypopigmentation, or hair tufts, as these could point to underlying diseases such as myelomeningocele or neurofibromatosis.

A significant portion of an assessment is the Adam's forward bend test (Fig. 6.2). The test is performed with the patient standing straight with feet a shoulder-width apart. The patient is then asked to bend forward creating 90° of flexion at the hip joint and allowing the arms to hang freely by their sides with palm facing the floor. To find any asymmetry put on by rotation or prominences, an inclinometer can be employed along the thoracolumbar spine. The patient is asked to move from a flexed to an upright posture and then to an extension posture at lumbar spine while thoroughly evaluating the patient from the side is another component of the examination. In case of any asymmetry, a radiographic evaluation is required, as a 7-degree or greater asymmetry on the exam often corresponds to a 20-degree scoliotic curve on X-rays [9]. Gait, range of motion, and limb length discrepancy must be documented along with a thorough neurological evaluation. Functional tests including the 6-min walk test, speed of walking, standing up from a chair, and the timed get-up-and-go test are of particular importance because evidence indicates that deteriorating kyphoscoliosis results from decrease in spinal extensor muscle strength.

6.4.3 Evaluation

A complete history-taking, physical examination, and functional assessment are all necessary for a thorough evaluation of kyphoscoliosis. The functional tests, like the 6-min walk test holds relevance owing to their strong correlation with the degree of spinal deformity in contrast to lab investigations like the arterial blood gas measures or pulmonary function tests [10]. A key stage in the evaluation procedure is radiographic imaging, which helps to ascertain the degree of spine curvature; 36-inch erect postero-anterior and lateral radiographs are required and may need to be taken repeatedly on a regular basis to track the advancement of curves (Fig. 6.3). A

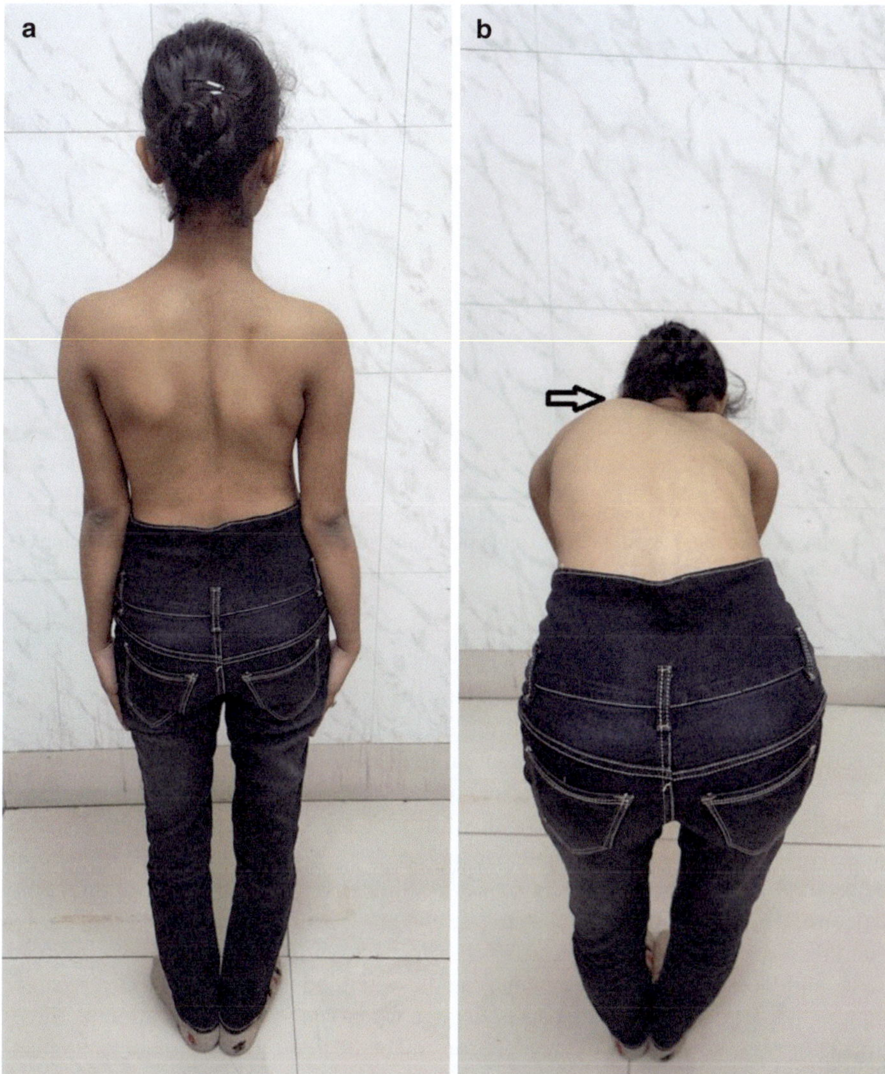

Fig. 6.2 Adam forward bend test (a screening tool used to detect functional or structural scoliosis). (**a**) Patient erect. (**b**) Patient bending forward at 90°. Look for asymmetry of the trunk and rib hump (arrow) indicative of rotational deformity

goniometer is utilized to measure the Cobb angles on these radiographs in both the lateral and anteroposterior orientations. The Cobb method determine the curve's coronal angle (Cobbs angle) by drawing lines perpendicular to the end plates of the most angulated vertebrae. The sagittal alignment is assessed by dropping a plum line on a lateral radiograph in an erect posture from the centre of the C7 vertebral body. This line should ideally cross the superior end plate of the S1 vertebral body

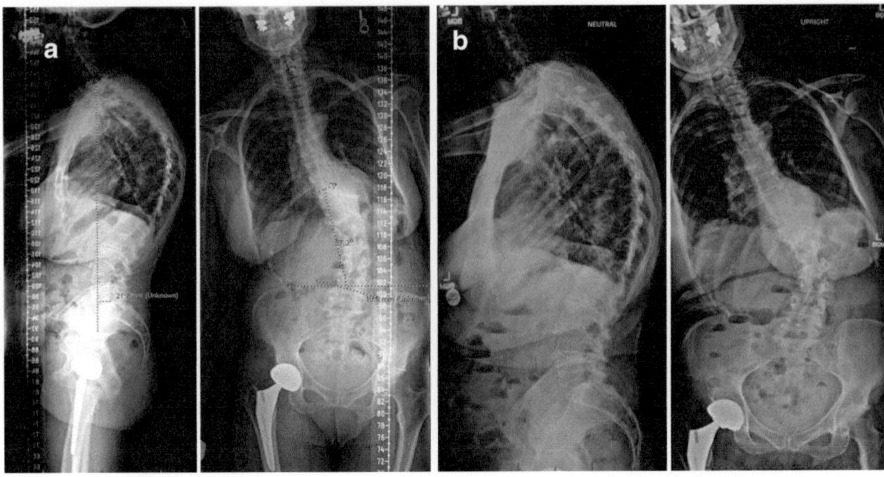

Fig. 6.3 Follow up of whole spine AP & Lateral X-ray in 2-year interval (**b**) showing significant curve progression and deterioration of spinal deformity (**a**: Cobb angle-37 & C7SVA-21 mm, **b**: Cobb angle-50 & C7SVA-68 mm).

at its posterior third, although the normal range varies from neutral to 4 cm anterior to the ideal position, that is, neutral [11].

To evaluate spinal instability and spondylolisthesis, flexion-extension dynamic views on lateral projections may be required. When surgical intervention is being considered, radiographic evaluation of curve flexibility is crucial. When selecting a surgical approach—posterior, anterior, or a combination method—bending films are utilized to assess the degree of flexibility of the curve and the compensating capacity of neighbouring segments of the spine [12]. CT scans, with or without myelographic assessment, can provide additional information concerning bone structure, central, and foraminal stenosis, and are frequently used as a preoperative planning aid [12]. Additional details regarding the soft tissues, disc hydration, vascular, and neurological components can be obtained using magnetic resonance imaging (MRI). However, because degenerative scoliosis is a complex three-dimensional condition, MRI interpretation can be difficult [6]. Although its application is still debatable, discography can also be used to locate painful areas, especially in the lumbar spine, which can help with the decision-making process for fusion surgery.

An internist, a physical medicine, and rehabilitation specialist, at least two members of the complex spine anaesthesiology team, coordinating nurses, and the operating surgeons participate in a monthly live conference as part of a planned multidisciplinary team review for adult spine deformity. Each patient's medical history and health concerns are thoroughly reviewed by the internists and anaesthesiologists prior to the meeting. They create a brief synopsis that is safely distributed to all parties and contains the patient's medical history, pertinent lab findings, and screening tests like echocardiograms and electrocardiograms. The team covers relevant preoperative and postoperative medical issues throughout the session, as well as the intended surgical repair. Nonoperative techniques are created for people whose medical circumstances make them unsuitable for surgery. Obesity, diabetes, osteoporosis, heart and lung disorders, and coagulopathy are important areas of concern for screening and treatment. For blood products, patients with normal preoperative coagulation and hematologic profiles are matched and cross-typed, whereas any abnormalities in haematocrit or coagulation prompt additional testing, possibly including haematology and internal medicine specialists [13].

6.4.4 Treatment/Management

The management of degenerative scoliosis requires a nuanced approach due to the condition's heterogeneity, diverse symptom presentation, and variable outcomes. Several factors, including medical comorbidities, social circumstances, and environmental conditions, significantly influence the treatment decision and prognosis. High risk patient and those carrying poor prognosis include cases with history of tobacco use, obstructive or restrictive pulmonary disease, cardiac ailments, cerebrovascular accidents (CVA), osteoporosis, lifestyle diseases like diabetes, and other significant stressful conditions.

The management plan should be tailored based on the patient's primary clinical complaints, their chronological development, and their expectations and social situation. Patients considered for surgical intervention undergo additional tests, including computed tomography (CT) scans of the spine and investigations pertaining to bone health (DEXA). The disability, overall well-being, and the functional status should also be quantified before the surgery by any of the established disability assessing questionnaire, like Oswestry Disability Index (ODI) or the Patient Reported Outcomes Measurement Information System (PROMIS). Given the complexity of the condition, detailed multidisciplinary counselling is essential to formulate an appropriate and effective treatment plan.

Treatment for degenerative scoliosis generally begins with conservative measures and may advance to surgical intervention if necessary. Kyphoscoliosis may be an incidental finding in young patients which does not compromise the functional abilities of the patient in any way. These patients need to be observed at regular intervals to look for any progression of deformity, occurrence of any neurological symptoms, or onset of pain, which may warrant a specialist referral.

6.4.5 Non-operative Management

Asymptomatic patients with degenerative scoliosis generally require no immediate treatment, although a periodic monitoring through X-rays is important for looking at the progression of the curve. When symptoms arise, it is essential to discuss the various non-operative treatment options with the patient, thoroughly reviewing their potential outcomes.

Non-surgical interventions are often selected based on empirical evidence and the options for treatments offered by the physician aiming at relieving pain and improving function. The treatment option ranges from yoga and physical therapy to pharmacologic agents and other alternative medicines like chiropractic. However, they do not change the natural progression of the curve. The primary goal of non-operative management is to provide transient symptomatic relief and serving as a preliminary step before considering surgical options. The effectiveness of these treatments should be tailor-made and not generalized as a trial of conservative management is recommended prior to the decision for surgical intervention.

Observation For asymptomatic cases or patients with a non-progressive curve, the patient can be kept on a regular follow-up keeping a close watch on radiological progression of curve or clinical worsening of symptoms including any onset of neurological symptoms.

Pain Management It often involves NSAIDs for pain relief. Stronger pain medications, such as narcotics, should be used cautiously due to potential respiratory risks. Muscle relaxants like cyclobenzaprine may be prescribed keeping in consideration their potential side effects. Tricyclic antidepressants can be helpful for managing night pain, while gabapentin may be used for neurogenic symptoms.

Bracing Convenient options for orthotic bracing ranging from soft to rigid supports as per the need may be used for various segments of the spine from the cervical to the sacral region. The choice of brace and its duration of use depend on the specific curvature of the spine and its needs. While bracing can provide temporary support and relief from pain, they do not have any role in preventing the progression of curve, rather it is presumed to have detrimental effect on muscle conditioning in long term.

Physical Therapy and Exercise Exercise programs that include stretching and strengthening exercises have shown significant benefits in improving thoracic kyphosis, although their effect on lumbar curvature is minimal. The physical therapy aims at stretching and strengthening of specific muscle groups which are shortened and have become weak.

Invasive Procedures Semi-invasive procedures such as blocks (Selective nerve root block (SNRB), caudal epidural analgesia, and facet injections) and trigger point injections can provide both diagnostic and therapeutic benefits, especially when there is uncertainty about the source of pain. Spinal cord stimulation (SCS) is another viable option for patients with back pain unresponsive to routine conservative treatment, those who are poor surgical candidates, or those who have experienced failed back surgery syndrome.

Lifestyle Changes Adopting a healthy and a disciplined lifestyle helps in improving the quality of life by causing reduction in the severity of symptoms.

Emotional There is a reasonable role of psychological component in the well-being of the patient. Physician must screen and counsel for anxiety and depression of the patient.

6.4.6 Surgical Management

The decision to pursue surgical treatment for degenerative scoliosis primarily hinges on the actual baseline severity of the curve which the patient is having. For older patients, pain and disability are the main factors guiding surgical decisions, while younger patients' surgical choices are more influenced by the degree of coronal deformity.

Surgical intervention is often considered when conservative treatments have failed, and the patient experiences persistent, intractable pain, neurologic changes, or ongoing progression despite bracing. Given the significant implications of spino-pelvic alignment, advancements in surgical techniques, and the limited effectiveness of non-operative treatments, surgery has become the preferred approach. Typically, curves greater than 45–50° are candidates for surgical management. However, it is important to note that adult spine deformity (ASD) surgeries are associated with extended recovery periods, notable complications, and substantial costs.

The primary aim of surgery in degenerative scoliosis is to achieve adequate neural clearance in involved segments and to restore the global spinal balance in sagittal and coronal plane maintaining the stability of the spine. For a successful surgical outcome, it is crucial to avoid a fat back syndrome and achieve a perfect or a positive sagittal balance not exceeding 4 cm [4, 11]. Surgical options typically involve either decompression alone or decompression combined with spinal fusion.

6.4.7 Decompression

Decompression-only surgery is considered for pure neurogenic claudication secondary to recess stenosis without underlying instability and disturbing axial back pain. One must also take into account the cases with progressive or worsening deformity where decompression alone surgery is not advisable. This approach typically involves procedures focused on clearance of specific neurological structures without creating much morbidity. This requires a good clinical judgement. These procedures are aimed at only relieving the neurological symptoms and are in no way aimed at addressing the deformity or preventing progression of the deformity and addressing the cause for axial low back pain [6]. Stand-alone decompression has limited indications and should be avoided at the apex of the curve due to increased risk of destabilizing and decompensating the spine putting the patient at risk of progression of deformity. Nonetheless, it may be considered for elderly patients with multiple comorbidities. Postoperatively, one must be watchful for the signs of deterioration like progression of deformity, worsening of axial back pain and instability.

6.4.8 Decompression with Spinal Fusion

The progression of scoliosis in a degenerative spine is typically evident by the increase in curvature leading to decompensation and instability between adjacent segments. To address these issues, surgical intervention often involves the fusion of affected spinal segments, with or without decompression. Recent literature highlights the benefits of combining decompression with fusion using fixation devices, which have shown positive outcomes in pain relief, improved mobility, and overall patient satisfaction. Fusion is generally recommended when back pain is predominant, with or without leg pain.

Pedicle screw and rod system is a versatile fixation device offering deformity correction in all the planes with single approach (posterior). A liberal release of ligaments and facetectomy is required in degenerative scoliosis as they are more rigid as compared to AIS (Adolescent Idiopathic Scoliosis). Extremely rigid curve requires more extensive release sometimes warranting anterior approach for releasing the anterior longitudinal ligament and the anterior disc osteophyte complex, which may hinder in achieving a decent kypho-scoliotic correction. A staged surgery may be opted looking into the physical state of the patient and associated morbidities. Various options for corrective osteotomies for kyphosis include the following:

- *Smith-Peterson Osteotomy*: A posterior column wedge osteotomy that opens the anterior column, used for Scheuermann kyphosis and flat-back syndrome.
- *Ponte Osteotomy*: A posterior closing wedge osteotomy, typically used for Scheuermann kyphosis.
- *Pedicle Subtraction Osteotomy*: A three-column closing-wedge posterior osteotomy, effective for kyphosis due to congenital or traumatic causes.
- *Vertebral Column Resection*: For more severe cases requiring extensive correction.

Anterior surgery is often accompanied by interbody fusion for which spacers in the form of auto or allograft or cages (titanium or polyetheretherketone) are used. It helps in fusion process and also solves the purpose of restoring disc height, indirect foraminal decompression, and improve lumbar lordosis (Fig. 6.4). While the traditional anterior retroperitoneal approach provides direct access to the intervertebral disc and vertebral bodies, thereby providing with the best fusion rates but at the same time carries risks of injury to great vessels and visceral organs. The LLIF (lateral lumbar interbody fusion) approach carries lesser risk being as it is a minimally invasive approach, but still carries a risk of injury to lumbar plexus. Invariably this requires a supplementary posterior instrumentation for stability all around, that

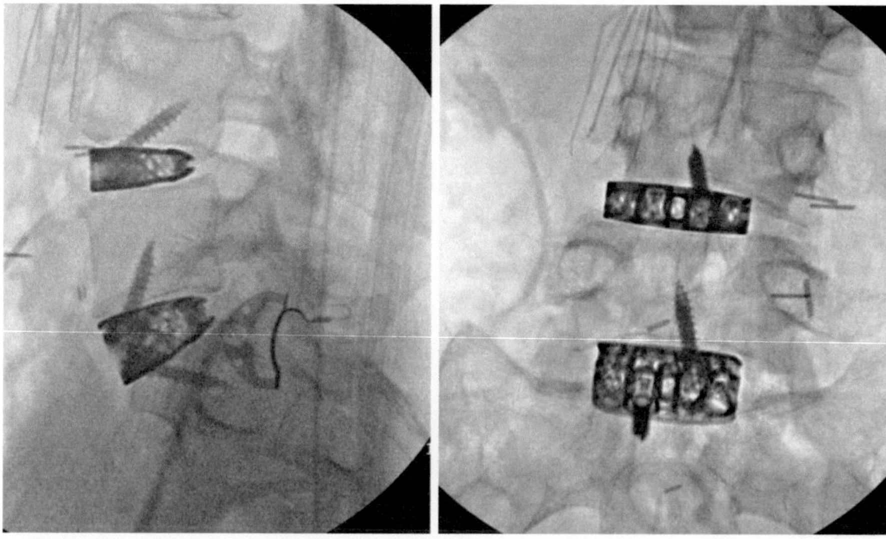

Fig. 6.4 Intraoperative X-ray image showing restoration of disc and foraminal height with improved lordotic curve after ALIF procedure at L4–5 and L5-S1 for adult spinal deformity correction surgery

is, 360-degree arthrodesis. (Fig. 6.5). Emerging concepts of selective/limited fusion are gaining popularity, especially in degenerative scoliosis owing to reduced morbidity and early rehabilitation [14]. Determining the appropriate levels for fusion can be challenging. Proximal junctional kyphosis (PJK) is a known complication of stopping the posterior constructs at the thoraco-lumbar junction, as it leads to decompensation and progressive kyphosis in long run, often necessitating additional surgeries.

Complications in degenerative spine deformity surgery are notably higher than in paediatric populations, with a pseudoarthrosis rate of up to 24%, particularly at the lumbo-sacral junction. Patients with thoraco-lumbar kyphosis, Osteo-arthritis (OA) of hip joint, and significantly high (>5 cm) positive sagittal balance are at increased risk of developing pseudoarthrosis. Osteoporosis, especially in postmenopausal women, further compounds these risks [6].

The surgical procedure for degenerative scoliosis carries a high complication rate ranging from 20% to 40%. Complications with frequent occurrence include infection, cerebrospinal fluid leak, pseudoarthrosis, implant failure, and increase in neurological symptoms [5].

6.5 Prognosis

Long-term outcomes and prognosis for surgical treatment of adult spine deformity (ASD) have shown promising results, particularly in enhancing the health-related quality of life (HRQOL). Studies indicate that operative treatment for ASD provides significant and durable improvements in HRQOL, even at a minimum 3-year

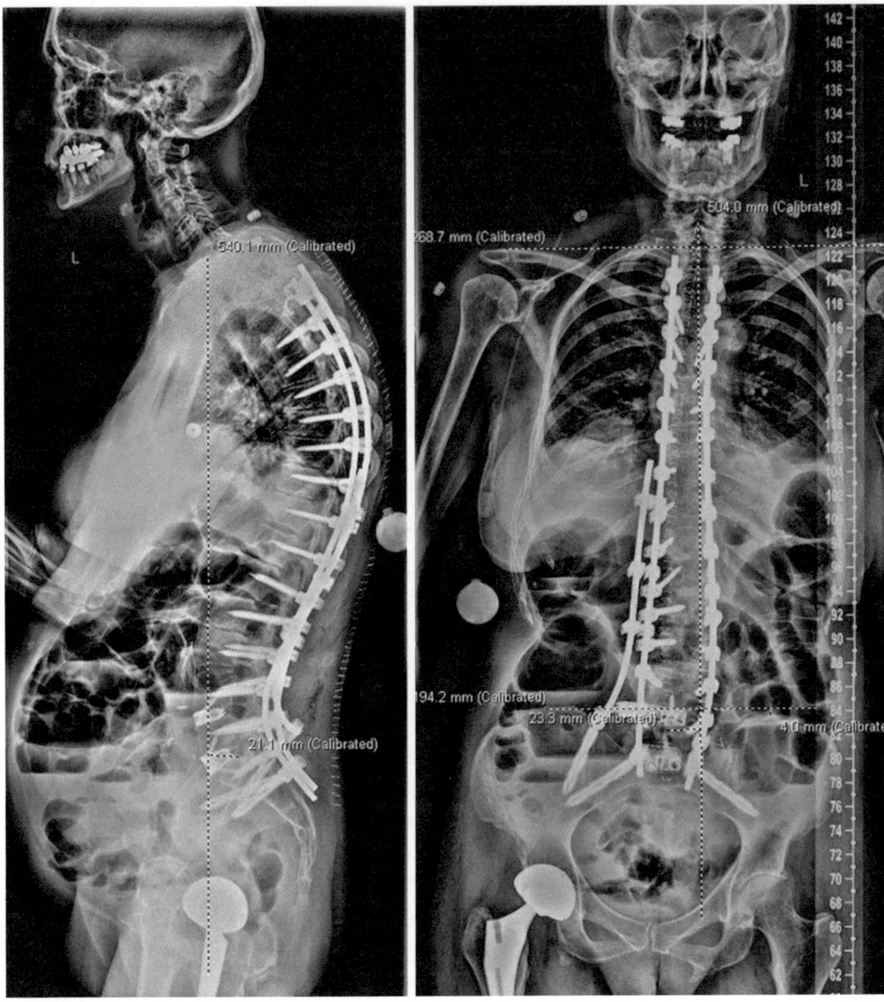

Fig. 6.5 Postoperative standing AP and Lateral X-ray showing well-balanced spine with deformity correction with a secure 360° circumferential arthrodesis

follow-up, with an average follow-up of 4.1 years [15]. This suggests that the benefits of surgery extend well beyond the short-term gains reported in earlier studies, offering sustained relief from pain and functional limitations.

However, the long-term prognosis has dependency on several factors like the severity of deformity, patient's physical status, surgical technique and expertise, and any associated complications. While surgery has proven effective in enhancing quality of life, the potential for complications, such as pseudoarthrosis or the need for revision surgeries, must be considered in the overall prognosis. Nonetheless, for many patients, the long-term benefits of surgical intervention in terms of pain relief, improved mobility, and overall satisfaction outweigh these risks, making it a viable option for managing adult spine deformity.

6.6 Futuristic Personalized Approach for Degenerative Spine Deformity

The future of adult spine deformity (ASD) treatment is bright. The medical and technological advancements have drastically reduced the peri-operative complication rates and enhanced patient's post op recovery. Artificial Intelligence and innovations like navigation, robotic spine surgery and patient-specific rods have enhanced preoperative planning and surgical precision, ultimately leading to greater patient satisfaction. Personalized treatment planning, which aligns preoperative disability with age and sex-matched postoperative outcome targets, may also play a crucial role in setting realistic goals for the management and outcome evaluation of the elderly population [16]. The adoption of computer-assisted navigation and robot-assisted surgeries has already improved the accuracy and safety of minimally invasive procedures, minimizing soft tissue trauma and facilitating quicker patient recovery. Additionally, the use of systemic bone-building agents such as teriparatide and abaloparatide is being explored to boost fusion success in spine surgeries. Another important area of research is paravertebral muscle health, particularly reducing fatty infiltration in the multifidus muscle, which has been associated with better surgical outcomes and reduced pain [17]. Strengthening these muscles could be key in preventing curve progression and maintaining correction post-surgery, further enhancing long-term outcomes for patients with ASD.

6.7 Conclusion

Adult degenerative kyphoscoliosis is a complex and increasingly prevalent condition that requires a nuanced and individualized approach to treatment. Unlike other spinal deformities, its slow progression over decades often results in a varied clinical presentation, necessitating tailored interventions that consider each patient's specific needs and resilience. The management spectrum ranges from palliative care to extensive corrective surgeries that carry inherent risks but offer significant potential benefits. For the spinal surgeon, a thorough and crystal-clear understanding of the intricate anatomy, radiology, and the associated risk-benefit profiles of various surgical options is essential. Unlike idiopathic scoliosis, for the decision making, the absolute Cobbs angle does not hold much importance rather stenosis, listhesis, and balance of spine in sagittal and coronal planes takes precedence for planning the surgery. Minimally invasive techniques provide valuable options with reduced risk, but larger, more complex procedures remain indispensable for significant corrections. Ultimately, the prognosis must be explained to the patient in detail helping him/her to foresee the outcomes and build realistic expectations accordingly. This is critical for achieving satisfactory post-operative outcome at the patient's as well at the surgeon's end. As the field continues to evolve, the integration of both minimally invasive and extensive surgical techniques will remain vital in delivering patient-specific care that optimizes outcomes for those with adult degenerative scoliosis.

References

1. Papaliodis DN, Bonanni PG, Roberts TT, Hesham K, Richardson N, Cheney RA, Lawrence JP, Carl AL, Lavelle WF. Computer Assisted Cobb Angle Measurements: A novel algorithm. Int J Spine Surg. 2017;11(3):21.
2. Ailon T, Shaffrey CI, Lenke LG, Harrop JS, Smith JS. Progressive Spinal Kyphosis in the Aging Population. Neurosurgery. 2015;77 Suppl 4:S164–72.
3. Johari J, Sharifudin MA, Ab Rahman A, Omar AS, Abdullah AT, Nor S, Lam WC, Yusof MI. Relationship between pulmonary function and degree of spinal deformity, location of apical vertebrae and age among adolescent idiopathic scoliosis patients. Singapore Med J. 2016;57(1):33–8.
4. Kotwal S, Pumberger M, Hughes A, Girardi F. Degenerative scoliosis: a review. HSS J. 2011;7(3):257–64. https://doi.org/10.1007/s11420-011-9204-5.
5. Benner B, Ehni G. Degenerative lumbar scoliosis. Spine. 1979;4:548. https://doi.org/10.1097/00007632-197911000-00018.
6. Ploumis A, Transfledt EE, Denis F. Degenerative lumbar scoliosis associated with spinal stenosis. Spine J. 2007;7(4):428–36. https://doi.org/10.1016/j.spinee.2006.07.015.
7. Ascani E, Bartolozzi P, Logroscino CA, Marchetti PG, Ponte A, Savini R. Idiopathic scoliosis after skeletal maturity. Spine. 1986;11(8):784–89. https://doi.org/10.1097/00007632-198610000-00007.
8. Faraj SS, Holewijn RM, van Hooff ML, et al. De novo degenerative lumbar scoliosis: a systematic review of prognostic factors for curve progression. Eur Spine J. 2016;25(8):2347–58.
9. Sheehan DD, Grayhack J. Pediatric Scoliosis and Kyphosis: An Overview of Diagnosis, Management, and Surgical Treatment. Pediatr Ann. 2017;46(12):e472–e480.
10. Menon B, Aggarwal B. Influence of spinal deformity on pulmonary function, arterial blood gas values, and exercise capacity in thoracic kyphoscoliosis. Neurosciences (Riyadh). 2007;12(4):293–8.
11. Oskouian RJ Jr, Shaffrey CI. Degenerative lumbar scoliosis. Neurosurg Clin N Am. 2006;17(3):299–315.
12. Ascani E, Bartolozzi P, Logroscino CA, Marchetti PG, Ponte A, Savini R, Travaglini F, Binazzi R, Di Silvestre M. Natural history of untreated idiopathic scoliosis after skeletal maturity. Spine. 1986;11(8):784–89.
13. Sethi RK, Pong RP, Leveque JC, Dean TC, Olivar SJ, Rupp SM. The Seattle Spine Team Approach to Adult Deformity Surgery: A Systems-Based Approach to Perioperative Care and Subsequent Reduction in Perioperative Complication Rates. Spine Deform. 2014;2(2):95–103. https://doi.org/10.1016/j.jspd.2013.12.002.
14. Boachie-Adjei O, Gupta MC. Adult scoliosis + deformity. AAOS Instructional Course Lectures. 1999;48(39):377–91.
15. Elias E, Bess S, Line B, et al. Outcomes of operative treatment for adult spinal deformity: a prospective multicenter assessment with mean 4-year follow-up. J Neurosurg Spine. 2022;37(4):607–16. https://doi.org/10.3171/2022.3.SPINE2295.
16. Kumar et al. Defining the normative level of functional low back pain disability in the American population: A crowdsourced evaluation of the Oswestry disability index. Spine J. https://doi.org/10.1016/j.spinee.2024.07.009.
17. D. Xie, J. Zhang, W. Ding, S. Yang, D. Yang, J. Zhang.Abnormal change of paravertebral muscle in adult degenerative scoliosis and its association with bony structural parameters. Eur Spine J. 2019;28(7):1626–37.

Facet Joint Arthritis: Degeneration of Spinal Joints

7

Vishal Kumar and Akashdeep Singh

7.1 Anatomy of Facet Joints

Facet joints are formed by the superior and inferior articular processes of two adjacent vertebrae, which extend vertically from where the pedicles and lamina meet (Fig. 7.1). These joints are an important part of the posterior spine and contribute to structural stability. As true synovial joints, facet joints are surrounded by a synovial membrane, fibrous capsule and synovial folds. They connect the lower and upper facets of the vertebrae and play a crucial role in spinal biomechanics [2]. The arterial blood supply to the spine comes from different sources: the ascending cervical artery, the thoracic aorta, and the abdominal aorta. Venous drainage is handled by the external and internal venous plexuses, as well as the basivertebral and intervertebral veins. Due to its lack of valves, the venous plexus can serve as a pathway for the spread of metastases and infections [3–5]. The articular cartilage does not contain nerves, but the capsules, synovium, and subchondral bone are well innervated. Each facet joint is innervated by a pair of nerves that branch from the medial branch of the spinal nerve, which include autonomic, nociceptive, and mechanoreceptor fibers [1, 6]. Table 7.1 depicts some common causes and pathophysiology of facet joint arthritis.

V. Kumar · A. Singh (✉)
Department of Orthopaedics, PGIMER, Chandigarh, India

V. Kumar, P. Mishra (eds.), *A Comprehensive Guide to Degenerative Spine Disorders*, https://doi.org/10.1007/978-981-96-9091-6_7

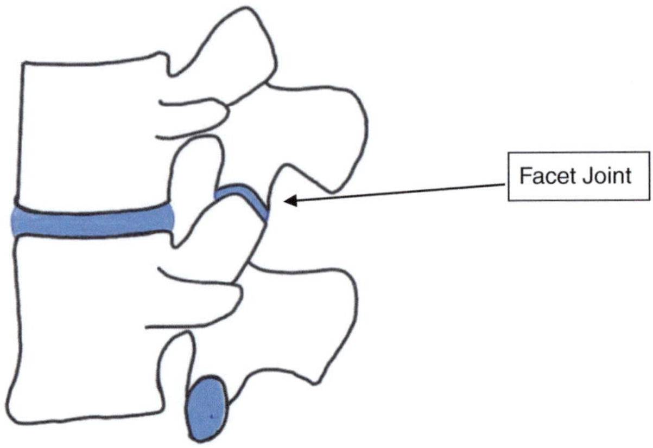

Fig. 7.1 Facet joint anatomy

Table 7.1 Pathophysiology of facet joint arthritis [2] (Fig. 7.2)

Osteoarthritis	Spinal stenosis	Degenerative spondylolisthesis	Trauma
Main causes/risk factors Biomechanical loading Increase in severity with age Disc degeneration Genetics Outcome Cartilage lesions and thinning Subchondral bone sclerosis Synovial and subchondral bone cysts Osteophytes and hypertrophy	Main causes/risk factors Hypertrophic spinal elements Advanced facet hypertrophy Development of facet osteophytes Facet joint inflammation Outcome Reduced spinal canal dimensions Compressed neural elements Neurogenic claudication	Main causes/risk factors Degeneration of facet joints/disc Facet orientation/tropism Outcome Translation of one vertebra in relation to another Vertebral body spur formation Sclerosis of cartilaginous end plate Hypertrophy and ossification of ligaments Further degeneration of the facet joint	Main cause/risk factor Abnormal motion of spine due to trauma Outcome Subluxation Dislocation Fracture Damaged facet capsule/disc/ligaments/cartilage Spinal instability Neurologic injury

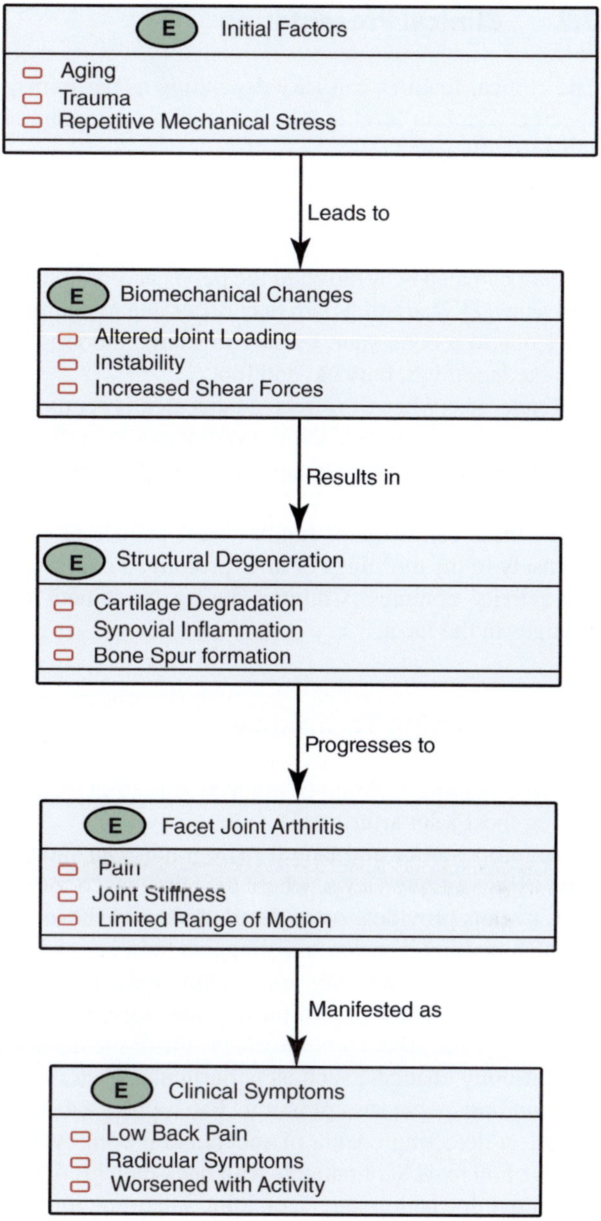

Fig. 7.2 Pathophysiology of facet joint arthritis

7.2 Clinical Presentation

The clinical features can vary depending as per joints, neural involvement, and the specific vertebral level involved. Common symptoms include localized pain, often felt as a dull ache [7].

Referred pain is another possible symptom, where the pain may spread to other areas such as the head, occiput, knees, hips, buttocks, or thighs, but it rarely extends below the knee [7].

Pain can also be referred to the pelvis and/or abdomen, typically usually felt as a dull ache [7]. Radiating pain may occur due to neural irritation or compression possibly due to a bone spur, leading to sharp, shooting pain (sciatica) that can extend into the leg, thigh, buttock, and foot.

Tenderness when the affected facet area is gently pressed is common, making the pain more pronounced. Pain severity can be influenced by posture and activity. Prolonged sitting can also aggravate the pain, while bending forward may provide some relief [1, 7].

Stiffness can occur if lumbar facet pain is related to arthritis, often felt more intensely in the mornings or after prolonged rest, and usually improves once physical activity resumes. Crepitus during movement can also result from arthritic changes in the facet.

7.3 Imaging Techniques

Various imaging techniques are available to detect radiologic findings when diagnosing facet joint arthritis [1].

Anteroposterior and lateral radiographs can show facet joints, but they are best seen using oblique views, where the classical "Scottie dog" sign appears [1].

CT scans provide a more detailed view of the anatomy of facet joints compared to MRI, making it easier to distinguish between various pathological conditions. To accurately assess the facet joint morphology, imaging should be done in all planes due to the oblique nature of the articular surfaces [1, 6].

MRI, on the other hand, excels in soft-tissue resolution and can reveal fine details of non-bony changes, such as periarticular cysts, soft-tissue edema, synovitis, and surrounding nerve compression. Fat-suppressed MRI sequences are particularly useful in detecting edema of subchondral bone, which is seen in the lumbar facet joints of up to 41% of patients with back pain [1, 6]. Additionally, SPECT scans can provide information on facet joint inflammation by showing increased uptake, though this finding is nonspecific [1].

7.4 Management of Chronic Facet Joint Arthritis

(a) Conservative management
(b) Operative management

(a) *Conservative Management*

When physical therapy or analgesics fail to relieve facet-related pain, other conservative treatments can be explored, such as medial branch blocks, radiofrequency denervation, and intra-articular injections.

Medial branch blocks/nerve blocks are primarily used to diagnose pain originating from the facet joints. These injections target the medial branch nerve, aiming to disrupt the transmission of pain signals. However, the effectiveness of these blocks can vary significantly, with less than 10% of patients experiencing pain relief beyond 1 year [8]. Due to their limited long-term effectiveness, medial branch blocks are primarily used for diagnostic purposes, and more research is needed to assess their therapeutic benefits.

Intra-articular facet joint injections, typically consisting of a mix of anesthetics and corticosteroids, are also used to reduce facet-related pain [9]. Recently, ultrasound-guided injections have gained popularity over fluoroscopy-guided injections, as ultrasonography appears to be more effective [12]. However, the effectiveness of these injections remains controversial, as current studies do not provide enough evidence to fully support their use [10, 11] (Fig. 7.3).

Radiofrequency denervation is another option for managing chronic facet-related pain [9]. This procedure uses radiofrequency energy applied through the skin to temporarily disrupt pain signals transmitted by the medial branch nerves through a heating effect [13]. The effects of radiofrequency denervation are temporary and can vary depending on the patient and the technique used [14].

(b) *Operative Management*

Facet Joint Excision (Facetectomy)

A partial facetectomy means removing medial part of the facet joint and lateral attachments of ligamentum flavum. In contrast, a complete facetectomy involves the

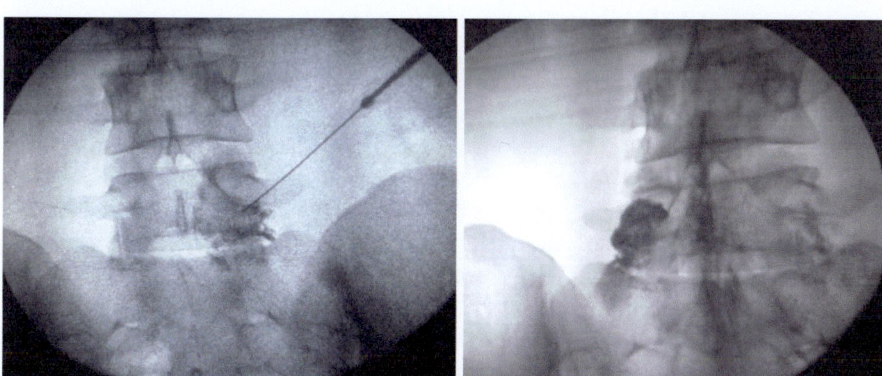

Fig. 7.3 Image-guided facet joint injections

removal of the entire facet joint, including the ligamentum flavum. Facetectomy is typically recommended for cases of persistent degenerative spine disease with neurological symptoms that do not respond to conservative treatments, particularly when there is significant facet joint hypertrophy and osteophyte formation [10, 15]. Since facetectomy is often done with other surgical maneuvers, its individual efficacy is difficult to assess, although it is considered an important adjunct in spine surgery [14].

A key concern after any type of facetectomy is the resulting spinal instability, which is directly related to the extent of the resection. Biomechanical analysis shows that resection can reduce the spine's failure strength by up to 50% [16]. To address this, facetectomy is usually combined with fusion techniques to restore spinal stability.

7.5 Facet Joint Fusion Systems

Facet joint fusion is beneficial as it provides spinal stability following facetectomy. It is generally regarded as a safe procedure [16]. Translaminar Facet Screws are inserted into the facet joints through the lamina, and Transfacet Pedicle Screws extend through the facet joint into the pedicle [17, 18]. Biomechanical studies suggest that both techniques offer comparable strength in stabilizing the thoracic and lumbar spine, but long-term studies are needed to evaluate their ability to achieve solid fusion and assess their safety [18].

7.6 Facet Replacement Systems

The Anatomic Facet Replacement System includes two implants fixed to the vertebrae with pedicle screws, connected by a cross-linking component. In finite-element models, this implant showed exactly normal kinematics, but no clinical study has been conducted to date [19].

The Total Facet Arthroplasty System is attached to the vertebral body using pegs and includes a sliding sphere and curved plate to preserve joint movement and articulation [20]. This system allows global motion compared to rigid fixation systems, but no clinical studies have been reported yet [20].

The Total Posterior Arthroplasty Prosthesis is a posterior dynamic fixation system in which the spinous process and facet joints are removed. Biomechanical studies suggest that this device can restore the axial rotation and lateral bending kinematics of an intact spine, but further research is needed to determine its potential role in managing facet joint degeneration [21].

All the operative techniques discussed above have limited clinical data supporting their use, and conclusions about their efficacy are primarily based on biomechanical studies, so any conclusions should be considered preliminary.

7.7 Future Directions and Research

The facet joint remains under-researched, with many aspects of its pain mechanisms and their relationship to degeneration still not fully understood. Further exploration into treatments such as platelet-rich plasma, new prosthesis designs, and facet tissue engineering is needed. Clinical studies in these areas could potentially offer long-term, motion-preserving solutions for facet joint pain.

7.8 Conclusion

Chronic low back pain originating from facet joints is a significant healthcare issue, representing a major socioeconomic burden due to its high prevalence. Facet joint pathology often mimics symptoms of spine root compression, leading to misdiagnosis and inappropriate treatment. The low specificity of facet joint syndrome and the suboptimal use of imaging techniques contribute to its misunderstanding. Improving knowledge of facet joint anatomy and biomechanics could help in providing more targeted ergonomic recommendations and lifestyle modifications. These approaches should be tested in randomized controlled trials to enhance the management of facet joint syndrome.

References

1. Perolat R, Kastler A, Nicot B, et al. Facet joint syndrome: from diagnosis to interventional management. Insights Imaging. 2018;9(5):773–89.
2. O'Leary SA, Paschos NK, Link JM, Klineberg EO, Hu JC, Athanasiou KA. Facet joints of the spine: structure–function relationships, problems and treatments, and the potential for regeneration. Annu Rev Biomed Eng. 2018;20(1):145–70.
3. Sioutas G, Kapetanakis S. Clinical anatomy and clinical significance of the cervical intervertebral foramen: a review. Folia Morphol (Warsz). 2016;75(2):143–8.
4. Gkasdaris G, Tripsianis G, Kotopoulos K, Kapetanakis S. Clinical anatomy and significance of the thoracic intervertebral foramen: a cadaveric study and review of the literature. J Craniovertebr Junction Spine. 2016;7(4):228–35.
5. Gkasdaris G, Kapetanakis S. Clinical anatomy and significance of the lumbar intervertebral foramen: a review. J Anat Soc India. 2015;64(2):166–73.
6. Gellhorn AC, Katz JN, Suri P. Osteoarthritis of the spine: the facet joints. Nat Rev Rheumatol. 2013;9(4):216–24.
7. Field R, Keene D, Abdi S. Radiofrequency treatment. In: Smith HS, editor. Current therapy in pain. Elsevier Health Sciences; 2009.
8. Manchikanti L, Pampati V, Bakhit CE, Rivera JJ, Beyer CD, et al. Effectiveness of lumbar facet joint nerve blocks in chronic low back pain: a randomized clinical trial. Pain Phys. 2001;4:101–17.
9. Staal JB, de Bie RA, de Vet HC, Hildebrandt J, Nelemans P. Injection therapy for subacute and chronic low back pain: an updated Cochrane review. Spine. 2009;34:49–59.
10. Carette S, Marcoux S, Truchon R, Grondin C, Gagnon J, et al. A controlled trial of corticosteroid injections into facet joints for chronic low back pain. N Engl J Med. 1991;325:1002–7.

11. Chou R, Loeser JD, Owens DK, Rosenquist RW, Atlas SJ, et al. Interventional therapies, surgery, and interdisciplinary rehabilitation for low back pain: an evidence-based clinical practice guideline from the American Pain Society. Spine. 2009;34:1066–77.
12. WuT ZWH, DongY SHX, Li JH. Effectiveness of ultrasound-guided versus fluoroscopy or computed tomography scanning guidance in lumbar facet joint injections in adults with facet joint syndrome: a meta-analysis of controlled trials. Arch Phys Med Rehabil. 2016;97:1558–63.
13. Maas ET, Ostelo RW, Niemisto L, Jousimaa J, Hurri H, et al. Radiofrequency denervation for chronic low back pain. Cochrane Database Syst Rev. 2015;10:CD008572.
14. Cohen SP, Huang JH, Brummett C. Facet joint pain—advances in patient selection and treatment. Nat Rev Rheumatol. 2013;9:101–16.
15. Garrido E, Connaughton PN. Unilateral facetectomy approach for lateral lumbar disc herniation. J Neurosurg. 1991;74:754–6.
16. Jacobs RR, Montesano PX, Jackson RP. Enhancement of lumbar spine fusion by use of translaminar facet joint screws. Spine. 1989;14:12–5.
17. Heggeness MH, Esses SI. Translaminar facet joint screw fixation for lumbar and lumbosacral fusion. A clinical and biomechanical study. Spine. 1991;16:S266–9.
18. Akbay A, İnceoğlu S, Milks R, Schlenk R, Palaoglu S, Benzel EC. Thoracic transfacet pedicle screw fixation: a new instrumentation technique. J Neurosurg Spine. 2005;3:224–9.
19. Goel VK, Mehta A, Jangra J, Faizan A, Kiapour A, et al. Anatomic facet replacement system (AFRS) restoration of lumbar segment mechanics to intact: a finite element study and in vitro cadaver investigation. SAS J. 2007;1:46–54.
20. Sjovold SG, Zhu Q, Bowden A, Larson CR, de Bakker PM, et al. Biomechanical evaluation of the Total Facet Arthroplasty SystemR (TFASR): loading as compared to a rigid posterior instrumentation system. Eur Spine J. 2012;21:1660–73.
21. WilkeHJ SH, Werner K, Schmolz W, Drumm J. Biomechanical evaluation of a new total posterior-element replacement system. Spine. 2006;31:2790–6.

Modic Changes: Vertebral Endplate Abnormalities

8

Vishal Kumar and Adarsh Tekumalla

Learning Objectives

- To accurately identify and classify the different types of Modic changes on MRI.
- To ascertain the etiology of Modic changes and its association with low back ache.
- To analyze the clinical association of Modic changes and its effect on treatment of low back pain.

8.1 Introduction

The first description of MRI signal changes adjacent to the degenerated intervertebral discs was by Roos et al. in 1987 [1]. These changes were attributed to the process of disc degeneration, instead of neoplasia or infection.

Subsequently, Modic et al. in 1988 gave a thorough description of three different types of changes noticed in the immediate vicinity of the disc (endplates) on magnetic resonance imaging (MRI) [2].

Whether this particular phenomenon is clinically relevant has been argued but there is a lack of clear consensus in regards to the clinical significance, etiology, pathophysiology, and surgical relevance of these changes. The relevance of this phenomenon in relation to degenerative spinal conditions is still controversial.

Modic changes (MC) are described as signal irregularities noted in the area of bone marrow of the vertebral bodies adjacent to the intervertebral discs on T1 & T2 MRI. They are usually found adjacent to an intervertebral disc undergoing degenerative disease.

This chapter attempts to describe, classify, and explain the association with low back pain in regards to the Modic changes.

V. Kumar · A. Tekumalla (✉)
Department of Orthopaedics, PGIMER, Chandigarh, India

V. Kumar, P. Mishra (eds.), *A Comprehensive Guide to Degenerative Spine Disorders*, https://doi.org/10.1007/978-981-96-9091-6_8

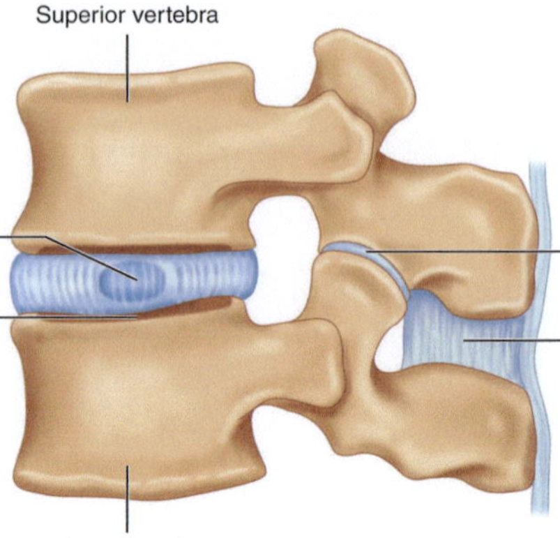

Fig. 8.1 Diagrammatic representation of a functional spinal unit (FSU)

8.2 Vertebral Endplates

The spine can be divided into functional spinal units (FSU), which represent the fundamental segmental structure. The components of the functional spinal units are the intervertebral disc and two vertebrae adjacent to the disc (Fig. 8.1).

The intervertebral disc comprises of the nucleus pulposus at the center and the annulus fibrosus at the periphery. Some authors consider endplates as an integral part of the intervertebral disc. The intervertebral disc is considered avascular with minimal nerve innervation and physiological studies show a lack of evidence for it being a primary pain generator [3]. Subsequently, attention has therefore been focused to other possible structures to look for an etiology for pain associated with degenerative disc disease.

The vertebral endplates are concave structures of 1 mm thickness, with two separate layers, namely, the cartilaginous endplate consisting of hyaline cartilage and the bony endplate made of cancellous bone. The endplates act as a regulator of the transport of essential nutrients to the disc and possess essential properties for the normal functioning of the spine [4]. Till skeletal maturity, the vertebral endplates show the presence of tiny perforating blood vessels from the adjacent vertebrae to the end plate that provide blood to the intervertebral disc during the growth phases of the spine. However, the endplate can act as a pain generator as it is abundant in neural elements.

8.3 Endplate Changes

Vertebral endplate changes refer to alterations in the areas of the vertebral endplates and adjacent bone marrow. They are commonly due to degenerative conditions, trauma, infection, or tumors [5].

Modic changes are considered as a subgroup of endplate changes.

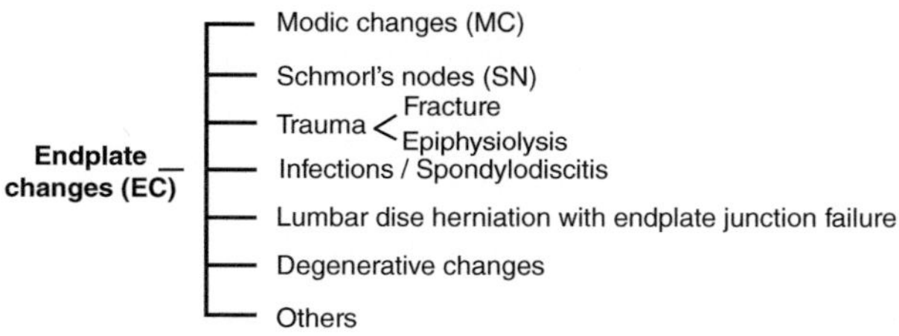

CT and MRI are used to visualize the endplate changes. MRI provides the necessary information and the level of detail on the vertebral bone marrow and the intervertebral disc. Computed tomography is useful in assessing the bony changes in the endplate.

8.4 Definition

Modic changes are defined as the signal intensity changes noted on magnetic resonance imaging (MRI) in the vertebral bone marrow that reflect pathologies, which are not related to malignancy, infection, or inflammatory disorders.

8.5 Grading

Three different types of Modic changes have been described based on their appearance on MRI in T1-weighted (T1w) and T2-weighted (T2w) images.

However, the identification and the subsequent classification can depend on the field strength of the MRI (Figs. 8.2, 8.3, and 8.4).

	T1 characteristics	T2 characteristics
Modic type 1 changes	Hypointense	Hyperintense
Modic type 2 changes	Hyperintense	Hyperintense
Modic type 3 changes	Hypointense	Hypointense

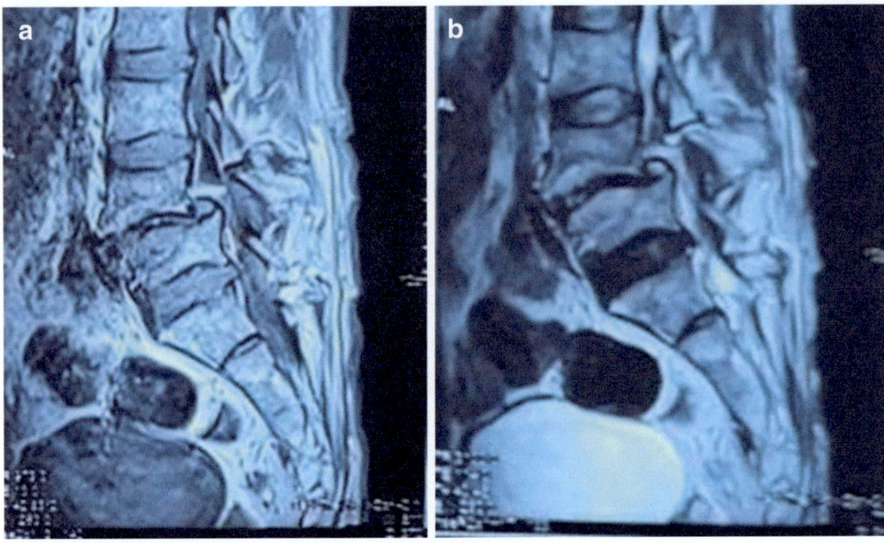

Fig. 8.2 MRI of 58/M with chronic low back ache with L4–5 listhesis with hypointense signal of T1W (**a**) and hyperintense signals on T2W (**b**)—*Modic Changes Type 1* [13]

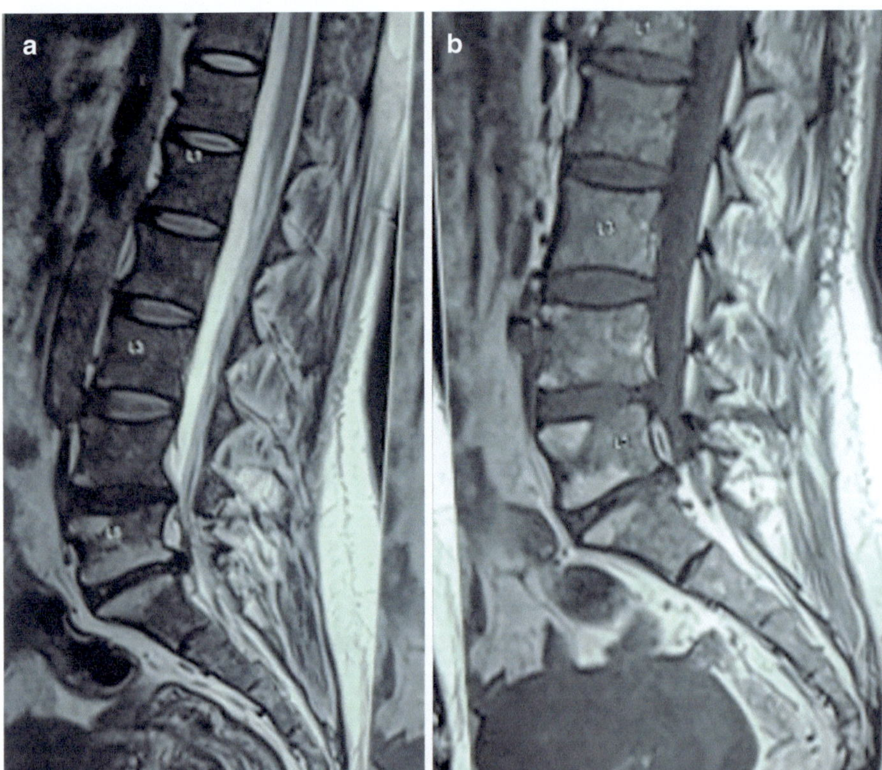

Fig. 8.3 MRI of a 42-year-old female with chronic low back ache with hyperintense signal changes noted on T2W (**a**) and T1W (**b**)—*Modic Changes Type 2* [13]

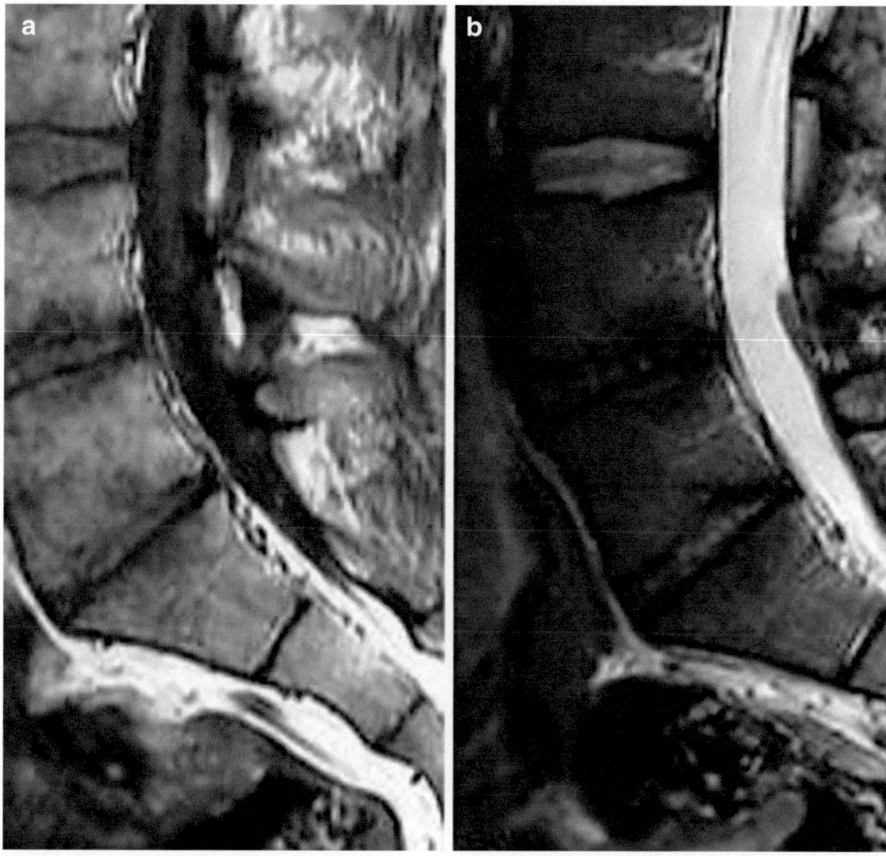

Fig. 8.4 Hypointense signal on both T1WI (**a**) and T2WI (**b**)—*Modic Changes Type 3*

8.6 Etiology

Modic changes have a high prevalence in low back ache patients (43%) compared to the asymptomatic individuals (6%).

Of the mentioned types of Modic changes, type 1 Modic changes have been associated with low back ache more than the others. Modic changes are most commonly seen at lumbar levels L4-S1 and are more pronounced at these levels as well.

They are found to be more prevalent in the anterior one third of the endplate, are generally symmetric above and below the affected disc, and have an association with severity of the disc degeneration and disc herniation [6].

The risk factors commonly associated include older age, male sex, diabetes mellitus, genetic factors, obesity, smoking, spinal deformities, and higher occupational stresses [7].

Type 1 Modic changes can change into Type 2 Modic changes and vice versa. They can also convert to MC3 eventually. About 20% of the lesions are of a mixed-type (MC1/2 or MC2/3).

In type 1 Modic changes, normal bone marrow is replaced by fibrous tissue between the thickened trabeculae, the disruption of endplates is seen, and vascularized granulation tissue fills the bone–disc junction, which is a sign of inflammation.

In type 2 Modic changes, the normal bone marrow is replaced by fatty marrow. The endplate shows disruption with fibrovascular granulation tissue (similar to MC1) at the junction of the disc and vertebral endplate.

In MC3, there is reactive sclerosis of the bone marrow.

The Modic changes possessing the property of interconvertibility and the existence of mixed-type (MC1/2 and MC2/3) changes suggests that the different types of Modic changes are representative of the same pathological process at different stages [8].

Modic type changes are not only isolated to the vertebra and endplates but are also to be found in the pedicles, which hints at an association with instability along with the significant association with degenerative disc disease.

The most commonly present risk factor for Modic type changes is the presence of degenerative disc disease. The probability of identifying Modic type changes in patients with other degenerative conditions like disc degeneration, disc herniation, and defects in the endplate is quite high.

Degenerative Disc Disease There appears to be a significant association of endplate damage and large disc herniations with Modic changes. Endplate damage leads to a series of degenerative events between vertebra and the disc. This subsequently leads to an increase in the intra-osseous pressure, thereby affecting the transport of nutrients and metabolites, causing hydraulic coupling of the intervertebral disc-vertebral body, and the flow of mediators of inflammation from disc to the bone marrow [9]. This leads to bone marrow lesions adjacent to the endplate.

Infective Discitis The plausibility of an infectious etiology of Modic changes is derived from the characteristics of the nature of disc such as poor vascularity, anaerobic environment, and a diminished healing capacity. Discitis can cause production of bacterial metabolites and proinflammatory cytokines, which subsequently leads to inflammatory changes within the adjacent bone marrow [10]. MC1 changes have been associated with elevated C-reactive protein (CRP). A few studies have questioned the supposed association between degenerative changes and infection, and have only shown a moderate support to the hypothesis of disc infection hypothesis in the pathology of MC.

Autoimmune Following the embryonic development of intervertebral disc, the nucleus pulposus never comes into direct contact with systemic circulation. After exposure to immune system, cells from the nucleus pulposus get recognized as "foreign" and results in the triggering of an autoimmune reaction [11].

To summarize, there is an inflammatory reaction in the disc secondary to damage, which leads to increased susceptibility to pathogens or immune-mediated reactions. These reactions lead to the formation of pain mediators and induce adipogenesis and recruitment of osteoclasts. The development of the described types of Modic type changes depends on the duration and severity of the inflammatory stimuli, as well as the response from the bone marrow.

8.7 Clinical Relevance

Although Modic type changes are strongly associated with degenerative disc disease, it remains uncertain why only some patients with degenerative disc disease develop the changes and why others do not.

There is a possibility that the propensity to develop Modic type changes is related to the composition and function of the bone marrow and its channels of communication with the disc through the endplates.

Type 1 Modic change are known to have an association with active low back ache and the resolution of these marrow changes has been shown to have an association with an improvement in patient reported outcomes [12].

Type 2 Modic changes appear to be more stable over time and a weaker association with low back pain [13].

There is a lack of conclusive evidence on the role of Modic type changes in the causation of chronic low back pain or any influence on the long-term outcome in patients with low back pain or disc herniation. Patients with Modic type changes generally tend to have less satisfactory outcomes following conservative treatment or discectomy, although there is a lack of clear evidence [14].

Modic changes are considered as incidental lesions on MRI and it is unclear if the presence of Modic changes itself is an indication for treatment in patients with chronic low back pain [15].

8.8 Summary

Modic changes are considered as important and clinically relevant findings on MRI. However, there is considerable variation as to the definition, classification, and uses in the clinical decision-making process.

There is a lack of conclusive evidence on the causative role of Modic type changes in chronic lower back pain or any influence thereof on the long-term outcome in low back pain patients.

Modic type changes are probably more than just a coincidental MRI finding in low back ache patients, but rather represent an underlying pathological process that should be a target for therapy.

References

1. MR imaging of marrow changes adjacent to end plates in degenerative lumbar disk disease [Internet]. Available from: www.ajronline.org.
2. Degenerative disk disease: assessment of changes in vertebral body marrow with MR imaging.
3. Kushchayev SV, Glushko T, Jarraya M, Schuleri KH, Preul MC, Brooks ML, et al. ABCs of the degenerative spine. Insights Imaging. Springer Verlag. 2018;9:253–74.
4. Moore RJ, Moore RJ. The vertebral end-plate: what do we know? Eur Spine J. 2000;9:92–6.
5. Zehra U, Bow C, Lotz JC, Williams FMK, Rajasekaran S, Karppinen J, et al. Structural vertebral endplate nomenclature and etiology: a study by the ISSLS spinal phenotype focus group. Eur Spine J. 2018;27(1):2–12.
6. Dudli S, Fields AJ, Samartzis D, Karppinen J, Lotz JC. Pathobiology of modic changes. Eur Spine J. Springer Verlag. 2016;25:3723–34.
7. Farshad-Amacker NA, Hughes AP, Aichmair A, Herzog RJ, Farshad M. Determinants of evolution of endplate and disc degeneration in the lumbar spine: a multifactorial perspective. Eur Spine J. 2014;23(9):1863–8.
8. Udby PM, Samartzis D, Carreon LY, Andersen MØ, Karppinen J, Modic M. A definition and clinical grading of Modic changes. J Orthop Res. John Wiley and Sons Inc. 2022;40:301–7.
9. Albert HB, Briggs AM, Kent P, Byrhagen A, Hansen C, Kjaergaard K. The prevalence of MRI-defined spinal pathoanatomies and their association with Modic changes in individuals seeking care for low back pain. Eur Spine J. 2011;20(8):1355–62.
10. Albert HB, Lambert P, Rollason J, Sorensen JS, Worthington T, Pedersen MB, et al. Does nuclear tissue infected with bacteria following disc herniations lead to Modic changes in the adjacent vertebrae? Eur Spine J. 2013;22(4):690–6.
11. Kaneyama S, Nishida K, Takada T, Suzuki T, Shimomura T, Maeno K, et al. Fas ligand expression on human nucleus pulposus cells decreases with disc degeneration processes. J Orthop Sci. 2008;13(2):130–5.
12. Herlin C, Kjaer P, Espeland A, Skouen JS, Leboeuf-Yde C, Karppinen J, et al. Modic changes—their associations with low back pain and activity limitation: a systematic literature review and meta-analysis. PLoS One. Public Library of Science. 2018;13:e0200677.
13. Määttä JH, Karppinen JI, Luk KDK, Cheung KMC, Samartzis D. Phenotype profiling of Modic changes of the lumbar spine and its association with other MRI phenotypes: a large-scale population-based study. Spine J. 2015;15(9):1933–42.
14. Viswanathan VK, Shetty AP, Rajasekaran S. Modic changes – an evidence-based, narrative review on its patho-physiology, clinical significance and role in chronic low back pain. J Clin Orthop Trauma. 2020;11(5):761–9.
15. Udby PM, Bendix T, Ohrt-Nissen S, Lassen MR, Sørensen JS, Brorson S, et al. Modic changes are not associated with long-term pain and disability: a cohort study with 13-year follow-up. Spine (Phila Pa 1976) [Internet]. 2019;44(17). Available from: https://journals.lww.com/spinejournal/fulltext/2019/09010/modic_changes_are_not_associated_with_long_term.7.aspx.

Ankylosing Spondylitis: Inflammatory Spine Disorder

9

Vishal Kumar and Ramesh Kalappagol Basappa

9.1 Introduction

Ankylosing spondylitis (AS) is a chronic, systemic, inflammation-related joint condition that usually starts in young adulthood [1]. AS mainly impacts the areas where ligaments and tendons connect to bones (entheses), resulting in inflammation and eventually calcification of ligaments, which results in pain and limited movement in the spine. This could progress to complete loss of spinal movement and fusion of the sacroiliac joints and spine [2]. Several additional symptoms, including low back pain (inflammatory back pain (IBP)), restricted spinal flexibility, peripheral arthritis, enthesitis, dactylitis, uveitis, psoriasis, and chronic inflammatory bowel disease (IBD), are characteristic of AS, one of the most severe forms of spondyloarthropathy [3]. "Ankylosing spondylitis" refers to the late stage of the illness characterized by ankylosis, while "axial spondyloarthropathy" encompasses the entire disease spectrum, including early stages without radiographic changes (pre-radiographic stage) and the advanced stages with full ankylosis. This terminology is preferred for a comprehensive classification of the disease [4, 5]. AS characteristically affects young adults, notably higher in males than in females [6].

9.2 Pathophysiology

In AS, enthesopathy mostly affects the subchondral bone and is characterized by an inflammatory infiltration that is erosive and consists of lympho-plasmocytes and occasionally polymorphonuclear cells. Fibrous tissue proliferates after this inflammatory process, resulting in cartilage and ultimately bone production. Destructive injuries are more likely when there is a restriction in the motion of the spine and the

V. Kumar · R. K. Basappa (✉)
Department of Orthopaedics, PGIMER, Chandigarh, India

V. Kumar, P. Mishra (eds.), *A Comprehensive Guide to Degenerative Spine Disorders*, https://doi.org/10.1007/978-981-96-9091-6_9

thoracolumbar fascia's capacity to affect the lumbar vertebrae's alignment, due to sacroiliac and spinal enthesitis. This restriction affects the myxoid subchondral bone marrow and shortens the visco-elastic part of the spinal ligaments [7]. As the disease advances, it damages surrounding articular or joint tissues.

A significant finding in 1973 by Brewerton et al. [8] showed a powerful link between human leukocyte antigen (HLA-B27) and AS. HLA-B27 is a class I antigen that displays antigenic peptides to T-cells and is located in the major histocompatibility complex (MHC) [8]. There are more than 40 variations of HLA-B27, and HLA-B2702, B2704, and B*2705 have the most significant link to AS. Two primary theories describe the connection between HLA-B27 and AS development: the canonical and noncanonical theories. In the canonical "arthritogenic peptide," theory, it is believed that the presentation of antigens by HLA-B27 plays a crucial role in the development of AS. It indicates that immune response by T-cells to self-antigens can lead to autoimmune reactions and inflammation [9]. Noncanonical theories include the "misfolded protein" hypothesis that involves the accumulation of improperly folded HLA-B27 proteins, and the "HLA-B27 surface homodimer" hypothesis that involves abnormal intracellular signalling due to HLA-B27 homodimers on the cell surface [10].

9.3 Clinical Presentation

Ankylosing spondylitis patients generally show symptoms such as back pain, extended morning stiffness, and a gradual decrease in movement in the central spine. Calin et al.'s 1977 criteria for inflammatory back pain involve onset before age 40, back pain lasting over 3 months, relief with exercise, morning stiffness, and gradual onset [11]. Distinguishing between AS-related IBP and mechanical lower back pain (MLBP) is essential for early AS diagnosis. Four important factors help to differentiate IBP from MLBP: enhancement through physical activity rather than rest, morning stiffness lasting over 30 min, waking up in the latter half of the night due to back discomfort, and alternating buttock pain [12].

Clinical examination for early ankylosing spondylitis is challenging because significant spinal deformities have typically not yet developed, and sacroiliitis and spondylitis are not easily detectable through clinical means alone. However, early diagnosis is critical for effective management and to slow disease progression. AS typically begins at the sacroiliac joints and progresses superiorly, eventually affecting the entire axial skeleton [13]. The main clinical findings include, reduced ability to move the spine, especially in forward and sideways directions, limited movement of the lower back, and restricted chest expansion. Early clinical signs include diminished sideways bending of the spine (below 10 cm), lessened chest expansion (under 4 cm), and restricted neck rotation (less than 70°) [14]. Stress tests (Fig. 9.1) for the sacroiliac joint are often positive, and the modified Schober test is used to assess spinal flexion. As the disease progresses individuals could experience more neck bending, curvature of the upper spine, and reduced typical curvature, leading to a stooped posture. Disease progression can be monitored by measuring height loss, limited chest expansion, spinal flexion, and occiput-to-wall distance (Fig. 9.2).

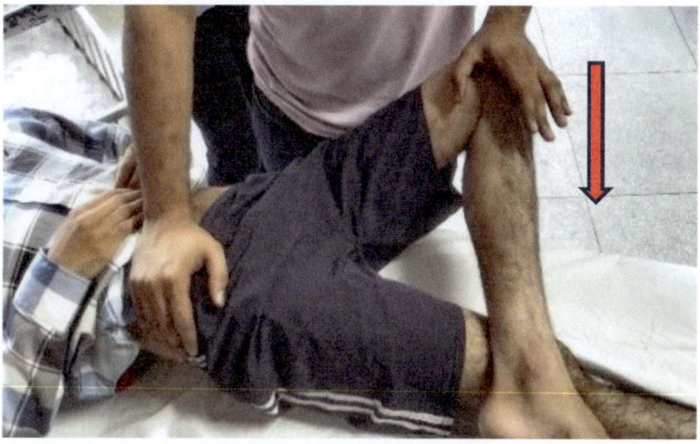

Fig. 9.1 FABER test: Flexion, abduction, and external rotation of the hip being tested, rest the ankle on the opposite knee, then apply pressure to the opposite ilium to stabilize the pelvis, and apply downward pressure to the affected knee. The test is considered positive if it recreates groin pain or pain in the gluteal region of the stressed side [15]

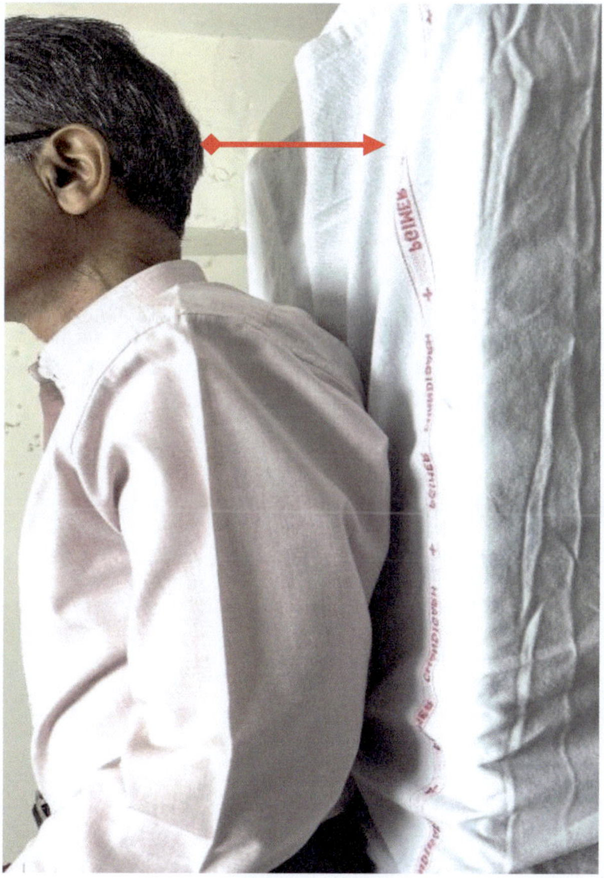

Fig. 9.2 Occiput-to-wall distance: The horizontal distance from the occiput to the wall is measured with the patient's buttocks and heels against the wall, with hips and knees extended [16]

The Bath Ankylosing Spondylitis Disease Activity Index (BASDAI) is a well-known tool for evaluating disease activity, while the Bath Ankylosing Spondylitis Functional Index (BASFI) measures limitations in daily activities [17]. Approximately 50% of AS patients will develop hip arthritis, and some may require surgery [18].

9.4 Imaging

Radiographic sacroiliitis, a hallmark of AS, develops over time and is influenced by the duration and severity of the disease [5, 19]. Prior to 1900, diagnosis was based only on the obvious clinical signs of spinal ankylosis. The introduction of conventional radiography demonstrated that sacroiliitis, as seen on radiographs, is a significant characteristic of AS. However, the inflammatory process that underlies AS starts before radiographic sacroiliitis or other signs like syndesmophytes or ankylosis are visible on X-rays.

Radiographs are essential for identifying, diagnosing, and tracking AS. Sacroiliitis, which can be seen early on, begins with bone erosion under the iliac part of the sacroiliac joint, then progresses to sclerosis and bone growth [20]. The radiographic grading of sacroiliitis is detailed in Table 9.1 [21].

Radiographic sacroiliitis is confirmed when reaching a grade of at least II bilaterally or III unilaterally. Early changes seen in the spine involve minor erosions at the edges of the vertebral bodies due to new bone formation around the bone surface. These erosions progress to the formation of syndesmophytes that connect vertebrae, leading to the characteristic "bamboo spine" appearance on X-rays (Fig. 9.5) [22]. The "dagger sign" occurs when the posterior interspinous ligament between the vertebrae ossifies [22].

Pseudoarthrosis is characterized by destruction and sclerosis of the disc-vertebral area and mimics vertebral discs infected under conditions like tuberculosis, yet it stems from unnoticed spinal fractures or segments that did not properly fuse [23].

Table 9.1 Radiographic grading of sacroiliitis [21]

Grade	Appraisal
I	Suspicious alterations
II	Minimal abnormality (specific spots with erosion or hardening, no change in the width of the joint)
III	Definite deviation (moderate or severe sacroiliitis with erosions, signs of sclerosis, expansion, constriction, or partial fusion) (Fig. 9.3)
IV	Complete fusion (Fig. 9.4)

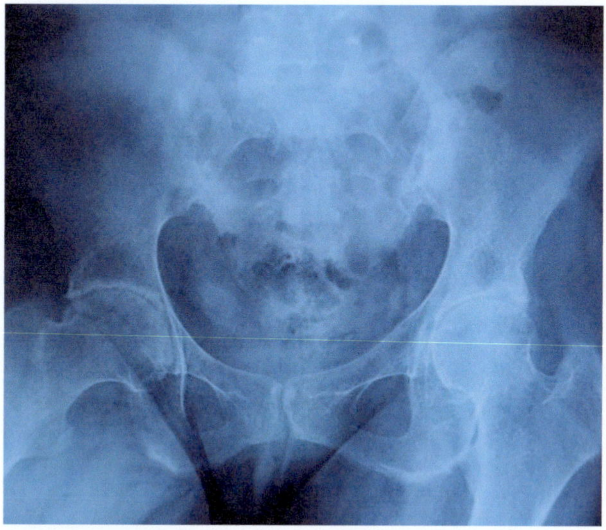

Fig. 9.3 Grade 3 sacroiliitis

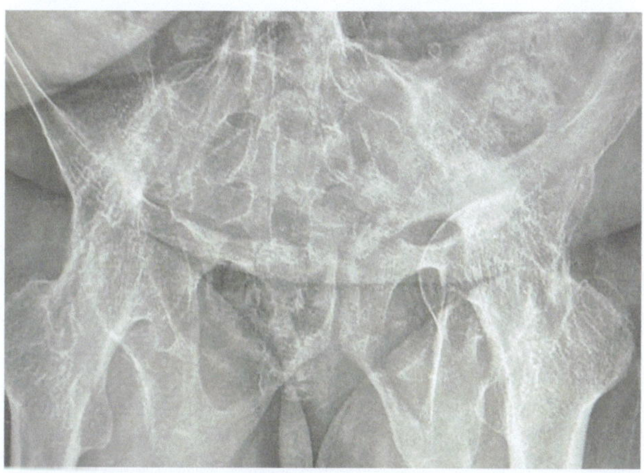

Fig. 9.4 Grade 4 sacroiliitis

X-rays are easily accessible and cost-effective, but they are not very sensitive for detecting early-stage AS. CT scans offer better visualization and localization of pathological findings, such as erosion, osteoporosis, sclerosis, and new bone formation. CT is the preferred method for evaluating cervical spine fractures in advanced AS [24].

Ultrasound (US) remains a major diagnostic tool due to its simplicity, cost-effectiveness, and availability. Color Doppler ultrasound (CDUS) has displayed excellent sensitivity and specificity in identifying clinically active sacroiliitis [25]. Active enthesitis, detected via ultrasonography, is highly suggestive of AS and is

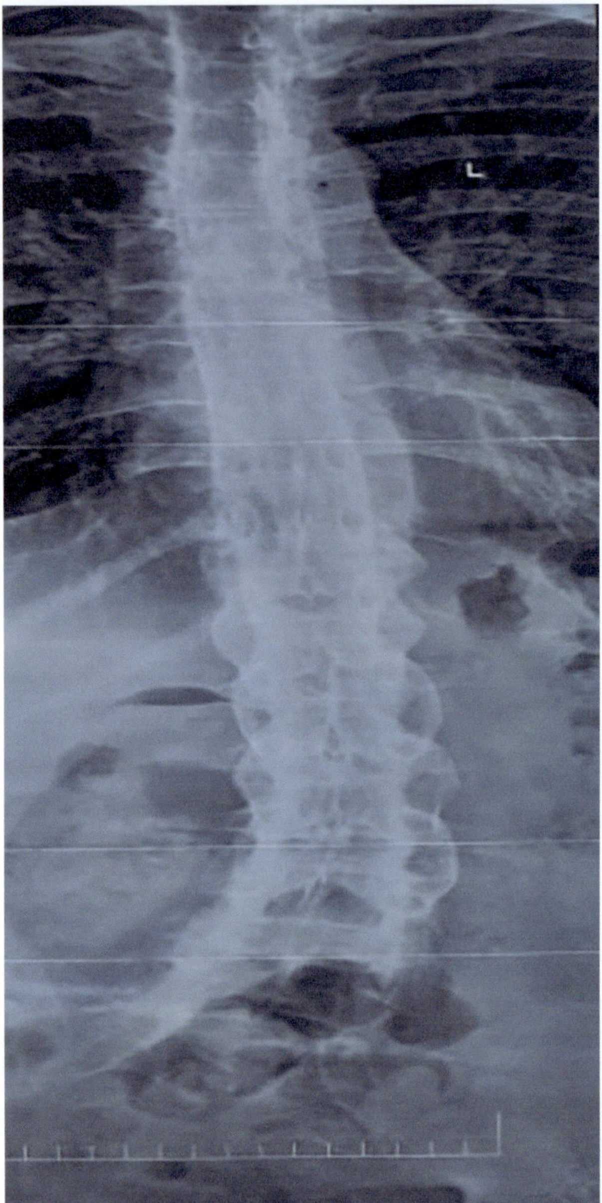

Fig. 9.5 Bamboo spine appearance on a radiograph

linked to higher vascularity caused by inflammation of the entheses. However, the ultrasound is limited by operator dependency, inter-observer variability, and the inability to visualize bone marrow inflammation [26].

In the initial stages of AS, when sacroiliitis is frequently invisible on traditional X-rays, MRI is the most effective method. MRI can identify acute inflammatory lesions at an early stage and display both ongoing inflammation and long-term structural modification [27]. The sensitivity of MRI is 97% in individuals with grade II sacroiliitis or higher on X-rays, and 76% in those with grade 0-I sacroiliitis. The MRI's fat-saturated short tau inversion recovery (STIR) method emphasizes inflammation, bone marrow swelling, and early erosions before they are visible on X-rays, especially in the sacroiliac joints. The lower iliac quadrant of the sacroiliac joints showed the same frequency of involvement in both AS and early axial spondyloarthropathy [28].

9.5 Laboratory Tests

The HLA-B27 genotype and C-reactive protein (CRP) levels are the main laboratory parameters typically utilized in the diagnosis of ankylosing spondylitis [14]. HLA B27 is still imperative, especially in the initial phase of the illness, as it is detected in about 89% of individuals with AS and shows high sensitivity (90%) and specificity (90%) in Caucasian populations. On the other hand, CRP is an acute-phase reactant that increases in response to inflammation [14]. Around 50% of patients with AS have high CRP levels, although its diagnostic value is limited due to inconsistent elevation. Despite a sensitivity of 50% and specificity of 80%, CRP can still help track disease activity and treatment response. Erythrocyte sedimentation rate (ESR) can be elevated in AS but is not consistently high in all patients, limiting its standalone diagnostic utility.

9.6 Diagnosis

Diagnosing ankylosing spondylitis poses significant challenges due to the lack of definitive diagnostic criteria, which contributes to an average diagnostic delay of 5–10 years. This delay often results in unnecessary procedures and increased morbidity. Early diagnosis is crucial to initiating effective therapy and improving patient outcomes.

The modified New York classification criteria (Table 9.2) [5] for AS requires X-ray proof of sacroiliitis plus at least one clinical indicator like inflammatory back pain (IBP), limited movement in the lower back, or reduced chest expansion. However, these criteria are more effective for later-stage diagnosis, not early detection.

The European Spondyloarthropathy Study Group (ESSG) introduced classification criteria in 1991, that emphasized factors such as inflammatory back pain (IBP) and asymmetric synovitis, in addition to family history, inflammatory bowel disease

Table 9.2 Modified New York criteria

Definite ankylosing spondylitis—Definite sacroiliitis (grade ≥ II bilaterally or unilateral grades II–IV) and any one of the following clinical criteria
Probable ankylosing spondylitis if 3 clinical criteria or radiologic criterion present without any signs or symptoms to satisfy clinical criteria
I. Clinical criteria
Persistent low back pain ≥3 months duration alleviated by physical activity not alleviated by rest.
Limitation of lumbar spine movements in sagittal and frontal planes.
Decreased chest expansion relative to normal values for age and gender-specific.
II. Radiologic criterion
Grade II sacroiliitis on both sides or grades III to IV sacroiliitis on one side.

(IBD), psoriasis, enthesopathy, alternating buttock pain, or a previous urogenital or enteric infection [29]. In 2009, the Assessment of Spondyloarthritis International Society (ASAS) developed criteria for axial spondyloarthritis, showing enhanced sensitivity (82.9%) and specificity (84.4%). According to the ASAS criteria, axial spondyloarthritis is classified into two types: non-radiographic axial spondyloarthritis and radiographic axial spondyloarthritis, also known as classic ankylosing spondylitis [30]. The concise criteria can be found in Fig. 9.6.

Historically, the Rome criteria (1963, updated 1968) [31] and the New York criteria (1984) [21] were the benchmarks but were inadequate for early diagnosis. The ASAS criteria have enabled a wider variety of diagnostic characteristics.

The differentiation between diagnostic and classification criteria for spondyloarthritis is unclear. So far, all established criteria mainly focus on classification and are better at detecting advanced stages of the illness rather than aiding in early detection.

Rudwaleit et al. [32] proposed a diagnostic algorithm for axial spondyloarthritis in 2004 among individuals suffering from chronic back pain. This algorithm recommends diagnosing axial spondyloarthritis in individuals who experience inflammatory back pain and exhibit three or more spondyloarthritis characteristics. Individuals who have inflammatory back pain and one or two characteristics of spondyloarthritis should undergo HLA-B27 testing as per guidelines. A confirmed HLA-B27 test result can help to confirm a diagnosis of axial spondyloarthritis. It is recommended to conduct HLA-B27 testing and MRI of the sacroiliac joints for patients presenting with isolated inflammatory back pain without other signs of spondyloarthritis. Confirmation of the diagnosis is achieved through the presence of HLA-B27 and MRI findings showing inflammation.

(applicable to individuals with ≥3 months of back pain with age onset <45years old)

Sacroiliitis on imaging* plus ≥1 axial spondyloarthritis feature**	OR	HLA-B27 positive plus ≥2 axial spondyloarthritis feature**

***Sacroiliitis on imaging**

- Active (acute) inflammation on MRI highly suggestive of axial spondyloarthritis-associated sacroiliitis
- Definite radiographic sacroiliitis according to the modified New York criteria

****Axial spondyloarthritis features**

- Inflammatory back pain
- Arthritis
- Enthesitis (heel)
- Anterior uveitis
- Dactylitis
- Psoriasis
- Crohn's disease or ulcerative colitis
- Good response to non-steroidal anti-inflammatory drugs
- Family history of axial spondyloarthritis
- HLA-B27 positive
- Elevated C-reactive protein levels (exclude other causes)

Fig. 9.6 The ASAS criteria for the classification of axial spondyloarthritis

9.7 Treatment

Treatment for ankylosing spondylitis encompasses various approaches aimed at managing inflammation, improving mobility, and addressing complications like spinal deformities.

9.8 Physical Therapy

Physical therapy is essential for managing AS, as it helps enhance muscle strength, mobility, and reduce pain. Different types of exercise therapies such as aquatic exercises, weight, and cardiovascular training are used in AS rehabilitation. Due to the significance of exercise in enhancing the quality of life and mobility of AS patients, home exercise programs are frequently recommended to patients for ongoing therapy after being discharged from the hospital [33]. Studies have indicated that combining physical therapy with anti-inflammatory drug treatments yields greater improvement in patient's conditions [34].

9.9 Treatment for Inflammation

For individuals with severe ankylosing spondylitis, the primary focus of anti-inflammatory therapy is to inhibit the activity of tumor necrosis factor α (TNF-α). TNF-α inhibitors are effective in decreasing inflammation associated with AS, especially in the initial phases to avoid skeletal abnormalities. There are two types of TNF-α inhibitor medications being used: anti-TNF antibodies like infliximab, adalimumab, [35] and TNF receptors such as etanercept [36]. These medications are approved for AS treatment and have shown success in reducing inflammation and improving symptoms.

Nonsteroidal anti-inflammatory drugs (NSAIDs) are frequently given to AS patients to treat back pain and stiffness. While their primary role is symptom management, studies have suggested that NSAIDs may also slow disease progression [37].

9.10 Surgical Intervention

Advancement of ankylosing spondylitis can result in abnormalities in the axial skeleton. A prevalent deformity seen in AS individuals is the fixed thoracolumbar kyphotic deformity (TLKD) of the spine. Surgical intervention becomes necessary to correct these deformities and prevent further complications. Currently, three surgical methods are utilized in spine surgery for correcting TLKD: opening wedge osteotomy (OWO), closing wedge osteotomy (CWO), and poly-segmental wedge osteotomy (PWO). The OWO method includes making osteotomies in vertebrae (such as L1, L2, and L3) and manually stretching the lumbar spine to form a wedge in the anterior column. The spine is stabilized by closing the posterior osteotomies. OWO aims to correct kyphotic deformity by increasing lordosis (forward curvature) in the spine [38]. The CWO method includes resecting posterior elements of a vertebra, and then extending the spine to close the posterior osteotomy by forming a gap in the anterior part of the column. The PWO procedure includes carrying out several wedge osteotomies in the posterior lumbar region. This technique allows for smaller closing angles of the osteotomies, leading to a more gradual extension of the spine and correction of deformity [39].

Another potential complication of AS is the occurrence of spinal fractures in the thoracic and lumbar regions. Spinal fractures can occur due to the weakened and fused vertebrae characteristic of AS. Surgery is essential to avoid additional fractures, support the spine, and possibly enhance neurological condition [40]. Surgical approaches for spinal fractures in AS may involve stabilization techniques such as instrumentation (e.g., screws, rods) and fusion procedures. The choice of surgical technique depends on the specific deformity or fracture pattern, aiming to achieve spinal realignment, stability, and improved functional outcomes for affected individuals.

References

1. Sieper J, Rudwaleit M, Khan MA, Braun J. Concepts and epidemiology of spondyloarthritis. Best Pract Res Clin Rheumatol. 2006 Jun;20(3):401–17.
2. Ghasemi-Rad M, Attaya H, Lesha E, Vegh A, Maleki-Miandoab T, Nosair E, et al. Ankylosing spondylitis: a state of the art factual backbone. World J Radiol. 2015 Sep 28;7(9):236–52.
3. Magrey MN, Danve AS, Ermann J, Walsh JA. Recognizing axial Spondyloarthritis: a guide for primary care. Mayo Clin Proc. 2020 Nov 1;95(11):2499–508.
4. Sieper J, Rudwaleit M, Baraliakos X, Brandt J, Braun J, Burgos-Vargas R, et al. The assessment of Spondylo arthritis international society (ASAS) handbook: a guide to assess spondyloarthritis. Ann Rheum Dis. 2009 Jun;68(Suppl 2):ii1-44.
5. van der Linden S, Valkenburg HA, Cats A. Evaluation of diagnostic criteria for ankylosing spondylitis. A proposal for modification of the New York criteria. Arthritis Rheum. 1984;27(4):361–8.
6. Crossfield SSR, Marzo-Ortega H, Kingsbury SR, Pujades-Rodriguez M, Conaghan PG. Changes in ankylosing spondylitis incidence, prevalence and time to diagnosis over two decades. RMD Open. 2021 Dec;7(3):e001888.
7. Willard FH. The muscular, ligamentous, and neural structure of the lumbosacrum and its relationship to low back pain. Mvmt Stabil Lumbopelvic Pain. 2007 Dec;31:5–45.
8. Brewerton DA, Hart FD, Nicholls A, Caffrey M, James DC, Sturrock RD. Ankylosing spondylitis and HL-A 27. Lancet. 1973 Apr 28;1(7809):904–7.
9. Benjamin R, Parham P. Guilt by association: HLA-B27 and ankylosing spondylitis. Immunol Today. 1990 Apr;11(4):137–42.
10. Mear JP, Schreiber KL, Münz C, Zhu X, Stevanović S, Rammensee HG, et al. Misfolding of HLA-B27 as a result of its B pocket suggests a novel mechanism for its role in susceptibility to spondyloarthropathies. J Immunol. 1999 Dec 15;163(12):6665–70.
11. Calin A, Porta J, Fries JF, Schurman DJ. Clinical history as a screening test for ankylosing spondylitis. JAMA. 1977 Jun 13;237(24):2613–4.
12. Rudwaleit M, Metter A, Listing J, Sieper J, Braun J. Inflammatory back pain in ankylosing spondylitis: a reassessment of the clinical history for application as classification and diagnostic criteria. Arthritis Rheum. 2006 Feb;54(2):569–78.
13. van der Linden S, van der Heijde D. Ankylosing spondylitis. Clinical features. Rheum Dis Clin N Am. 1998 Nov;24(4):663–76,vii.
14. Braun J, Sieper J. Early diagnosis of spondyloarthritis. Nat Clin Pract Rheumatol. 2006 Oct;2(10):536–45.
15. Castro MP, Stebbings SM, Milosavljevic S, Pedersen SJ, Bussey MD. Assessing the construct validity of clinical tests to identify sacroiliac joint inflammation in patients with non-radiographic axial spondyloarthritis. Int J Rheum Dis. 2019 Aug;22(8):1521–8.
16. Viitanen JV, Kokko ML, Heikkilä S, Kautiainen H. Neck mobility assessment in ankylosing spondylitis: a clinical study of nine measurements including new tape methods for cervical rotation and lateral flexion. Br J Rheumatol. 1998 Apr;37(4):377–81.
17. Agrawal P, Tote S, Sapkale B. Diagnosis and treatment of ankylosing spondylitis. Cureus. 16(1):e52559.
18. Saglam Y, Ozturk I, Cakmak MF, Ozdemir M, Yazicioglu O. Total hip arthroplasty in patients with ankylosing spondylitis: midterm radiologic and functional results. Acta Orthop Traumatol Turc. 2016 Aug 1;50(4):443–7.
19. Braun J, Sieper J, Bollow M. Imaging of sacroiliitis. Clin Rheumatol. 2000;19(1):51–7.
20. Resnick D, Niwayama G, Goergen TG. Comparison of radiographic abnormalities of the sacroiliac joint in degenerative disease and ankylosing spondylitis. AJR Am J Roentgenol. 1977 Feb;128(2):189–96.
21. Goie The HS, Steven MM, van der Linden SM, Cats A. Evaluation of diagnostic criteria for ankylosing spondylitis: a comparison of the Rome, New York and modified New York crite-

ria in patients with a positive clinical history screening test for ankylosing spondylitis. Br J Rheumatol. 1985 Aug;24(3):242–9.
22. Jacobson JA, Girish G, Jiang Y, Resnick D. Radiographic evaluation of arthritis: inflammatory conditions. Radiology. 2008 Aug;248(2):378–89.
23. Karasick D, Schweitzer ME, Abidi NA, Cotler JM. Fractures of the vertebrae with spinal cord injuries in patients with ankylosing spondylitis: imaging findings. AJR Am J Roentgenol. 1995 Nov;165(5):1205–8.
24. Geijer M, Sihlbom H, Göthlin JH, Nordborg E. The role of CT in the diagnosis of sacro-iliitis. Acta Radiol. 1998 May;39(3):265–8.
25. Unlü E, Pamuk ON, Cakir N. Color and duplex Doppler sonography to detect sacroiliitis and spinal inflammation in ankylosing spondylitis. Can this method reveal response to anti-tumor necrosis factor therapy? J Rheumatol. 2007 Jan;34(1):110–6.
26. Chary-Valckenaere I, d'Agostino MA, Loeuille D. Role for imaging studies in ankylosing spondylitis. Joint Bone Spine. 2011 Mar;78(2):138–43.
27. Ai F, Ai T, Li X, Hu D, Zhang W, Morelli JN. Value of diffusion-weighted magnetic resonance imaging in early diagnosis of ankylosing spondylitis. Rheumatol Int. 2012 Dec;32(12):4005–13.
28. Weber U, Pfirrmann CWA, Kissling RO, Hodler J, Zanetti M. Whole body MR imaging in ankylosing spondylitis: a descriptive pilot study in patients with suspected early and active confirmed ankylosing spondylitis. BMC Musculoskelet Disord. 2007 Feb 27;8:20.
29. Dougados M, van der Linden S, Juhlin R, Huitfeldt B, Amor B, Calin A, et al. The European Spondylarthropathy study group preliminary criteria for the classification of spondylarthropathy. Arthritis Rheum. 1991 Oct;34(10):1218–27.
30. Taurog JD, Chhabra A, Colbert RA. Ankylosing spondylitis and axial Spondyloarthritis. N Engl J Med. 2016 Jun 30;374(26):2563–74.
31. Moll JM, Wright V. New York clinical criteria for ankylosing spondylitis. A statistical evaluation. Ann Rheum Dis. 1973 Jul;32(4):354–63.
32. Rudwaleit M, van der Heijde D, Khan MA, Braun J, Sieper J. How to diagnose axial spondyloarthritis early. Ann Rheum Dis. 2004 May;63(5):535–43.
33. Brophy S, Davies H, Dennis MS, Cooksey R, Husain MJ, Irvine E, et al. Fatigue in ankylosing spondylitis: treatment should focus on pain management. Semin Arthritis Rheum. 2013 Feb;42(4):361–7.
34. Stockdale J, Selfe J, Roddam H. An exploration of the impact of anti-TNFα medication on exercise behaviour in patients with ankylosing spondylitis. Musculoskeletal Care. 2014 Sep;12(3):150–9.
35. Sfikakis PP. The first decade of biologic TNF antagonists in clinical practice: lessons learned, unresolved issues and future directions. Curr Dir Autoimmun. 2010;11:180–210.
36. Baji P, Péntek M, Szántó S, Géher P, Gulácsi L, Balogh O, et al. Comparative efficacy and safety of biosimilar infliximab and other biological treatments in ankylosing spondylitis: systematic literature review and meta-analysis. Eur J Health Econ. 2014 May;15(Suppl 1):S45–52.
37. Wanders A, van der HD, Landewé R, Béhier JM, Calin A, Olivieri I, et al. Nonsteroidal antiinflammatory drugs reduce radiographic progression in patients with ankylosing spondylitis: a randomized clinical trial. Arthritis Rheum. 2005;52(6):1756–65.
38. Scudese VA, Calabro JJ. Vertebral wedge osteotomy. Correction of rheumatoid (ankylosing) spondylitis. JAMA. 1963 Nov;16(186):627–31.
39. Van Royen BJ, De Gast A. Lumbar osteotomy for correction of thoracolumbar kyphotic deformity in ankylosing spondylitis. A structured review of three methods of treatment. Ann Rheum Dis. 1999 Jul;58(7):399–406.
40. Lu ML, Tsai TT, Lai PL, Fu TS, Niu CC, Chen LH, et al. A retrospective study of treating thoracolumbar spine fractures in ankylosing spondylitis. Eur J Orthop Surg Traumatol. 2014 Jul;24(Suppl 1):S117–23.

10 Osteoporosis and Vertebral Compression Fracture

Vishal Kumar and Ramesh Kalappagol Basappa

10.1 Introduction

Osteoporosis (OP) is a significant global public health problem, impacting more than 200 million individuals globally, with its frequency rising as the population ages [1]. It is a bone disorder related to metabolism that causes weaker bones and increases the likelihood of fractures in areas such as the hip, spine, and other skeletal regions [2].

10.2 Definition

The understanding of osteoporosis has changed over the years. At first, in 1984, it was defined as an age-related condition with lower bone density and higher fracture risk without a known cause [3]. By 2001, it was redefined to emphasize reduced bone strength due to a combination of bone density and quality, increasing susceptibility to fractures [4]. It is better described as a progressive skeletal disorder, marked by an overall decrease in bone density (quantitative) primarily resulting from deterioration in the quality of bone tissue structure (qualitative), leading to greater vulnerability to fractures due to greater bone fragility [5].

The World Health Organization (WHO) has established guidelines for evaluating bone health and identifying the likelihood of fractures. The T-score is used to determine how far a patient's test result differs from the average of a young, healthy

V. Kumar · R. K. Basappa (✉)
Department of Orthopaedics, PGIMER, Chandigarh, India

V. Kumar, P. Mishra (eds.), *A Comprehensive Guide to Degenerative Spine Disorders*, https://doi.org/10.1007/978-981-96-9091-6_10

Table 10.1 Defining osteoporosis by BMD: the WHO classification by T-score [6]

Diagnosis	T-Score
Normal	−1.0 and above
Osteopenia	Between −1.0 and − 2.5
Osteoporosis	At or below −2.5
Severe osteoporosis	At or below −2.5 plus fragility fractures

reference group in terms of standard deviations. Osteoporosis is defined by the WHO using bone mineral density (BMD) measurements collected from DEXA (dual-energy X-ray absorptiometry) scans. According to the WHO guidelines (Table 10.1), a BMD T-score lower than −2.5 indicates osteoporosis, while a T-score between −1 and − 2.5 indicates osteopenia [6].

10.3 Pathophysiology

Normal bone remodeling involves balancing bone breakdown by osteoclasts through acidification and proteolytic digestion with the creation of new bone in the resorption cavity by osteoblasts [7]. Reduced BMD characterizes osteoporosis and results from an imbalance between bone resorption and bone formation, marked by decreased osteoblastic activity and increased osteoclastic activity. The lack of estrogen, especially after menopause in women, worsens this imbalance. Lower estrogen levels lead to more bone resorption by extending osteoclasts' lifespan and less bone formation by reducing osteoblasts' lifespan. This causes progressive bone loss and a higher likelihood of fractures (Fig. 10.1a and b) [8].

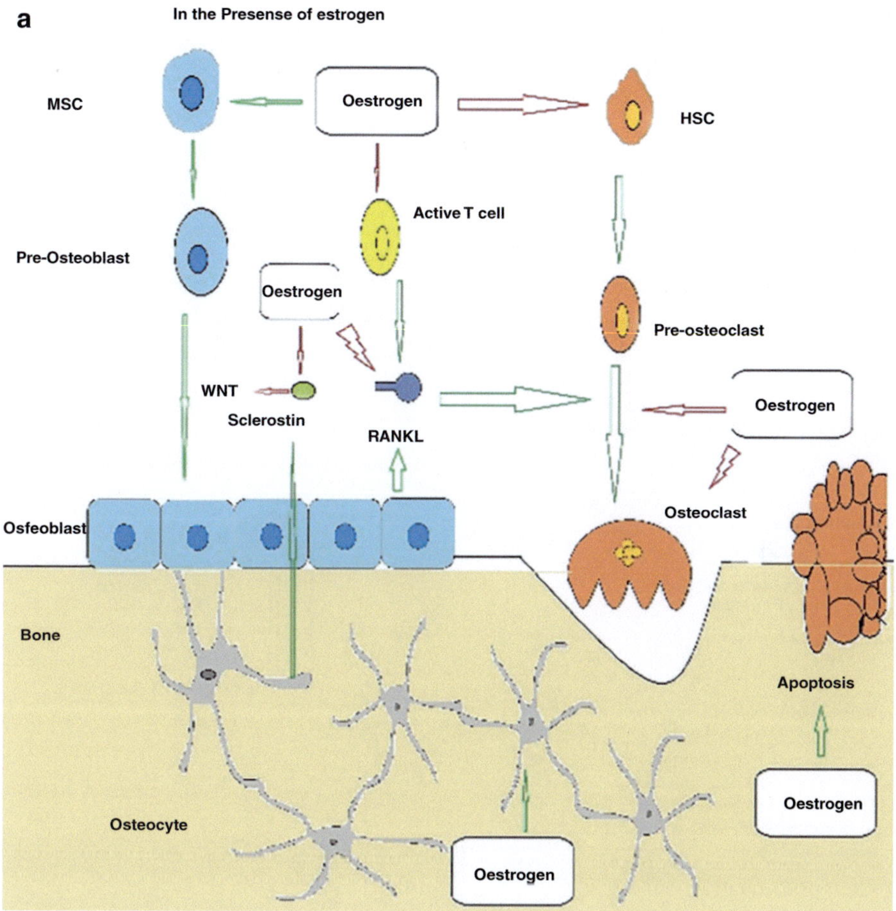

Fig. 10.1 Pathophysiology (**a**) Physiological bone remodelling: estrogen boosts bone formation by promoting the differentiation and function of osteoblasts and inhibiting the differentiation and activity of osteoclasts through direct effects on cells and decreased production of receptor activator of nuclear factor-κB ligand (RANKL) by activated T cells, mesenchymal stem cells (MSC), osteoblasts, and osteocytes. (**b**) Estrogen deficiency: Increased production of RANKL leads to an elevation in osteoclast count and function. At the same time, the activity of each osteoblast is hindered, in part due to an increase in the WNT inhibitor sclerostin, while the overall amount of osteoblasts goes up. HSC, hematopoietic stem cell

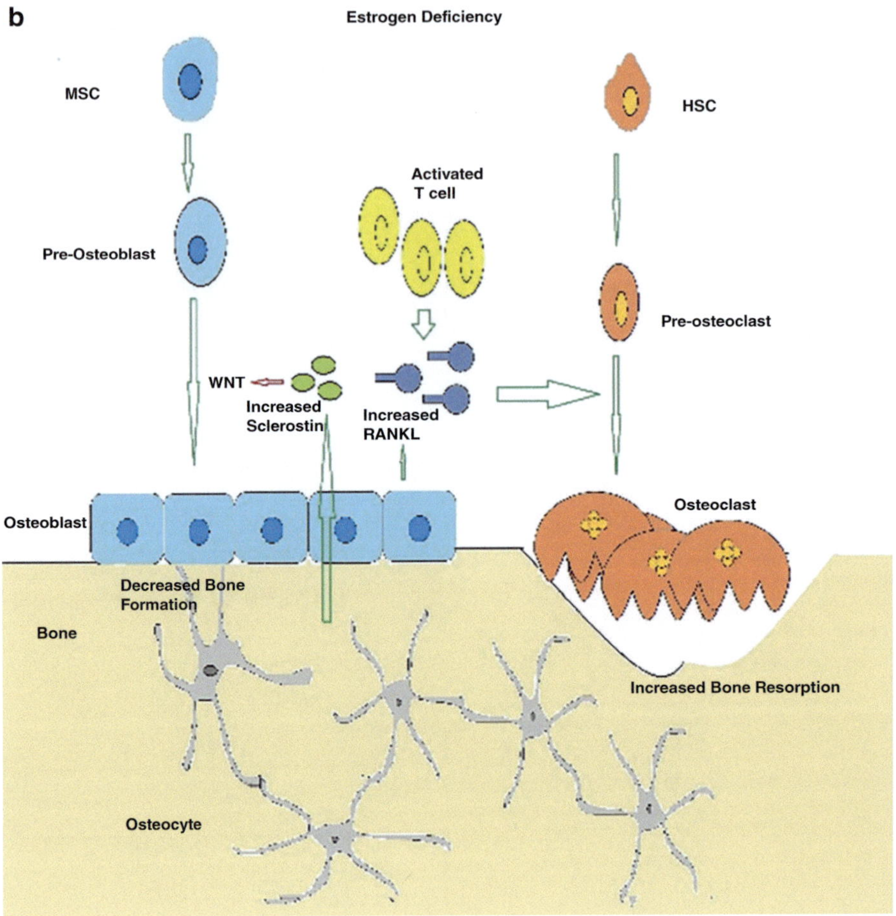

Fig. 10.1 (continued)

10.4 Clinical Signs and Symptoms

Acute back pain during rest or routine activities like bending or lifting is the earliest symptom of osteoporosis. Common sequelae include vertebral body compression fractures (Fig. 10.2a) and fractures in the hips (Fig. 10.2b), humerus, and distal radius. Pathologic fractures, often resulting from falls, are prominent clinical manifestations. Thin patients who experience hip fractures likely have reduced resistance and low bone density [9].

Both modifiable and nonmodifiable elements contribute to decreased bone density [10]. Table 10.2 provides a list of both modifiable and nonmodifiable

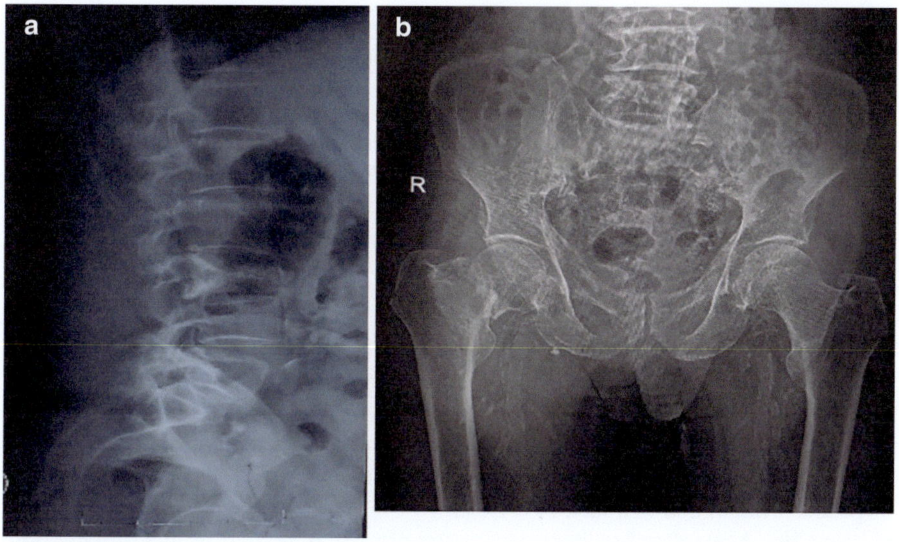

Fig. 10.2 Osteoporotic bone. (**a**) and (**b**) | Radiographs showing vertebra fractures (**a**) and proximal femur (**b**)

Table 10.2 Risk factors for osteoporosis [10]

Nonmodifiable	Modifiable
Advanced age Female Early menopause(<45 years) Low peak bone mass Parental history of fragility fracture History of previous fracture	Smoking Hyperthyroidism and hyperparathyroidism Inadequate calcium and vitamin D intake Low body weight (BMI <21 kg/m2) Estrogen deficiency Prolonged immobility Chronic glucocorticoid therapy

Table 10.3 Risk factors for falls [10]

Balance and gait disorders
Cognitive impairment
Neurodegenerative disorders of the central nervous system
Epilepsy
Vitamin D deficiency
Visual impairment
Impaired hearing
Medications affecting postural stability

elements. Recognizing risk factors for falls is equally crucial to determining BMD in preventing nonvertebral fractures [10]. Table 10.3 provides a list of risk factors for falls.

Table 10.4 Common causes of secondary osteoporosis [12]

Endocrine	Chronic drug therapy	Nutritional	Others
Hypogonadism Thyrotoxicosis Cushing's Hyperprolactinemia	Steroids Anticoagulants Anticonvulsants Gonadotropin-releasing hormone agonists, aromatase inhibitors	Malabsorption syndromes, vitamin-D deficiency, and calcium deficiency	Multiple myeloma, alcohol intake, and malnutrition

10.5 Classification

Osteoporosis has been categorized into primary and secondary forms [11].

Primary osteoporosis is classified into three types:

- Type I—Postmenopausal osteoporosis: osteoporosis that occurs in postmenopausal women due to a lack of estrogen.
- Type II—Age-related osteoporosis: osteoporosis is related to age, affects both men and women as their bone density declines due to aging.
- Type III—Idiopathic osteoporosis: osteoporosis without a known cause.

Secondary osteoporosis is seen in patients who have an identifiable cause or disease process (Table 10.4) [12].

10.6 Bone Strength and Quality

Bone strength is determined by the merging of bone density and bone quality [4]. It is influenced by both structural and material factors that contribute to overall bone quality. Bone strength is greatly affected by the structural characteristics of bone, including its geometry, microarchitecture, and cortical thickness. Material properties, including mineralization, collagen composition, and the accumulation of microfractures, also contribute [8].

10.7 Estimating the Likelihood of Fractures in Women After Menopause

10.7.1 FRAX Tool

The Fracture Risk Assessment Tool, abbreviated as FRAX, offers a numerical prediction of fracture risk for individuals with decreased bone density. This is important because most fragility fractures happen in individuals with osteopenia, not osteoporosis. The FRAX model, supported by the WHO, uses clinical risk factors and can incorporate femoral neck BMD to predict an individual's 10-year absolute risk of fractures related to osteoporosis [13]. FRAX is beneficial for pinpointing individuals with decreased bone density who face a higher chance of fractures and are likely to see improvements with treatment. FRAX aids in making clinical decisions to manage fracture risk to decrease disability, expenses, and death related to fractures.

FRAX has been confirmed to be suitable for men and postmenopausal women between 40 and 90 years old who have not received treatment for osteoporosis before. The clinical risk factors included in FRAX can be found in Table 10.5 [14]. While FRAX does not substitute for clinical judgment, it offers a numerical assessment of the actual risk of fractures, facilitating conversations between physicians and patients and enhancing fracture risk management. To learn more about determining fracture risk, check out the official FRAX tool website (https://frax.shef.ac.uk/FRAX/) [15].

FRAX has several notable limitations: it can only be applied to patients not currently undergoing osteoporosis treatment [16]. It does not adequately account for the increased risk of fracture following a prior fracture. Specifically, it does not adjust for the compounded risk associated with multiple fractures compared to a single fracture, which may lead to an underestimation of the true fracture risk in these patients [13]. It does not consider the dosage and duration of glucocorticoid therapy [17]; and it mainly focuses on BMD of the femoral neck, neglecting BMD readings from other important areas like the lumbar vertebrae [16].

Table 10.5 Risk factors used in FRAX [14]

Risk factors
Current age
Gender
Weight (kg)
Height (cm)
Prior osteoporotic fracture
Parent fractured hip
Current smoking
Oral glucocorticoid use
Rheumatoid arthritis
Secondary causes of osteoporosis
Alcohol intake (≥3 drinks per day)
Femoral neck BMD

10.8 Fracture Risk Reduction

The National Osteoporosis Foundation (NOF) in 2008 recommends conducting a comprehensive history assessment to identify risk factors and assist in making clinical decisions. The NOF suggests utilizing the FRAX model to assess fracture by considering clinical risk factors and BMD readings. The NOF [18] recommends pharmacotherapy for postmenopausal women and men over 50 years old who have any of these traits:

- A past occurrence of hip or vertebral fracture, whether clinically diagnosed or morphometrically identified.
- Osteoporosis is confirmed when the BMD T-score is equal to or less than −2.5 after ruling out other potential causes.
- Low bone density with FRAX 10-year chance of hip fracture of ≥3% or of major osteoporotic fracture of ≥20%, using the US version of the WHO algorithm.

10.9 Diagnosis

10.9.1 Candidates for Assessment

The NOF advises conducting BMD testing to determine treatment plans, considering the patient's risk factors [16]. BMD testing is advised for females 65 years old and above, males 70 and above, postmenopausal women younger than 65, males 50–69 years old with fracture risk factors, and those with fractures at or after age 50. Recent research conducted by the study of osteoporotic fractures has identified various common, significant, and clinically beneficial risk factors in women. This list consists of factors like weak BMD, a fracture occurring after age 40, a fracture in a close relative's hip, wrist, or vertebra, or current smoking [19].

Diagnostic evaluation includes measuring BMD through DEXA or QCT (quantitative computed tomography), evaluating bone turnover markers, and conducting laboratory tests to identify underlying causes.

10.9.2 Radiologic Assessments

The Singh index (SI) [20] is a classification system used to assess the bone density of the femoral neck based on the appearance of trabecular patterns visible in plain radiographs. It is a straightforward, semi-quantitative tool for diagnosing osteoporosis, especially useful in settings where routine and mass screening is required, as X-ray films are readily accessible in most outpatient clinics.

The grades of the Singh index are as follows:

- Grade 1: Only thin principal compression trabeculae are visible.
- Grade 2: Principal compression trabeculae are present, with other trabeculae nearly resorbed.

- Grade 3: Principal tensile trabeculae are thinned, and continuity is broken.
- Grade 4: Principal tensile trabeculae are thinned, but continuity is maintained.
- Grade 5: Principal tensile and compression trabeculae are readily visible, with prominence of Ward's triangle.
- Grade 6: All trabeculae are visible and have normal thickness.

Grade 3 and below typically indicate definite osteoporosis. The index ranges from 1 (severe osteoporosis) to 6 (normal bone density).

According to the WHO protocol, the method for diagnosing osteoporosis is through DEXA scans that measure areal BMD at key skeletal sites like the spine or hip [21]. Bone densitometry can detect bone weakening early on, indicating the need for timely treatment, and estimating the risk of future fractures [21]. QCT offers volumetric BMD along with more information on bone shape and structure, especially useful for evaluating the spine and differentiating between cortical and trabecular bone. Its ability to detect changes in BMD due to trabecular bone turnover makes it a valuable tool for monitoring skeletal changes and disease progression or treatment outcomes in osteoporosis [21].

10.10 Laboratory Studies

Common laboratory tests may consist of a full blood count with leukocyte differentiation; levels of calcium, albumin, phosphorus, alkaline phosphatase, blood urea nitrogen, and creatinine in the blood; as well as a 24-h urine sample to assess calcium and creatinine levels [10].

Additional diagnostic tests are needed to identify potential underlying conditions that could be causing bone loss if secondary causes of osteoporosis are suspected. These tests help tailor the treatment approach and manage any contributing disorders effectively. Thyroid function tests for diagnosing primary or iatrogenic hyperthyroidism, and parathyroid hormone levels for evaluating hyperparathyroidism, while serum protein electrophoresis, urinary immunoelectrophoresis, and bone marrow aspirate may be required to identify multiple myeloma. Testing the serum 25-hydroxyvitamin D level can aid in identifying a possible deficiency in vitamin D. Osteopenic or osteoporotic men should undergo testing for their serum testosterone levels as they often have no symptoms of low testosterone that can contribute to bone loss [10].

10.11 Biochemical Markers of Bone Turnover

BMD measurements do not accurately reflect bone remodelling markers and are not useful for measuring bone loss rates; so bone turnover rates are currently evaluated with different methods. Alterations in markers suggest an ongoing bone metabolism process. Postmenopausal women have higher levels of markers indicating bone formation and breakdown compared to premenopausal women, indicating increased

Table 10.6 Bone turnover biochemical indicators [23]

Markers of bone resorption	Markers of bone formation
Urinary collagen cross-links (pyridinoline deoxypyridinoline) Urinary calcium and hydroxyproline Type I collagen telopeptides N-terminal crosslinking telopeptide (NTX-1) C-terminal crosslinking telopeptide (CTX-1) Tartrate-resistant acid phosphatase (TRAP)	Serum osteocalcin Bone-specific alkaline phosphatase (BSAP) Propeptide of type I procollagen N-terminal propeptide of type I procollagen C-terminal propeptide of type I procollagen

bone turnover due to estrogen deficiency [22]. These markers can also be used to evaluate drug effectiveness, anticipate bone mass gains, and help in choosing appropriate treatment for patients (Table 10.6) [23].

10.12 Prevention and Management

10.12.1 Reduction of Risk Factors and Nutritional Modifications

The primary goal in treating osteoporosis is to prevent osteoporotic fractures. Effective management of osteoporosis involves a combination of lifestyle modifications, dietary adjustments, physical activity, and preventive measures to reduce the risk of fractures and improve overall bone health. It is essential to adopt healthy habits such as keeping a balanced diet, participating in consistent physical activity, abstaining from tobacco and excessive alcohol consumption, following the recommended calcium and vitamin D intake, and taking precautions to avoid falls [24].

Adults aged 65 and above are advised to consume 1500 mg of calcium daily, preferably from dairy products to improve absorption. A daily dose of 700–800 IU of vitamin D is advised for older adults, as it reduces the risk of hip fractures and improves muscle strength and balance [25]. Ensuring normal vitamin D levels is critical.

Phosphorus: Essential for bone development and mineralization, the suggested daily intake is 700 mg. However, about 10–15% of elderly individuals may not meet this requirement, especially those taking calcium supplements that can bind phosphorus and cause deficiencies [26].

10.13 Pharmacologic Treatments

10.13.1 Anti-Resorptive Drugs

10.13.1.1 Bisphosphonates

Most prescribed bisphosphonates today are nitrogen-containing, inhibiting farnesyl pyrophosphate synthase that is crucial for osteoclast attachment to bone. This inhibition detaches osteoclasts, reducing bone resorption. Non-nitrogen bisphosphonates are rarely used due to their potential to impair bone mineralization and cause osteomalacia [27].

Drugs like alendronate (70 mg/week) and risedronate (35 mg/week) inhibit osteoclast activity, reducing bone turnover and increasing bone density, which lowers fracture risk by 20% to 50% [28]. Proper ingestion techniques are crucial to avoid oesophageal and gastric complications. Osteonecrosis, especially postdental procedure, is a noted risk, primarily in high IV doses.

10.13.1.2 Denosumab

Denosumab, a human monoclonal antibody, targets and inhibits the cytokine receptor activator of nuclear factor kappa-B ligand (RANKL). Denosumab stops RANKL from binding to its receptor on osteoclasts and their precursors by attaching to RANKL. This blockage leads to a decrease in osteoclast development, activity, and longevity, causing a reduction in bone breakdown and an increase in bone density. It is administered subcutaneously every 6 months. Denosumab can cause hypersensitivity reactions, hypocalcemia, and excessive suppression of bone turnover as common side effects. Research has shown that using denosumab can lower hip fractures by as much as 40% and result in a 68% decrease in vertebral fractures [29].

10.13.1.3 Sclerostin Inhibitor (Romosozumab)

Romosozumab is a drug prescribed for osteoporosis treatment, especially for postmenopausal women with a high risk of fractures. A monoclonal antibody blocks sclerostin, a protein that hinders bone growth. Romosozumab encourages bone formation and decreases bone resorption by inhibiting sclerostin. This two-fold process assists in boosting bone density and decreasing the likelihood of fractures. It is injected once a month subcutaneously, at a dose of 210 mg [30].

10.14 Selective Estrogen Receptor Modulators (SERMs)

Raloxifene boosts bone mineral density and decreases vertebral compression fracture risk by up to 60%. However, it does not affect hip fracture rates and carries risks of thromboembolism and vasomotor symptoms [31].

10.15 Calcitonin

Calcitonin decreases bone resorption, moderately increasing spinal BMD and reducing vertebral fracture rates, though it does not prevent hip fractures. Calcitonin is usually reserved for patients intolerant to other medications and helps to alleviate bone pain from vertebral compression fractures [32].

10.16 Hormone Replacement Therapy (HRT)

Estrogen therapy (ET) effectively boosts bone mineral density (BMD) and helps prevent fractures in postmenopausal women. It can increase BMD by 2%–7% and helps prevent vertebral and hip fractures, but prolonged use presents higher risks of heart attack, stroke, blood clotting, and breast cancer. Due to the associated risks, it should be used for short-term and primarily for women experiencing severe menopausal symptoms [33]. For postmenopausal women under 60 at fracture risk or within 10 years of menopause, ET could be the first-line treatment, but not advisable for women over 60 due to heightened breast cancer risk [34].

10.17 Anabolic Agents

10.17.1 PTH (Parathyroid Hormone)

10.17.1.1 PTH Analogues (Teriparatide, Abaloparatide)

Teriparatide

Teriparatide, a synthetic form of human *parathyroid hormone* (PTH), is a substance that promotes the creation of bone cells. Increasing BMD by 3%–9% and reducing vertebral fractures by up to 65%. It is given through subcutaneous injection for a maximum of 2 years; it lowers nonvertebral fractures by half; although it has not been proven to specifically reduce hip fractures [35].

Abaloparatide

Abaloparatide is a synthetic peptide similar to parathyroid hormone-related protein (PTHrP) and acts as a specific agonist for parathyroid hormone receptor type 1 (PTH1R) [36]. It is typically given to patients via subcutaneous injection at a daily dose of 80 mcg. According to the American College of Endocrinology's clinical practice guidelines, abaloparatide is recommended for treating postmenopausal osteoporosis as it can improve BMD and reduce the risk of vertebral and nonvertebral fractures in women with this condition. Abaloparatide is often given to patients who cannot tolerate or have not benefitted from traditional osteoporosis therapies [37].

10.18 Addressing a Lack of Vitamin D

Many older individuals often suffer from a lack of vitamin D. It is advised to regularly measure serum 25-hydroxyvitamin D levels as they have a longer half-life and consistent levels in comparison to 1,25-dihydroxyvitamin D. The aim is to keep 25-hydroxyvitamin D levels above 30 ng/ml and PTH levels below 42 pg/ml. Deficiencies may be addressed by supplementing with vitamin D3 for 8 weeks, either through a daily intake of 6000 IU or a weekly intake of 50,000 IU. After reaching the target serum 25-hydroxyvitamin D levels, it is advised to take a daily maintenance dose of 1000 to 2000 IU to maintain sufficient levels. If the deficiency

Table 10.7 Risk factors—VCFs influenced by multiple risk factors include [41]

Osteopenia and osteoporosis
Older age
Previous VCFs
Inactivity
Administration of corticosteroids (more than 5 mg per day for duration for 3 months)
Weighing under 53 kg
Women
Consumption of more than two alcoholic drinks per day for women or more than three per day for men
Tobacco use
Insufficient levels of vitamin D
Depression

continues even after treatment with vitamin D2 (ergocalciferol) or D3 (cholecalciferol), calcitriol can be an option [38]. It is important to closely monitor serum calcium levels in patients taking calcitriol to prevent hypercalcemia risks.

10.19 Vertebral Compression Fractures

Vertebral compression fractures (VCFs) are frequently occurring fragility fractures and are often a sign of osteoporosis (OP) [39]. The occurrence and seriousness of VCFs can indicate the likelihood of new fractures regardless of BMD tests. These fractures can cause issues like back pain, difficulty in sleeping, reduced activity, further bone weakening, higher risk of fractures, spinal deformities, reduced lung function, impaired abilities, more health problems, and eventually death [40]. Risk factors for VCFs are outlined in detail in Table 10.7 [41].

10.20 Epidemiology

VCFs are more common in older adults, particularly women over 70 years old. Females aged 50 years and over experienced a rate of 10.7 new VCFs per 1000 people, while males in the same age group had a rate of 5.7 new VCFs per 1000 people. The rate increased from 3% in females under 60 years to 20% in females over 70 years, and from 7.5 to 20% in males of the same age range [42].

10.21 Symptoms and Signs

Over two-thirds of patients with VCFs are asymptomatic and often diagnosed by chance. Typical symptoms consist of abrupt start of spine discomfort, worsened by coughing, sneezing, standing, or walking, alleviated by rest [43]. Pain usually persists for 4 to 6 weeks during bone recovery in an osteoporotic VCF. After the initial phase, patients may experience restricted spinal movement, height loss, physical deformity, and reduced functionality. VCFs most frequently occur in the lower thoracic spine and are typically stable, rarely causing nerve root irritation or spinal cord damage [43].

Physical examination results are frequently within normal limits, though there may be kyphosis and midline spinal tenderness, as well as noticeable muscle spasms and tenderness at the site of the fracture. Persistent vertebral compression fractures can result in a decrease in height and also cause kyphosis. Compression fractures in the front part of the thoracic spine can cause thoracic kyphosis (Dowager's hump), the stooped posture often observed in people with osteoporosis [11].

A large portion of patients with cluster fractures suffer severe pain after their initial fracture and any subsequent fractures, leading to the need for additional investigation into potential causes of osteopenia. Each fracture results in a decrease in axial height, leading to a difference between standing height and arm span. Individuals with advanced spinal compression may develop a shortened trunk and stature noticeable when standing [11]. Long-term consequences include reduced dimensions in thoracic and abdominal cavities, decreased ability to exercise, feeling full and bloated after small meals, and potential abdominal protrusion and thickened skin folds due to severe lower back collapse [11].

10.22 Diagnostic Evaluation

VCFs may be asymptomatic but may cause sudden or long-lasting back pain [44]. The initial diagnosis relies on evaluating the patient's risk factors.

10.23 Evaluation of Risks

Risk evaluation includes a thorough case history, physical examination, lab tests, and comprehensive imaging. A thorough case history includes medical history, age when menopause began (for women), lifestyle habits, and individual risk factors. As stated in the "guidelines for the management of osteoporosis and fragility fractures," examining the patient's stance is necessary to look for signs of heightened kyphosis or lost height, which could suggest the presence of vertebral compression fractures [45].

FRAX tool can be utilized in clinical settings to determine the risk of fractures, assist in diagnosing VCFs, and guide treatment and prevention plans for osteoporosis [14].

Diagnostic imaging of osteoporosis (OP) and fragility fractures involves traditional X-rays to assess spinal fractures, DEXA bone density testing, computed tomography (CT), MRI, bone scans (if needed), and ultrasound (QUS). Bone scintigraphy can assist in determining the cause of back pain in osteoporotic patients with symptoms.

X-ray is a primary way to assess spinal fractures. Compression fractures are usually identified through side view X-rays of the spine (Fig. 10.3), with or without

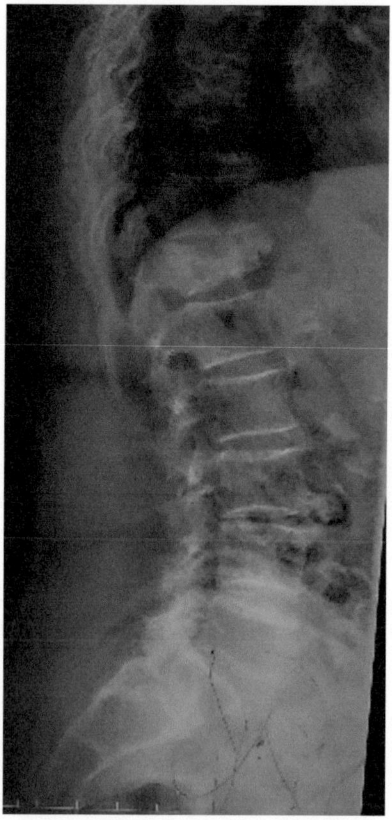

Fig. 10.3 Radiograph showing osteoporotic fracture of D12 vertebra

anteroposterior views. A VCF is described as a 15%–20% decrease in vertebral height or a 4-mm reduction from baseline [46].

MRI differentiates between benign and malignant fractures, detects edema to determine fracture timing, and identifies complications such as retropulsion, posterior column fractures, and spinal cord involvement [46, 47]. CT is valuable for assessing complex fractures in more detail [47, 48]. DEXA scan is used post-VCF diagnosis to assess the severity of osteoporosis [34].

10.24 Prevention and Treatment

Treatment aims to alleviate pain, restore function, and avoid future fractures. Even without vertebral compression fractures, it is important to remember that osteoporosis-related bone resorption can still lead to back pain. Symptoms usually heal within 6–8 weeks as the body heals. These patients typically receive treatment through medication, restricting activities/rest, back braces, physical therapy, or a mix of these methods [49].

10.24.1 Conservative Care

Encouraging early mobility is important in conservative treatment as soon as it is possible. Bed rest may be advised initially for severe pain, but it can result in bone and muscle loss, pressure sores, and blood clots [50]. All patients must ensure they have enough vitamin D and calcium, and follow appropriate exercise and fall prevention plans.

Commonly used medications for pain relief include nonsteroidal anti-inflammatory drugs, acetaminophen, narcotics, and muscle relaxants. These medications help patients to move and participate in physical therapy and should be gradually reduced as pain improves [51]. In patients with intact neurological function and vertebral compression fractures, calcitonin can reduce pain and improve mobility for up to 4 weeks [52].

A study on thoracolumbar bracing showed enhancements in posture, strength, and quality of life in a small sample group. While bracing is often recommended for a period of 6 to 8 weeks following a VCF, there is only limited evidence to support this practice [53].

Physical therapy and exercise have the potential to benefit individuals with vertebral compression fractures (VCFs) and osteoporosis. There is less evidence supporting home exercise programs, but small trials show they can reduce pain, enhance balance, and improve quality of life. Strengthening back extensors may also increase strength and bone density while lowering the chance of future VCFs [54].

10.24.2 Vertebroplasty and Kyphoplasty

Discomfort caused by a spinal fracture typically persists for 1–3 weeks before gradually decreasing and vanishing in a couple of months. Nevertheless, in certain situations, a biomechanical instability could arise and continue because of the seriousness and location of the VCF. Vertebral augmentation procedures like vertebroplasty and kyphoplasty are commonly recommended for patients experiencing severe and disabling pain [45]. Vertebroplasty involves injecting liquid cement (PMMA) into a compressed vertebra using a needle inserted through the pedicle. Kyphoplasty entails creating a cavity with the inflation of a balloon tamp followed by the injection of PMMA [48, 50].

Vertebroplasty is indicated for painful osteoporotic VCFs that persist despite 2–3 weeks of conservative treatment. It is also considered for patients suffering from painful primary bone tumors, such as aggressive hemangiomas or giant cell tumors, as well as lytic metastatic tumors accompanied by a pathological fracture or an impending fracture. Absolute contraindications for vertebroplasty include asymptomatic fractures, allergies to bone fillers or contrast agents, and irreversible coagulopathy. Relative contraindications include radicular pain, more than 70% collapse of vertebral body height, and bone fragments pressing against neural structures [55]. Both treatments could alleviate pain and disability and enhance alignment. Longo et al. state that it is not possible to determine if cementoplasty techniques are better than conservative management [56]. Possible complications include cement extravasation (more frequent with vertebroplasty), embolism, neurologic damage, bleeding, hematoma, infection, and a higher risk of VCFs at different levels [48, 50].

References

1. Lin JT, Lane JM. Osteoporosis: a review. Clin Orthop Relat Res. 2004 Aug;425:126–34.
2. Genant HK, Cooper C, Poor G, Reid I, Ehrlich G, Kanis J, et al. Interim report and recommendations of the World Health Organization task-force for osteoporosis. Osteoporos Int. 1999;10(4):259–64.
3. Consensus conference: Osteoporosis. JAMA. 1984 Aug 10;252(6):799–802.
4. NIH consensus development panel on osteoporosis prevention, diagnosis, and therapy. Osteoporosis prevention, diagnosis, and therapy. JAMA. 2001 Feb 14;285(6):785–95.
5. Consensus development conference: diagnosis, prophylaxis, and treatment of osteoporosis. Am J Med. 1993 Jun;94(6):646–50.
6. Kanis JA, Cooper C, Rizzoli R, Reginster JY. Scientific advisory Board of the European Society for clinical and economic aspects of osteoporosis (ESCEO) and the committees of scientific advisors and National Societies of the international osteoporosis foundation (IOF). European guidance for the diagnosis and management of osteoporosis in postmenopausal women. Osteoporos Int. 2019 Jan;30(1):3–44.
7. Manolagas SC. Birth and death of bone cells: basic regulatory mechanisms and implications for the pathogenesis and treatment of osteoporosis. Endocr Rev. 2000 Apr;21(2):115–37.
8. Seeman E. The structural and biomechanical basis of the gain and loss of bone strength in women and men. Endocrinol Metab Clin N Am. 2003 Mar;32(1):25–38.
9. Kaplan FS. Prevention and management of osteoporosis. Clin Symp. 1995;47(1):2–32.
10. Wilkins CH. Osteoporosis screening and risk management. Clin Interv Aging. 2007;2(3):389–94.
11. Glaser DL, Kaplan FS. Osteoporosis. Definition and clinical presentation. Spine (Phila Pa 1976). 1997;22(24 Suppl):12S–6S.
12. Fitzpatrick LA. Secondary causes of osteoporosis. Mayo Clin Proc. 2002 May;77(5):453–68.
13. Kanis JA, Johnell O, Oden A, Johansson H, McCloskey E. FRAX and the assessment of fracture probability in men and women from the UK. Osteoporos Int. 2008 Apr;19(4):385–97.
14. Unnanuntana A, Gladnick BP, Donnelly E, Lane JM. The assessment of fracture risk. J Bone Joint Surg Am. 2010 Mar;92(3):743–53.
15. Kanis JA, Johansson H, Harvey NC, McCloskey EV. A brief history of FRAX. Arch Osteoporos. 2018 Oct;13:118.
16. Cosman F, de Beur SJ, LeBoff MS, Lewiecki EM, Tanner B, Randall S, et al. Clinician's guide to prevention and treatment of osteoporosis. Osteoporos Int. 2014 Oct;25(10):2359–81.
17. Watts NB, Ettinger B, LeBoff MS. FRAX facts. J Bone Miner Res. 2009 Jun;24(6):975–9.
18. Kanis JA, Harvey NC, Cooper C, Johansson H, Odén A, McCloskey EV, et al. A systematic review of intervention thresholds based on FRAX : a report prepared for the National Osteoporosis Guideline Group and the international osteoporosis foundation. Arch Osteoporos. 2016 Dec;11(1):25.
19. Cummings SR, Nevitt MC, Browner WS, Stone K, Fox KM, Ensrud KE, et al. Risk factors for hip fracture in white women. Study of osteoporotic fractures research group. N Engl J Med. 1995 Mar 23;332(12):767–73.

20. Singh M, Nagrath AR, Maini PS. Changes in trabecular pattern of the upper end of the femur as an index of osteoporosis. J Bone Joint Surg Am. 1970 Apr;52(3):457–67.
21. Brunader R, Shelton DK. Radiologic bone assessment in the evaluation of osteoporosis. Am Fam Physician. 2002 Apr 1;65(7):1357–64.
22. Garnero P, Sornay-Rendu E, Chapuy MC, Delmas PD. Increased bone turnover in late postmenopausal women is a major determinant of osteoporosis. J Bone Miner Res. 1996 Mar;11(3):337–49.
23. Seibel MJ. Biochemical markers of bone turnover part I: biochemistry and variability. Clin Biochem Rev. 2005 Nov;26(4):97–122.
24. Gillespie LD, Robertson MC, Gillespie WJ, Sherrington C, Gates S, Clemson LM, et al. Interventions for preventing falls in older people living in the community. Cochrane Database Syst Rev. 2012 Sep 12;2012(9):CD007146.
25. Bischoff-Ferrari HA, Willett WC, Wong JB, Giovannucci E, Dietrich T, Dawson-Hughes B. Fracture prevention with vitamin D supplementation: a meta-analysis of randomized controlled trials. JAMA. 2005 May 11;293(18):2257–64.
26. Bischoff HA, Stähelin HB, Dick W, Akos R, Knecht M, Salis C, et al. Effects of vitamin D and calcium supplementation on falls: a randomized controlled trial. J Bone Miner Res. 2003 Feb;18(2):343–51.
27. Ganesan K, Goyal A, Roane D. Bisphosphonate. In: StatPearls [internet]. Treasure Island: StatPearls Publishing; 2024.
28. Barrionuevo P, Kapoor E, Asi N, Alahdab F, Mohammed K, Benkhadra K, et al. Efficacy of pharmacological therapies for the prevention of fractures in postmenopausal women: a network meta-analysis. J Clin Endocrinol Metab. 2019 May 1;104(5):1623–30.
29. Cummings SR, San Martin J, McClung MR, Siris ES, Eastell R, Reid IR, et al. Denosumab for prevention of fractures in postmenopausal women with osteoporosis. N Engl J Med. 2009 Aug 20;361(8):756–65.
30. Cosman F, Crittenden DB, Adachi JD, Binkley N, Czerwinski E, Ferrari S, Hofbauer LC, Lau E, Lewiecki EM, Miyauchi A, Zerbini CA, Milmont CE, Chen L, Maddox J, Meisner PD, Libanati C, Grauer A. Romosozumab treatment in postmenopausal women with osteoporosis. N Engl J Med. 2016 Oct 20;375(16):1532–43.
31. Ettinger B, Black DM, Mitlak BH, Knickerbocker RK, Nickelsen T, Genant HK, et al. Reduction of vertebral fracture risk in postmenopausal women with osteoporosis treated with raloxifene: results from a 3-year randomized clinical trial. Multiple outcomes of Raloxifene evaluation (MORE) investigators. JAMA. 1999 Aug 18;282(7):637–45.
32. Chesnut CH, Silverman S, Andriano K, Genant H, Gimona A, Harris S, et al. A randomized trial of nasal spray salmon calcitonin in postmenopausal women with established osteoporosis: the prevent recurrence of osteoporotic fractures study. PROOF Study Group. Am J Med. 2000 Sep;109(4):267–76.
33. Lindsay R, Gallagher JC, Kleerekoper M, Pickar JH. Bone response to treatment with lower doses of conjugated estrogens with and without medroxyprogesterone acetate in early postmenopausal women. Osteoporos Int. 2005 Apr;16(4):372–9.
34. Yong EL, Logan S. Menopausal osteoporosis: screening, prevention and treatment. Singapore Med J. 2021 Apr;62(4):159–66.
35. Neer RM, Arnaud CD, Zanchetta JR, Prince R, Gaich GA, Reginster JY, et al. Effect of parathyroid hormone (1-34) on fractures and bone mineral density in postmenopausal women with osteoporosis. N Engl J Med. 2001 May 10;344(19):1434–41.
36. Miller PD, Hattersley G, Riis BJ, Williams GC, Lau E, Russo LA, Alexandersen P, Zerbini CA, Hu MY, Harris AG, Fitzpatrick LA, Cosman F, Christiansen C, ACTIVE Study Investigators. Effect of Abaloparatide vs placebo on new vertebral fractures in postmenopausal women with osteoporosis: a randomized clinical trial. JAMA. 2016;316(7):722–33.

37. Camacho PM, Petak SM, Binkley N, Diab DL, Eldeiry LS, Farooki A, Harris ST, Hurley DL, Kelly J, Lewiecki EM, Pessah-Pollack R, McClung M, Wimalawansa SJ, Watts NB. American Association of clinical endocrinologists/American college of Endocrinology clinical practice guidelines for the diagnosis and treatment of postmenopausal osteoporosis- 2020 update *executive summary*. Endocr Pract. 2020 May;26(5):564–70.
38. Holick MF, Binkley NC, Bischoff-Ferrari HA, Gordon CM, Hanley DA, Heaney RP, et al. Evaluation, treatment, and prevention of vitamin D deficiency: an Endocrine Society clinical practice guideline. J Clin Endocrinol Metab. 2011 Jul;96(7):1911–30.
39. Griffith JF. Identifying osteoporotic vertebral fracture. Quant Imaging Med Surg. 2015 Aug;5(4):592–602.
40. Dionyssiotis Y. Management of osteoporotic vertebral fractures. Int J Gen Med. 2010 Jul 21;3:167–71.
41. Whooley MA, Kip KE, Cauley JA, Ensrud KE, Nevitt MC, Browner WS. Depression, falls, and risk of fracture in older women. Study of osteoporotic fractures research group. Arch Intern Med. 1999;159(5):484–90.
42. Li Y, Yan L, Cai S, Wang P, Zhuang H, Yu H. The prevalence and under-diagnosis of vertebral fractures on chest radiograph. BMC Musculoskelet Disord. 2018 Jul 18;19(1):235.
43. Ong T, Kantachuvesiri P, Sahota O, Gladman JRF. Characteristics and outcomes of hospitalised patients with vertebral fragility fractures: a systematic review. Age Ageing. 2018 Jan 1;47(1):17–25.
44. Waterloo S, Søgaard AJ, Ahmed LA, Damsgård E, Morseth B, Emaus N. Vertebral fractures and self-perceived health in elderly women and men in a population-based cross-sectional study: the Tromsø study 2007–08. BMC Geriatr. 2013 Sep 30;13:102.
45. Nuti R, Brandi ML, Checchia G, Di Munno O, Dominguez L, Falaschi P, et al. Guidelines for the management of osteoporosis and fragility fractures. Intern Emerg Med. 2019 Jan;14(1):85–102.
46. Old JL, Calvert M. Vertebral compression fractures in the elderly. Am Fam Physician. 2004 Jan 1;69(1):111–6.
47. Prather H, Hunt D, Watson JO, Gilula LA. Conservative care for patients with osteoporotic vertebral compression fractures. Phys Med Rehabil Clin N Am. 2007;18(3):577–91,xi.
48. McConnell CT, Wippold FJ, Ray CE, Weissman BN, Angevine PD, Fries IB, et al. ACR appropriateness criteria management of vertebral compression fractures. J Am Coll Radiol. 2014 Aug;11(8):757–63.
49. Chandra RV, Maingard J, Asadi H, Slater LA, Mazwi TL, Marcia S, et al. Vertebroplasty and Kyphoplasty for osteoporotic vertebral fractures: what are the latest data? AJNR Am J Neuroradiol. 2018 May;39(5):798–806.
50. Barr JD, Jensen ME, Hirsch JA, McGraw JK, Barr RM, Brook AL, et al. Position statement on percutaneous vertebral augmentation: a consensus statement developed by the Society of Interventional Radiology (SIR), American Association of Neurological Surgeons (AANS) and the Congress of Neurological Surgeons (CNS), American College of Radiology (ACR), American Society of Neuroradiology (ASNR), American Society of Spine Radiology (ASSR), Canadian interventional radiology Association (CIRA), and the society of NeuroInterventional surgery (SNIS). J Vasc Interv Radiol. 2014 Feb;25(2):171–81.
51. Longo UG, Loppini M, Denaro L, Maffulli N, Denaro V. Osteoporotic vertebral fractures: current concepts of conservative care. Br Med Bull. 2012 Jun;102:171–89.
52. Lyritis GP, Ioannidis GV, Karachalios T, Roidis N, Kataxaki E, Papaioannou N, et al. Analgesic effect of salmon calcitonin suppositories in patients with acute pain due to recent osteoporotic vertebral crush fractures: a prospective double-blind, randomized, placebo-controlled clinical study. Clin J Pain. 1999 Dec;15(4):284–9.

53. Esses SI, McGuire R, Jenkins J, Finkelstein J, Woodard E, Watters WC, et al. The treatment of symptomatic osteoporotic spinal compression fractures. J Am Acad Orthop Surg. 2011 Mar;19(3):176–82.
54. Sinaki M, Itoi E, Wahner HW, Wollan P, Gelzcer R, Mullan BP, et al. Stronger back muscles reduce the incidence of vertebral fractures: a prospective 10 year follow-up of postmenopausal women. Bone. 2002 Jun;30(6):836–41.
55. Röllinghoff M, Zarghooni K, Schlüter-Brust K, Sobottke R, Schlegel U, Eysel P, Delank KS. Indications and contraindications for vertebroplasty and kyphoplasty. Arch Orthop Trauma Surg. 2010 Jun;130(6):765–74.
56. Longo UG, Loppini M, Denaro L, Maffulli N, Denaro V. Conservative management of patients with an osteoporotic vertebral fracture: a review of the literature. J Bone Joint Surg Br. 2012 Feb;94(2):152–7.

Diagnostic Imaging in the Degenerative Spine Disorder

11

Shah Waliullah, Priyank Pratap, Mayank Mahendra, Santosh Kumar Sharma, and Deepak Kumar

11.1 Introduction

The aging process causes natural, progressive morphological changes in the spine but can also be influenced by genetic factors, lifestyle, and injury [1]. Aging also increases the chance of developing osteoarthritis of the spine, which frequently manifests as the earliest signs of degeneration of the intervertebral discs, vertebral bodies, ligaments, and facet joints [2, 3].

The most common degenerative spine conditions include the following:

Osteoarthritis (Spondylosis)
This condition involves the degeneration of cartilage in the facet joints and can lead to bone spurs. Symptoms often include localized pain, stiffness, and reduced range of motion.

Degenerative Disc Disease (DDD)
DDD is characterized by the breakdown of intervertebral discs, which can result in loss of disc height, disc bulging, or herniation. This condition can cause back pain, radiculopathy (pain radiating to the limbs), and spinal instability.

Spinal Stenosis
Spinal stenosis involves narrowing the spinal canal, which can compress the spinal cord and nerves. Symptoms include pain, numbness, and weakness in the limbs, and in severe cases, loss of bladder or bowel control.

S. Waliullah (✉) · P. Pratap · M. Mahendra · S. K. Sharma · D. Kumar
Department of Orthopaedic Surgery, King George's Medical University, Lucknow, India

V. Kumar, P. Mishra (eds.), *A Comprehensive Guide to Degenerative Spine Disorders*, https://doi.org/10.1007/978-981-96-9091-6_11

Spondylolisthesis

A deformity or fracture in the pars interarticularis is frequently the cause of spondylolisthesis, a disorder in which one vertebra slides forward over the one underneath it. It may result in symptoms of nerve compression and back discomfort.

Herniated Disc

A herniated disc can compress surrounding nerves when the nucleus pulposus, the disc's inner gel-like core, pushes through an annulus fibrosus rip in the outer layer. This may cause severe discomfort, weakness, and numbness.

Facet Joint Syndrome

Degeneration of the facet joints can lead to inflammation and pain, which may be localized to the affected joints or referred to other areas.

The key imaging modalities include the following:

X-Ray

It provides a clear image of the bones and is useful for identifying bone spurs, vertebral alignment issues, and advanced degenerative changes such as significant disc space narrowing and spondylolisthesis.

Magnetic Resonance Imaging (MRI)

MRI is the gold standard for evaluating soft tissues, including intervertebral discs, spinal cord, and nerves. It can detect disc herniations, spinal stenosis, and inflammation of soft tissues. MRI is particularly valuable for visualizing nerve root compression and assessing the severity of degenerative changes.

Computed Tomography (CT) Scan

CT scans are great for evaluating bone structures and offer detailed cross-sectional images of the spine. They are helpful in assessing spinal canal constriction, bone spurs, and complicated fractures.

Myelography

This technique involves injecting a contrast dye into the spinal canal followed by X-ray or CT imaging. It is beneficial for identifying spinal cord compression and nerve root impingement that may not be visible on standard imaging.

Bone Scan

A bone scan can detect areas of increased bone activity, which can indicate inflammation, infection, or malignancy. It is sometimes used to differentiate between degenerative and other pathological conditions.

Anatomy of the Spine

The spine is one of the most important parts of the body. It makes many different functions possible, including movement and balance. The spine also ensures an upright posture, protects the spinal cord, and absorbs shocks.

The spine and vertebrae are made up of various elements, all of which protect the spinal cord and communicate with the brain. These elements also provide sensations throughout the body via a complex interplay of the bones, ligaments, and muscle structures of the back and the nerves surrounding them.

11.2 Sections

The spinal column consists of 33 bones, known as vertebrae, which are divided into five sections: the cervical, thoracic, and lumbar spine sections, as well as the sacrum and coccyx bones.

The cervical section of the spine consists of the upper seven vertebrae, C1 to C7, and is connected to the base of the skull. The two uppermost vertebrae, the atlas, and the axis, form the joint that connects the skull to the spine. The cervical section is responsible for the mobility and normal function of the neck and protects the spinal cord, arteries, and nerves leading from the brain to the body.

The thoracic section of the spine is located at chest level, between the cervical and lumbar spine. The vertebrae in this section are labeled T1 to T12 and serve as an attachment for the rib cage.

The lumbar vertebrae are located between the thoracic vertebrae and the sacrum. The five lumbar vertebrae, labeled L1 to L5, are the most important weight-bearing section of the spine.

The sacrum is the section located at the base of the spine. As its five levels, S1 to S5, are fused together, it has no intervertebral discs separating the vertebrae. The pelvis is connected to the spine in the area of the sacrum.

The coccyx is located at the base of the spine and consists of four fused vertebrae (Fig. 11.1).

Spinal Curvature

Viewed from behind, the spine is normally a straight line. If it curves to one side or the other, this indicates scoliosis.

However, when viewed from the side, the spine has some normal, gradual curves. The neck and lumbar spine have a lordotic curve, which means that they curve inwards.

The thoracic spine has a kyphotic curve, which means that it curves outwards.

These curves in the spine help to maintain balance in an upright position and support the weight of the head and upper body. However, too much curvature can lead to an imbalance in the spine, causing spinal problems that can lead to pain or loss of mobility.

In order to prevent muscular strain from an upright posture, the normal adult spine is positioned above the pelvis. On the other hand, spinal abnormalities can result from changes in the posture of the spine that put strain on the muscles. It can be extremely uncomfortable or even result in disability if the spine is injured and unable to function normally.

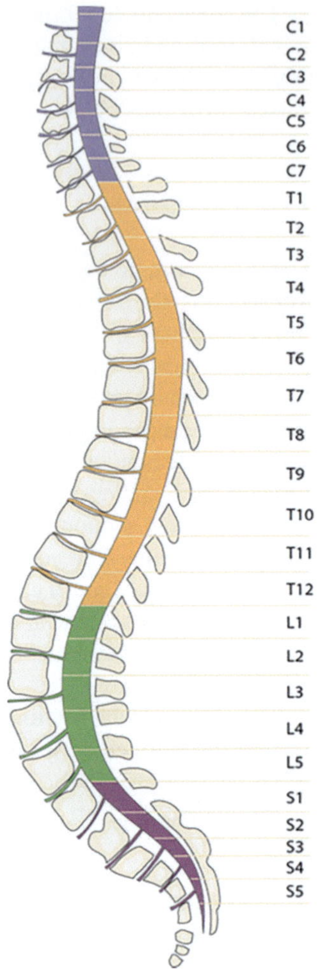

Fig. 11.1 Spinal cord anatomy (spinal cord anatomy by Servier Medical Art is licensed under creative commons attribution-non commercial 4.0 international)

Parts of the Spine

The spine consists of many parts that protect the spinal cord, facilitate movement, and support the body.

1. Spinal Cord

Nerve pathways in the spinal cord provide messages from the arms, legs, and body to the brain, including pain.

2. Nerve Roots

Information is transferred from the spinal cord to various body parts, including the arms, legs, and organs, via nerve roots.

3. Vertebral Body

The vertebrae's weight-bearing structure is the cylinder-shaped vertebral body (Fig. 11.2).

4. Lamina

The lamina's flat plates serve as the spinal canal's outside wall and shield the spinal cord.

5. Vertebral Canal

The lamina and vertebral body form the vertebral canal in which the spinal cord rests.

6. Pedicles

The lamina and the vertebral body are joined by pedicles.

7. Discs

The vertebrae are separated from one another by the intervertebral discs. Because of their sturdy, elastic construction, the spine can naturally bend and twist.

8. Articular Facet

Two adjacent vertebrae attach to the articular surfaces.

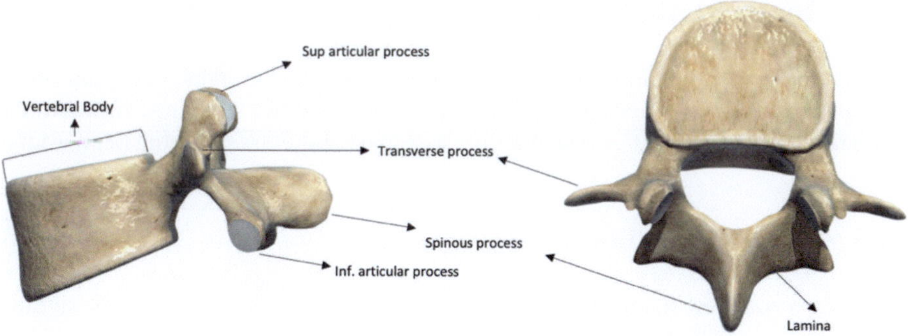

Fig. 11.2 Vertebral body anatomy

9. Spinous Process

Each vertebra has a spinous process that extends from the rear. The spinous processes are attached to the muscles and ligaments that move and stabilize the vertebrae.

10. Transverse Process

Each vertebra has two transverse processes that extend from its sides. The transverse processes, which move and support the vertebrae, are attached to muscles and ligaments.

11.3 Pathophysiology of Degenerative Spine Disease

Compression of the nerve roots in the spinal canal caused by one or more of the following factors is considered to be the cause of back pain radiating from disc disease [4].

- Disc herniation material (herniated nucleus pulposus).
  1. Different degrees of HNP are distinguished, from disc protrusion (the annulus remains intact) to extrusion (the annulus is affected, but the herniated material remains in the disc space) to sequestration-free fragments.
  2. HNP material is predictably resorbed over time, with the sequestered fragment having the highest resorption potential.
- In general, 90% of patients experience symptomatic improvement in radicular symptoms within 3 months when only non-surgical protocols are used.

11.4 Hypertrophy/Expansion of Degenerative Tissue

The ligamentum flavum and the facet joint are common sources. Like any other joint in the body, the facet joint is subject to degenerative changes. In addition, synovial enlargement and/or associated cysts can endanger neighboring nerve roots.

11.5 Imaging Modalities

Magnetic resonance imaging and basic X-rays of the spine are the two most significant and commonly performed imaging techniques.

Conventional spinal radiographs remain useful as an initial examination to identify major abnormalities, including narrowing of the disc space (associated with discopathy), osteophytes, degenerative sclerosis, scoliosis, spondylolisthesis, and other congenital spinal abnormalities. When degenerative spine disease is minimal, radiography may be the sole imaging test performed [5–7]. It is best to use magnetic resonance imaging (MRI) if a patient has neurological impairment, radicular symptoms, or chronic discomfort [8].

At the moment, additional methods are also used. Computed tomography (CT) was the primary diagnostic method for degenerative spinal disease in the 1990s, but MR has mostly surpassed CT. In addition to MR, CT is utilized, especially when bony spinal canal stenosis is progressing [9]. Conventional myelography, radiculography, and CT myelography—all of which have been virtually discontinued—all need the intrathecal administration of contrast media. CT discography and other intrusive examinations like discography can only be performed in specialized facilities. They are commonly carried out in tandem with therapeutic procedures like nucleolysis or nucleoplasty. Nuclear medicine methods such as PET/CT and bone scintigraphy are employed when it is important to differentiate between malignant lesions and degenerative spinal disease. Vascular tests (Doppler sonography, CT angiography, MR angiography) should be considered for patients exhibiting cerebellar symptoms, which may be caused by osteophytes or disc herniations pressing on the vertebral arteries) [10–12].

More recently, efforts have been made to use additional cutting-edge methods, such as functional imaging (motion), MR spectroscopy, diffusion-weighted imaging (DWI) diffusion tensor imaging (DTI), and functional magnetic resonance imaging (fMRI). Since DTI enables both qualitative and quantitative evaluation of degenerative myelopathy, it is the most promising of these methods. Since motion imaging, which offers functional evaluations of spinal structures, necessitates vertical MR equipment that is currently unavailable in the majority of MR departments, the alternative technique of axial weight-bearing imaging is more frequently utilized. Despite offering intriguing scientific insights into degenerative myelopathy, MR spectroscopy, and functional magnetic resonance imaging have not yet been used in clinical practice because of technical difficulties primarily brought on by the tiny size of the spinal cord [13, 14].

11.6 Imaging Characteristics of Particular Types of Degenerative Changes

11.6.1 Intervertebral Disc Degeneration

Degeneration of the intervertebral disc can frequently be identified by conventional radiographs that demonstrate sclerotization and osteophytes of adjacent regions of the vertebral bodies along with narrowing of the intervertebral space. These findings make it impossible to differentiate disc herniation or bulging from simple degeneration. Because it may detect early signs of degeneration, such as a diminished signal on T2 and T2*-weighted images (black disc disease) brought on by the disc's degenerative dehydration, MR is the recommended method (Fig. 11.3) [5, 6].

A symmetrical displacement of more than 180° of the disc circumference is indicative of a disc protrusion on axial magnetic resonance imaging (MRI). On the other hand, a localized displacement of the disc fragment outside of the

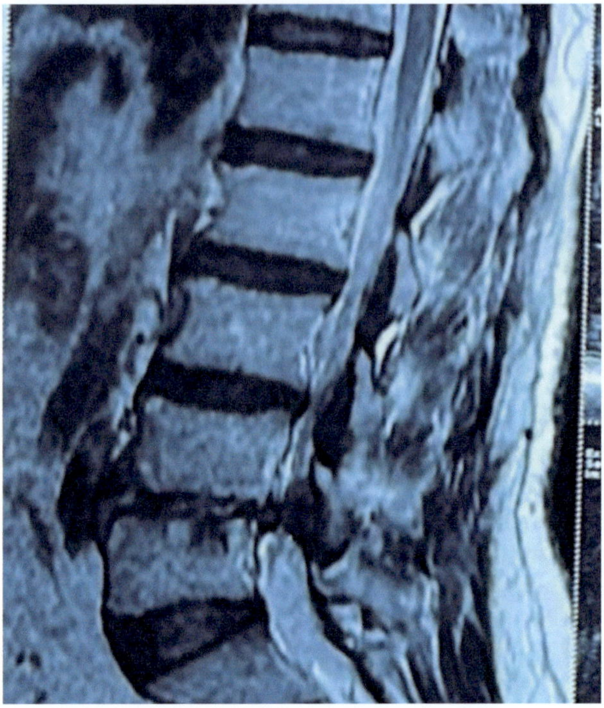

Fig. 11.3 MR, T2-weighted image, sagittal plane. The decreased signal in the L4/L5 intervertebral disc is consistent with the degenerative process. At the L4/L5 level, herniation of the degenerative disc is also visible

intervertebral region indicates a herniated disc. Several writers view disc bulging as a separate disorder from disc herniation, which is typically regarded as the initial stage, even though the majority of bulging discs are asymptomatic. On T2-weighted MR scans, high-intensity zones (HIZ) are regions of increased signal that are indicative of annulus fibrosus tears in a number of protruding discs (Fig. 11.4) [10].

There are four different kinds (stages) of herniated discs (Fig. 11.5):

1. Disc bulge.
2. Protrusion is the nucleus pulpous's localized displacement into the annulus fibrosus without full rupture.
3. Extrusion occurs when the annulus fibrosus is totally ruptured by the localized displacement of the nucleus pulposus into it.
4. The movement of an intervertebral disc fragment without any continuity with the intervertebral disc is known as the sequestration.

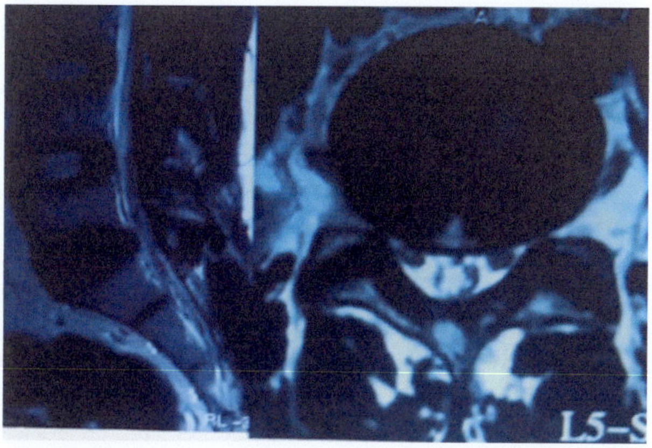

Fig. 11.4 MR, T2-weighted image, axial plane. The disc protrusion with a high-intensity zone in the posterior part probably represents an annular tear.

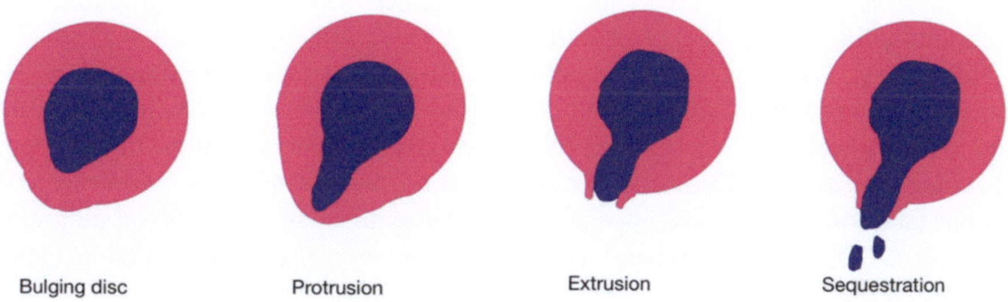

Fig. 11.5 Stages of disc prolapse

11.7 Intervertebral Disc

MR makes it possible to distinguish between different kinds of disc herniation based on their morphology and connection to the posterior longitudinal ligament. Additionally, younger, active disc herniations can be distinguished from older, non-active ones due to the partial enhancement of their inflammatory response in signal on T2-weighted and T1-weighted postcontrast imaging. However, because of fibrosis and dehydration, the latter appears black.

Magnetic resonance imaging (MR) can also easily show the relationship between a herniated disc and the surrounding spinal canal and intervertebral foramina structures, namely compression of the spinal cord and nerve roots. Each of the MR skills listed here is crucial for disc herniation diagnosis and therapy planning [5, 6, 7, 15, 16, 17].

CT can also diagnose disc bulging and disc herniation; however, most of the previously mentioned information is absent. However, when it comes to identifying particular indications of disc degeneration, such as disc calcifications and the vacuum phenomenon (a gas generated during the degenerative process), CT is more effective than MR. On CT, these alterations are observed as extremely low and high-density foci; on MR, vacuums, and calcifications are only sometimes evident as low-signal areas [10].

11.8 Vertebral Bodies Degeneration

Osteophytes and Modic lesions (types 1, 2, and 3) are the most common degenerative changes in the vertebral bodies. CT, especially MR, can assess their relationship to the spinal cord, nerve roots, intervertebral foramina, dural sac, and spinal canal, while basic X-rays can easily diagnose the latter [5, 6, 18].

Since magnetic resonance imaging (MR) can detect increased water content in the regions of the vertebral bodies adjacent to the endplates (as indicated by an increased signal on T2-weighted and fat saturation pictures and a lower signal on T1-weighted images), it is the only method that can be used to diagnose Modic type 1 lesions (aseptic spondylodiscitis). It is believed that Modic type 1 lesions, particularly those located at the L5/S1 level, are associated with radicular symptoms and persistent pain.

Modic type 2 lesions (fatty degeneration) can only be seen using magnetic resonance imaging (MRI). Increased fat content is compatible with areas of increased signal on T1-weighted images and decreased signal on fat saturation images, both of which can be seen by MRI (Fig. 11.6). In all pulse sequences, Modic type 3 lesions (sclerotic alterations) appear as hyperdense areas on conventional radiography and CT and as hypointense regions on magnetic resonance imaging (MR) [18–21].

Figure 11.6.MR.sagital plane, T1-weighted image. Multiple hyperintense areas in the numerous vertebral bodies adjacent to the intervertebral disc are consistent with Modic type-2 degenerative changes.

Erosive osteochondrosis (endplate degeneration) is a unique kind of vertebral body degeneration. It appears as abnormalities in the outlines of the endplates and can be seen on CT and conventional radiography, although MR is still the best modality. Similar to Modic changes, erosive osteochondrosis is typically accompanied by degeneration of the nearby intervertebral discs (Fig. 11.7) [6].

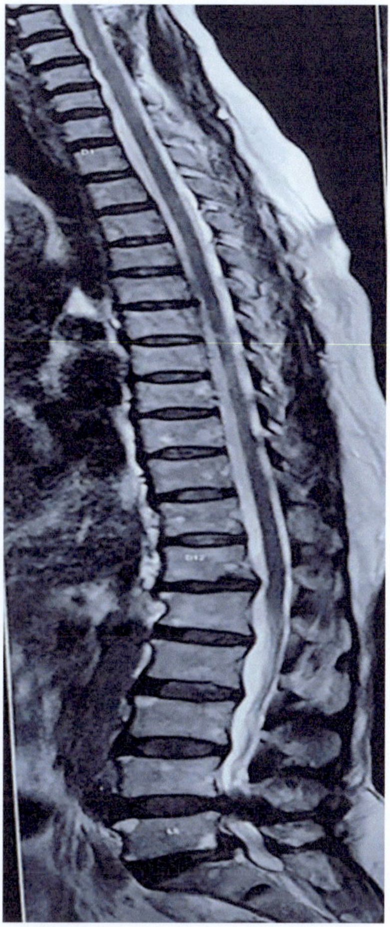

Fig. 11.6 MR, sagittal plane, T1-weighted image illustrating anterolisthesis (grade 2) of L5 on S1

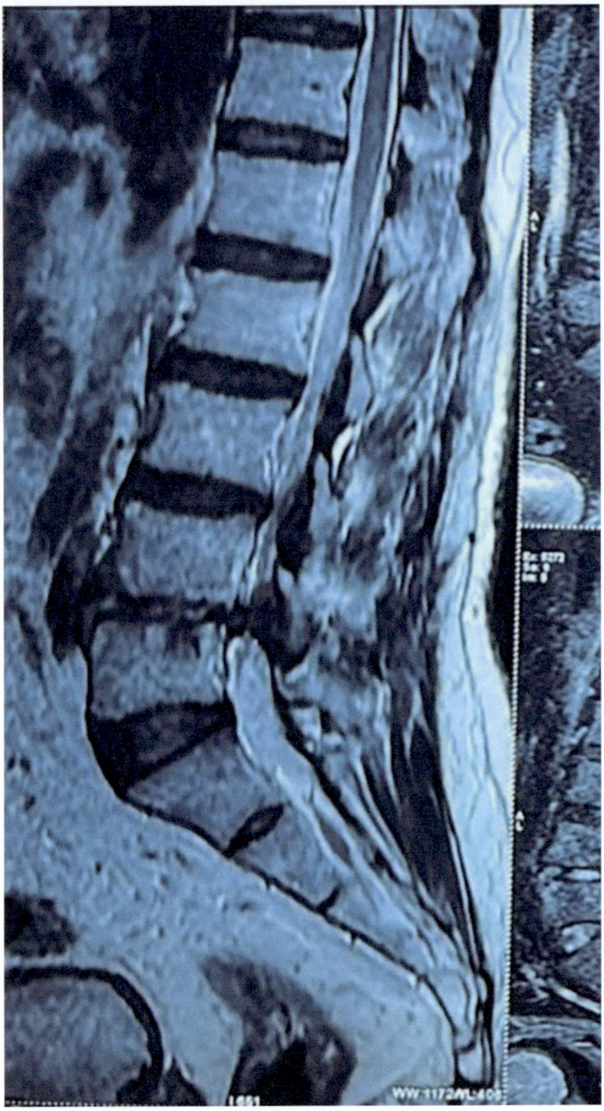

Fig. 11.7 MR, sagittal plane, T1-weighted. There are irregularities of the vertebral end plate at the L4/L5 level, with a low signal in the adjacent intervertebral disc.

11.9 Facet Joints Degeneration

Osteophytes and articular process hypertrophy are signs of facet joint degeneration. The vacuum phenomenon (gas in the joint space) and facet joint synovial cysts are far less prevalent signs. Both axial MR and CT scans make it simple to evaluate facet degeneration and its effects on the spinal canal (stenosis, compression of the dural sac) [6, 10].

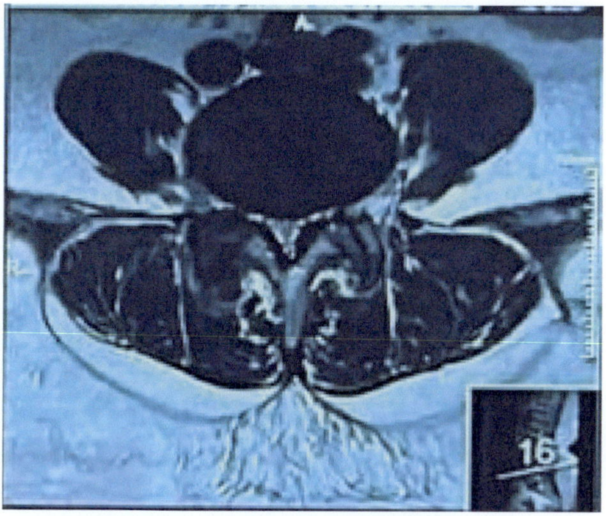

Fig. 11.8 MR, T2-weighted image, axial plane showing hypertrophied ligamentum flavum

11.10 Ligamentum Flavum Degeneration

Ligamentum flavum degeneration is typically associated with facet joint degeneration and is detected on axial MR and CT imaging as a ligament thickness of more than 4 mm (Fig. 11.8.).

11.11 Degenerative Spondylolisthesis

Spine radiography and CT easily detect degenerative spondylolisthesis; nevertheless, MR offers the most accurate assessment of its effect on spinal canal structures (Fig. 11.9). Nevertheless, X-rays play a crucial role, especially Flexion and extension views, which are advised to assess instability (Fig. 11.10). Standing X-rays provide a more accurate assessment of instability in comparison to lying down posture.

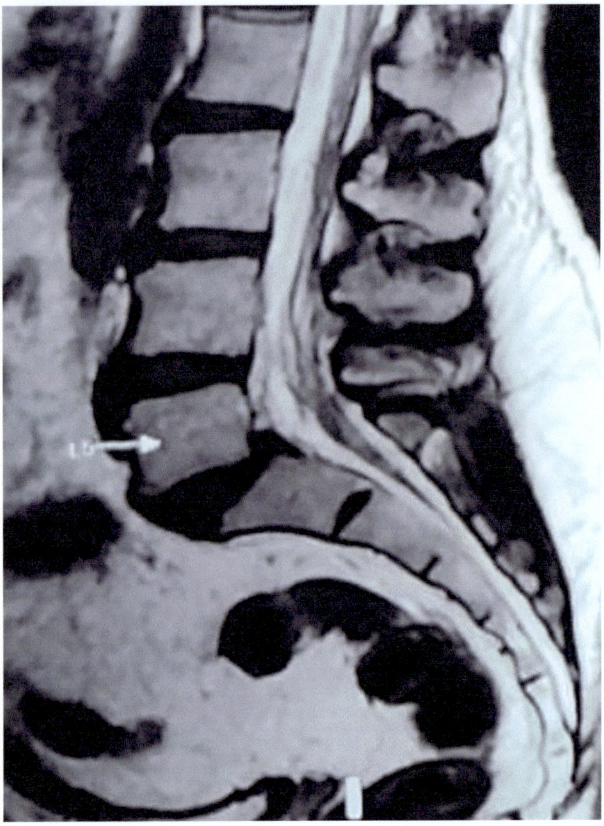

Fig. 11.9 MR, sagittal plane, T1-weighted. Anterolisthesis of L5 vertebrae over S1 vertebrae intervertebral disc.

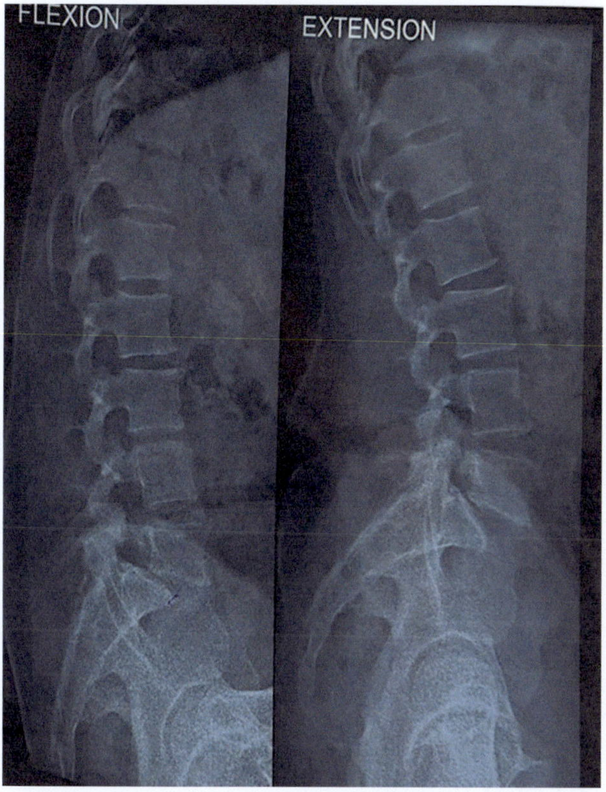

Fig. 11.10 X-ray Lumbo sacral spine lateral view in Flexion and Extension showing forward displacement of L5 vertebrae over S1. Displacement is more marked in the Flexion view, depicting instability

11.12 Spinal Canal Stenosis

Spinal canal stenosis may be associated with any of the degenerative alterations of the disco-vertebral unit, including disc bulging or herniation, osteophytes of the posterior borders of the vertebral bodies, facet joint hypertrophy, osteophytes, and/or ligamentum flavum thickening (Fig. 11.11).

There are two types of stenosis: central spinal stenosis, which affects the middle part of the spinal canal, and lateral spinal canal stenosis, which affects the lateral recesses of the spinal canal and the intervertebral foramina.

Central canal stenosis is easily visible on both MR and CT axial images, although lateral stenosis is best evaluated on parasagittal MR imaging. Compression of the spinal canal's components is usually the basis for visual evaluation of stenosis. Another method is to measure the canal; for instance, if the canal's sagittal diameter is less than 12 m, central spinal stenosis in the lumbar region is detected [5–7, 15, 22].

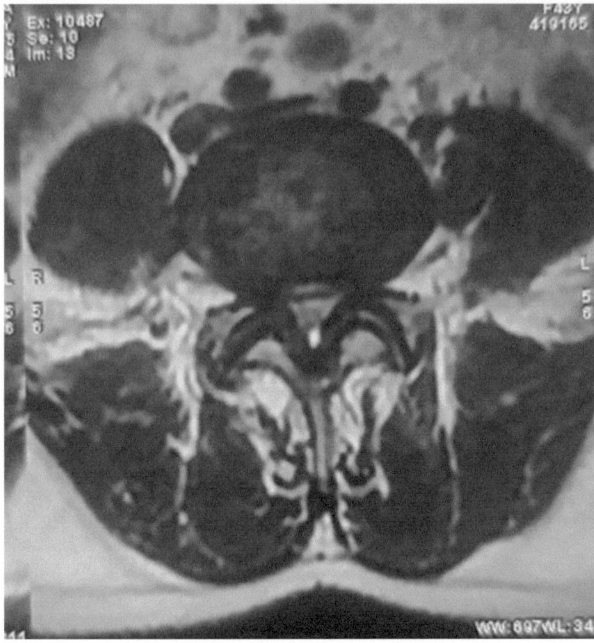

Fig. 11.11 MR, T2-weighted image, axial plane. Marked spinal stenosis with compression of the dural sac by a bulging disc, facet joint degenerative changes and thickened ligamentum flavum

11.13 Spinal Cord Changes

During the degenerative phase, the spinal cord alters as a result of osteophytes or disc herniation causing chronic compression. Magnetic resonance imaging (MR), which displays foci of enhanced signals at the compression level on T2-weighted images, is the only imaging modality that can detect these changes (Fig. 11.12).

The spinal cord is frequently found to be unchanged despite clinical indications of myelopathy. The identification of variations in fractional anisotropy (FA) at the compression level in spinal cords that seem normal has demonstrated the usefulness of diffusion tensor imaging in these circumstances [23–25].

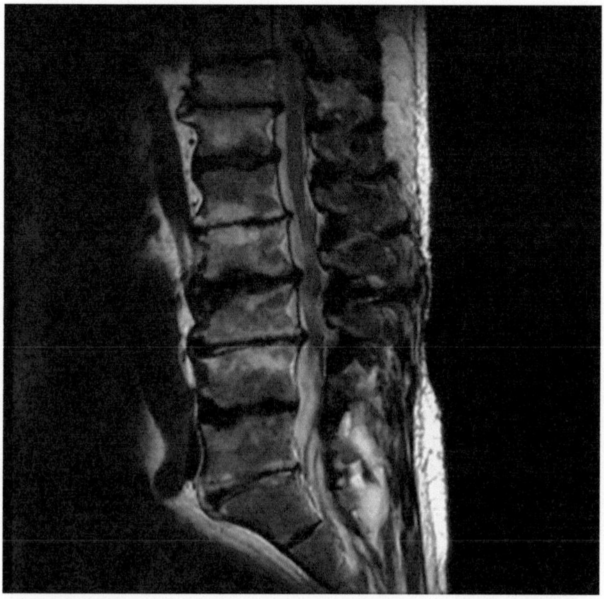

Fig. 11.12 MR, T2-weighted image, saggital plane. Marked spinal stenosis with compression of the dural sac by a bulging disc at multiple levels with area of altered signals

References

1. Brinjikji W, Luetmer PH, Comstock B, et al. Systematic literature review of imaging features of spinal degeneration in asymptomatic populations. AJNR Am J Neuroradiol. 2015;36:811–6. [PMC free article] [PubMed] [Google Scholar]
2. Kushchayev SV, Glushko T, Jarraya M, et al. ABCs of the degenerative spine. Insights Imaging. 2018;9:253–74. [PMC free article] [PubMed] [Google Scholar]
3. Sasiadek MJ, Bladowska J. Imaging of degenerative spine disease–the state of the art. Adv Clin Exp Med. 2012;21:133–42. [PubMed] [Google Scholar]
4. Donnally CJ III, Hanna A, Varacallo M. Lumbar degenerative disk disease. In: StatPearls [Internet]. Treasure Island: StatPearls Publishing; 2024. Available from: https://www.ncbi.nlm.nih.gov/books/NBK448134/.
5. Gallucci M, Puglielli E, Splendiani A, Pistoia F, Spacca G. Degenerative disorders of the spine. Eur Radiol. 2005;15:591–8.
6. Sąsiadek M, Konopka M. Choroby kręgosłupa. In: Walecki J, editor. Polska Fundacja Upowszechniania Nauki. Wydział Nauk Medycznych PAN, Warszawa Postępy neuroradiologii: wydanie multimedialne; 2007. p. 397–428.
7. Sąsiadek M, Hendrich B. Diagnostyka obrazowa kręgosłupa z uwzględnieniem nowych technik obrazowania. Pol Przegl Neurol. 2010;5(1):38–9.
8. Wojtek P, Ziółko E, Adamczyk T, Trejtowicz D, Liszka J, Kwiatkowska A, Brodziak A. Results of magnetic resonance imaging of the vertebral column in patients with myelodysplastic syndrome. Pol J Radiol. 2009;74(2):44–7.
9. Bartynski WS, Lin L. Lumbar root compression in the lateral recess: MR imaging, conventional myelography, and CT myelography comparison with surgical confirmation. AJNR Am J Neuroradiol. 2003;24(3):348–60.

10. Sąsiadek M. Degenerative conditions of the spine. In: Baert AL, editor. Encyclopedia of diagnostic imaging. Berlin: Springer; 2008. p. 611–5. ISBN 978-3-540-35278-5 (Print); 978-3-540-35280-8 (Online).
11. Reul J, Gievers B, Weis J, et al. Assessment of the narrow cervical spinal canal: prospective comparison of MRI, myelography and CT-myelography. Neuroradiology. 1995;37:187.
12. Hartel M, Kluczewska E, Simka M, Ludyga T, Kostecki J, Zaniewski M. Magnetic resonance venography of chronic cerebrospinal venous insufficiency in patients with associated multiple sclerosis. Pol J Radiol. 2011;76(1):59–62.
13. Kubas B, Łebkowski W, Łebkowska U, Kułak W, Tarasów E, Walecki J. Proton MR spectroscopy in mild traumatic brain injury. Pol J Radiol. 2010;75(4):7–10.
14. Tarasów E, Kochanowicz J, Brzozowska J, Mariak Z, Walecki J. MR spectroscopy in patients after surgical clipping and endovascular embolization of intracranial aneurysms. Pol J Radiol. 2010;75(4):24–9.
15. Sozański T, Sokolska V, Gomułkiewicz M, Magdalan J, Trocha M, Bladowska J, Merwid-Ląd A. Filmless radiology–digital radiography systems. Adv Clin Exp Med. 2009;18:641–8.
16. Hendrich B, Bladowska J, Sąsiadek M. Znaczenie badań obrazowych w diagnostyce nieurazowych zespołów bólowych kręgosłupa. Pol Przegl Neurol. 2010;6(2):92–100.
17. Kraemer J, Koester O. MRI of the lumbar spine. New York: Georg Thieme Verlag, Stuttgart; 2003.
18. Vroomen PCAJ, Wilmink JT. de Krom MCTFM: prognostic value of MRI findings in sciatica. Neuroradiology. 2002;44:59–63.
19. Sąsiadek M, Bladowska J. Hyperintense vertebral lesions. Neuroradiology. 2011;53(Suppl 1):S169–74.
20. Zhang YH, Zhao CQ, Jiang LS. Modic changes: a systematic review of the literature. Eur Spine J. 2008;17:1289–99.
21. Fayad F, Lefevre-Colau MM, Drape JL. Reliability of a modified Modic classification of bone marrow changes in lumbar spine MRI. Joint Bone Spine. 2009;76:286–9.
22. Vitzthum HE, Kaech DL. Modic changes in patients with degenerative diseases of the lumbar spine. ArgoSpine J. 2009;21:57–61.
23. Sipola P, Leinonen V, Niemeläinen R, Aalto T, Vanninen R, Manninen H, Airaksinen O, Battié MC. Visual and quantitative assessment of lateral lumbar spinal canal stenosis with magnetic resonance imaging. Acta Radiol. 2011;52(9):1024–31.
24. Sąsiadek M, Szewczyk P. Imaging of the spine: new possibilities and its role in planning and monitoring therapy. Pol J Radiol. 2009;74:52–8.
25. Vargas MI, Delavelle J, Jlassi H, et al. Clinical application of diffusion tensor tractography of the spinal cord. Neuroradiology. 2008;50:25–9.

Symptoms and Clinical Presentation in Degenerative Spine Disorders

12

Abhinav Bhute, Sameer Nagpal, and Siddharth Aiyer

12.1 Introduction

Degenerative spine disorders represent a broad range of conditions resulting from the gradual wear of spinal structures, including intervertebral discs, facet joints, ligaments, and vertebrae. This decline, which may involve the cervical, thoracic, and lumbar regions, presents unique clinical symptoms according to the affected area. As degeneration advances, individuals commonly experience pain, restricted mobility, and neurological complications. Recognizing the diverse clinical presentations across spinal regions is critical for accurate diagnosis and tailored management strategies.

In the cervical spine, degenerative changes, often categorized as cervical spondylosis, involve a spectrum of alterations impacting the neck area. Diagnosing these cervical disorders necessitates a comprehensive, exclusionary approach to avoid misdiagnosing other serious conditions like vascular events or demyelinating diseases. Symptoms can vary widely, from localized stiffness and pain to neurological deficits when neural involvement occurs. Effective management of cervical degeneration hinges on identifying the affected area and understanding the scope of the condition through thorough patient history and clinical evaluation.

Thoracic, or dorsal, spine degeneration is comparatively rare due to the stabilizing role of the rib cage. When degeneration in this region does occur, it often affects structures such as intervertebral discs, facet joints, and vertebral bodies. Factors such as aging and osteoporosis further contribute to degeneration in the thoracic spine, particularly among postmenopausal women, who are at increased risk of compression fractures. These fractures can exacerbate degenerative processes, leading to kyphosis, chronic pain, and decreased mobility, which substantially affect quality of life.

A. Bhute · S. Nagpal · S. Aiyer (✉)
Sancheti Institute for Orthopaedics and Rehabilitation, Pune, India

V. Kumar, P. Mishra (eds.), *A Comprehensive Guide to Degenerative Spine Disorders*, https://doi.org/10.1007/978-981-96-9091-6_12

Due to its load-bearing function, the lumbar spine is especially prone to degenerative changes. Symptoms commonly include lower back pain, radiating leg pain, and neurological impairments, such as motor weakness and sensory disturbances, which restrict mobility and function. Chronic lumbar pain and functional limitations impact not only physical abilities but also impose considerable psychosocial and economic strain. Early diagnosis and management of lumbar degeneration are crucial to prevent progression and enhance outcomes.

12.2 Cervical Degenerative Spinal Disorders

12.2.1 Axial Neck Pain and Cervical Radiculopathy

The degenerative cervical disc often starts to lose its elasticity secondary to radial annular tears, loss of hydration, and cartilage degeneration. Facet joints and uncovertebral joints also undergo degenerative changes due to altered weight bearing of the spinal column in the form of synovitis and micro-tears in articular cartilage and capsule. Biomechanical models have shown that, in a healthy spine 80 percent of compressive load is transferred through intervertebral discs and the remaining 20 percent is transferred through the facets. The cervical spine does have the most variable facet orientation in the spinal column C2-C3 and C5-C6 facets are most susceptible to degeneration due to their high mobility [39, 42].

But with progressive degeneration of the disc, the facet joints are loaded for up to 70% of loads leading to degenerative changes in the facet in the form of articular damage and capsular tears resulting in loss of joint space, hypertrophy, and synovitis. Nociceptors, free and encapsulated substance-P-containing nerves in the synovial membrane and the subchondral bone, when stimulated generate the sensation of pain [9].

In the cervical spine, facets of C3-T1 do have a similar dual nerve supply pattern as the lumbar spine. The medial branch curves around the articular pillar of the cervical facet and supplies the facet articular at the same level and the level below. These nerves when stimulated have a unilateral pain distribution not extending beyond shoulder level. However, the rami of C2 and C3 have major branches, namely, greater occipital, lesser occipital, and third occipital nerve. When involved, these are the major causes of occipital headaches. This pain is usually sharp, and throbbing in nature with episodic exacerbation. It starts from the base of the skull and radiates upward along the posterior and lateral aspect of the scalp up to the back of the eyes.

Acute disc herniations are common during this dysfunction stage as the biomechanical strength of the annulus becomes compromised and the microtears, when subjected to the sudden excessive load microtears might extend as complete tears with protrusion or herniation of nucleus pulposus into the spinal canal. The clinical presentation of cervical disc herniation is a sudden onset of axial neck pain with ipsilateral upper extremity pain and paraesthesia in the affected dermatome. It can be associated with weakness.

Axial neck pain is generated via the activation of nociceptors in the PLL and posterior annulus supplied with sinu-vertebral or recurrent meningeal nerves. Radicular symptoms are associated with the mechanical compression of the nerve root during its course from the canal to the outer aspect of the foramen. Clinically the arm pain is invariably present in cases of cervical radiculopathy with sensory deficits being the second most common clinical sign and symptom. Other clinical features associated with radiculopathy are reflex deficit, motor deficit, axial neck pain, and periscapular and anterior chest pain in the order of decreasing association.

Differentiating radiculopathy from mononeuropathy requires a thorough neurological examination. The mononeuropathy does have motor and sensory involvement depending upon the level of entrapment. However, radiculopathy has a very uniform involvement of sensory, motor, and reflex involvement with the presence of nerve tension signs [41]. Nerve root tension signs are provocative tests that cause replication of symptoms after performing certain manoeuvrers which further compromise the area of affected intervertebral foramen thereby confirming the pathology [22].

12.2.2 Cervical Myelopathy

Cervical myelopathy results from the compression of the spinal cord in the spinal canal. The most common cause of cervical myelopathy is degenerative cervical myelopathy which includes a range of static changes such as varying degrees of disc herniations, ligamentous hypertrophy or ossification, facet hypertrophy, and cord dysfunction at multiple levels. Gradually the micro instability develops leading to facet subluxation facet cysts and osteophyte formation at end plates which further compress the spinal cord. Myelopathy can occur secondary to a dynamic cord compression when the sagittal diameter is in extreme flexion/extension when there is angular instability of >11 degrees or translation of >3.5 mm. Repeated compression of the cord causes ischemia and cell membrane permeability dysfunction leading to apoptosis of oligodendrocytes and therefore myelopathy. Anterior horn cells are most sensitive to these changes [13].

Soft cervical disc herniations account for almost 20–25% percent of cervical myelopathy. Central disc herniation compromising >30 percent of the cervical canal cross-sectional area is more likely to cause myelopathy. Patients with primary canal stenosis, i.e., Torg-Pavlov ratio < 0.8 are most susceptible to myelopathy secondary to cervical disc herniation.

Bajwa et al. reported that patients having a primary bony canal stenosis have a higher incidence of myelopathy even in the absence of major compressive elements as the sagittal diameter in the sub-axial spine is <13 mm in primary canal stenosis compared to 18 mm in a control population [3]. Unlike lumbar degenerative disorders, cervical degenerative myelopathy rarely improves without an intervention. The natural history of this disease shows a gradual progression of symptoms. Duration of compression and degree of compression have a negative impact on the prognosis.

Men contribute to 70% of the affected population and present in the fifth to seventh decade of life with varying degrees of myelopathy and diverse symptoms. The most common presentation is the paraesthesia of non-dermatomal pattern, wasting of the intrinsic muscle of the hand, and loss of fine motor skills in the upper extremity (Fig. 12.1). Pain may be an accompanying complaint in some patients due to degenerative cervical spine.

An examination should include a comprehensive assessment of power grading in all 4 limbs, especially in the intrinsic muscles of the hand. An increase in tone and hyperreflexia are other consistent features of cervical myelopathy. Pyramidal signs associated with myelopathy include hyperreflexia, Hoffman's sign, Babinski sign, and ankle clonus. These signs have a utility in early diagnosis of myelopathy when the patient has apparently no complaints. Hyperreflexia, Hoffmann, Babinski, and clonus are the most sensitive tests for myelopathy in order of maximum to minimum sensitivity. Therefore patellar tendon reflex and Hoffman test can be used as screening tests for myelopathy [8].

Vibration and proprioception are most frequently involved in cervical myelopathy. Patterns of sensory involvement can predict and localize the level of lesion. The involvement of sensations is often the most reliable for the localization of the level of maximum involvement among the other clinical features such as motor weakness and reflexes [20].

Bowel and bladder involvement is usually late and relatively less frequent in compressive cervical myelopathy. Misawa et al. reported that 28% of all individuals with a urinary disturbance with cervical myelopathy had confirmation of neurological involvement of the bladder upon urodynamic studies [32].

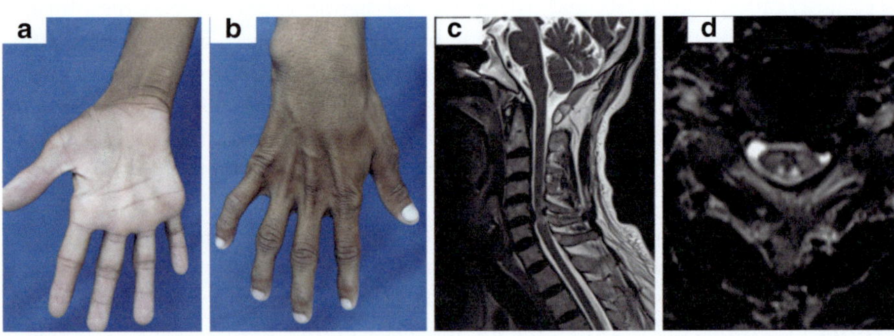

Fig. 12.1 A 45-year-old male. (**a**) Clinical photo showing palmar aspect wasting noted on the thenar and hypothenar musculature (**b**) Wasting of the dorsal interossei muscles. (**c**) MRI T2-weighted sagittal section showing a C56 level disc extrusion and canal stenosis with cord edema resulting in a clinical presentation of cervical myelopathy. (**d**) Axial T2-weighted cuts at the C5–6 level showing the cord signal changes in the form of hyperintense signal

12.2.3 Gait Impairment in Cervical Myelopathy

Gait impairment is the most important clinical predictor of myelopathy. Gait analysis studies have shown hyper-extension of the knee in the stance phase and loss of ankle plantar flexion in the swing phase. An overall increase in the stance phase is observed with the shortening of the single-level stance phase. There is a shortening of stride length and a widening of steps to balance the body [31]. Patients often have difficulty in maintaining balance, especially during climbing steps. This gait instability increases in the evening as the visual compensation starts to deteriorate with low light resulting in frequent falls and loss of confidence in walking. This often makes patients wheelchair-bound. Loss of fine motor skills and dexterity secondary to loss of proprioception, intrinsic muscle weakness, and spasticity results in an inability to perform buttoning and unbuttoning of a shirt, shaving, combing, writing, driving, and maintaining hygiene.

12.2.4 Impact on Quality of Life and Morbidity

The impact of cervical spondylotic myelopathy on quality of life is far greater compared to other chronic illnesses such as diabetes, chronic lung disease, hypertension, and cancer. Inability to ambulate, loss of hand coordination, and inability to write are the major contributors to the impact of myelopathy on quality of life.

Patients with cervical degeneration causing myelopathy are eight fold more likely to suffer mortality and 1.8 times more likely to face adverse events following surgical intervention compared to patients with clinically significant cervical degeneration without myelopathy [30]. The incidence of morbid psychiatric illnesses such as anxiety and depression is 6–8 times higher in patients with severe myelopathy.

12.2.5 Differential Diagnosis

A few conditions which can present as a differential diagnosis for degenerative cervical myelopathy include amyotrophic lateral sclerosis which is the most prevalent motor neuron disease. One can differentiate between these two by assessing the involvement of the sensory system which is invariably spared in motor neuron disease. Another organic condition that might present as a differential is multiple sclerosis which does have cranial nerve involvement and visual dysfunction. Any space-occupying lesion in the brain might present with focal, generalized neurological deficit with headaches. One can differentiate such pathology by thoroughly examining the cranial nerves, and assessing the consciousness level and lateralizing features.

Weakness and paraesthesia can also be the presenting feature of peripheral entrapments but there will be an absence of upper motor neuron involvement and lack of axial neck pain. Vitamin B12 deficiency can lead to subacute combined degeneration of the cord, presenting with spastic paraparesis, positive Romberg sign and gait instability. Differentiating factors include the presence of glossitis, cognitive involvement, and signs of anemia secondary to vitamin B12 deficiency [26].

It is very common to encounter patients with tandem cervical and lumbar canal stenosis. They may have features of mixed upper and lower motor neuron lesions, intermittent claudication, and complex gait disturbances. This scenario becomes a diagnostic dilemma [46] [48].

12.2.6 Degenerative Atlanto-Axial Disorders

Studies suggest that the craniovertebral junction is less amenable to degeneration than the atlanto-axial and the sub-axial spine. The atlanto-occipital joint is among the most stable joints of the human skeleton and it is rare to find cases of instability or degeneration of this joint in the absence of a high-energy trauma.

Degenerative atlantoaxial joint is a rare disorder and is less common compared to atlantoaxial instability occurring secondarily to a traumatic injury, inflammatory process, or congenital occurrence such as os-odontoideum [25].

Clinically, the patients have continuous unilateral suboccipital pain mimicking a headache. This pain does increase on flexion-extension, lateral bending, and especially on rotary movements.

12.3 Dorsal Spine Degenerative Disorders

12.3.1 Axial Thoracic Pain

A common early manifestation of dorsal degenerative spine conditions is axial thoracic pain. This pain is typically localized to the mid-back area and is often described by patients as dull, aching, or deep. It is usually exacerbated by activities that involve thoracic movement, such as twisting, bending, or lifting, and can be relieved by rest. Axial thoracic pain often arises due to degenerative changes in the intervertebral discs, which lose their hydration and elasticity over time. These changes decrease the disc's biomechanical integrity increasing mechanical stress on surrounding structures [12].

The facet joints, which provide stability and allow for controlled movements between the vertebrae, also undergo degenerative changes. Cartilage loss, osteophyte formation, and inflammation in the facet joints contribute significantly to localized pain. The richly innervated nature of these joints makes them a potent source of discomfort when they degenerate. Additionally, the degeneration of the thoracic discs can cause vertebral endplate changes, further contributing to pain as the nerve endings in the endplates become sensitized to mechanical stress [21].

Muscle spasms in the paraspinal muscles frequently accompany axial thoracic pain. These spasms occur as a protective response to the instability caused by disc and joint degeneration. The chronic nature of these muscle spasms can lead to persistent pain and stiffness, further limiting the patient's range of motion. The pain from these spasms may radiate to adjacent areas, such as the shoulders or upper abdomen, adding complexity to the clinical presentation [14].

12.3.2 Radicular Pain or Girdle Pain

Although less common than in the lumbar spine, radicular pain can occur in thoracic degenerative conditions due to nerve root compression. The thoracic spinal nerves, which emerge between the vertebrae and run along the ribs, can be compressed by herniated discs or osteophytes, leading to radicular symptoms. Radicular pain is typically described as sharp, shooting, or electric-like and follows the path of the affected nerve. The specific distribution of the pain depends on the level of the nerve root involved, manifesting as pain radiating around the rib cage or along the upper abdomen.

Thoracic disc herniations can be categorized into four types based on their location:

1. *Central Herniations:* These are most prone to causing spinal cord compression, leading to myelopathic symptoms such as increased muscle tone, hyperreflexia, abnormal gait, and potential urinary or bowel incontinence.
2. *Centrolateral Herniations:* These may result in ipsilateral muscle weakness combined with contralateral pain or sensory disturbances, resembling Brown-Séquard syndrome.
3. *Lateral Herniations:* Primarily cause radicular pain by compressing spinal nerves as they exit the intervertebral foramen, with pain radiating along the affected nerve's dermatome [12].

For example, compression at the T4–T5 level may cause pain that radiates around the chest, mimicking conditions like intercostal neuralgia or even cardiac pain. Lower thoracic nerve root compression can result in pain that wraps around the abdomen, leading to symptoms that could be confused with gastrointestinal conditions. Patients with radicular pain often report increased discomfort with activities that increase intrathoracic pressure, such as coughing, sneezing, or straining during bowel movements. This can help differentiate radicular pain from other types of thoracic pain. Persistent nerve compression can result in chronic neuropathic pain, which is more challenging to treat and can significantly impact a patient's quality of life [47].

12.3.3 Thoracic Myelopathy

Myelopathy is a critical and potentially disabling feature of advanced dorsal degenerative spine conditions. It arises when there is compression of the spinal cord within the thoracic region, often due to central canal stenosis. Thoracic myelopathy is of particular concern because the thoracic spine houses a portion of the spinal cord that controls the motor and sensory functions of the lower body. Unlike lumbar stenosis, which primarily affects nerve roots, thoracic stenosis can directly impact the spinal cord, leading to widespread neurological deficits.

Patients with thoracic myelopathy may present with a range of symptoms, including motor weakness, spasticity, and sensory changes in the lower extremities. These motor symptoms often manifest as difficulty walking, a sense of heaviness or stiffness in the legs, and unsteady gait. Spasticity can cause tightness in the muscles, making movements jerky and uncoordinated (Fig. 12.2). Sensory disturbances, such as numbness, tingling, or a "band-like" sensation around the chest or abdomen, are also common.

A hallmark of myelopathy is hyperreflexia, which reflects the involvement of upper motor neurons. This can be assessed through clinical tests such as the plantar reflex and the presence of a Babinski sign. In severe cases, patients may develop bladder or bowel dysfunction, indicating significant spinal cord involvement. Thoracic myelopathy is a progressive condition, and without timely surgical intervention, the neurological deficits can become permanent. Therefore, early recognition and appropriate imaging, such as MRI, are essential for identifying the extent of spinal cord compression and planning the appropriate intervention [2, 43, 44].

12.3.4 Postural Changes and Deformity

Degenerative changes in the thoracic spine often lead to progressive postural changes, most notably increasing thoracic kyphosis. This condition, commonly known as hyperkyphosis, is characterized by an exaggerated forward curvature of the upper spine. As the intervertebral discs lose height and the vertebral bodies develop wedge-shaped deformities due to osteoporotic changes, the natural curve of the thoracic spine becomes more pronounced. This alteration in spinal alignment

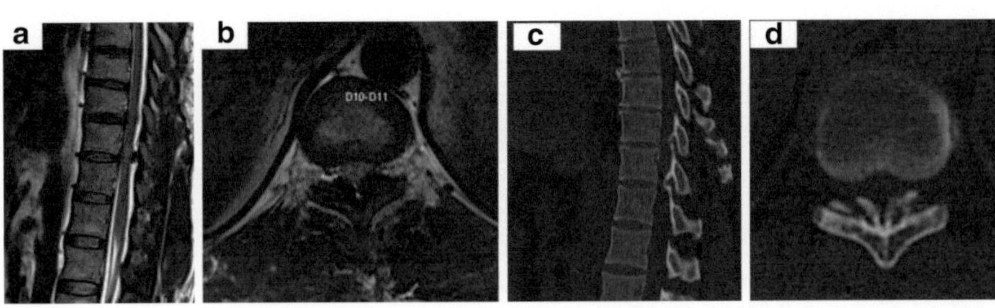

Fig. 12.2 (**a**, **b**) T2 weighted sagittal and axial section of thoracolumbar MRI showing an ossified and hypertrophied ligamentum flavum at T10-T11 with spinal cord compression and hyperintense signal seen in the cord. The patient presented with unsteady gait, hyperreflexia, spasticity and myelopathy features. (**c**, **d**) CT scan showing that the flavum hypertrophy is accompanied with significant calcification

shifts the body's center of gravity forward, making it difficult for patients to maintain an upright posture.

Hyperkyphosis can lead to a range of secondary complications, including back pain, reduced lung capacity, and impaired sagittal balance. The increased curvature compresses the thoracic cavity, limiting the expansion of the lungs during respiration. This reduction in pulmonary function can result in symptoms such as shortness of breath, particularly during physical exertion. Patients with severe kyphosis may also experience gastrointestinal symptoms due to the pressure exerted on abdominal organs, further complicating their clinical picture.

The forward-leaning posture associated with kyphosis places additional stress on the lower back and the muscles of the upper back and shoulders. This can lead to chronic muscular pain and fatigue, as the muscles work overtime to support the altered posture. Over time, patients may develop compensatory changes in their lumbar and cervical spine to accommodate the shift in posture, which can lead to further degenerative changes in these regions. The progressive nature of kyphosis makes early detection and intervention, including physical therapy and appropriate bracing, crucial to preventing further deterioration [6, 23].

12.4 Lumbar Degenerative Spine Disorders

12.4.1 Axial Low Back Pain

Low back pain (LBP) is among the most prevalent health issues globally and is often one of the earliest symptoms of lumbar spine degeneration. Approximately 70–85% of individuals experience LBP at some point during their lives. Globally, LBP is the primary cause of activity limitation for individuals under 45 years of age. It also ranks as the second most common reason for physician visits and the third leading cause of surgical interventions which suggests a significant economic impact of LBP on individuals and society.

Chronic low back pain (CLBP), defined as pain persisting beyond 7–12 weeks or the expected healing period, often becomes a recurring issue, substantially affecting individuals over extended periods. LBP was the leading cause of work-related absenteeism, accounting for 11–19% of sick days, and globally, LBP is a leading cause of long-term disability in many developed countries [1].

Axial or localized low back pain is often one of the initial indicators of lumbar spine degeneration. This type of pain frequently serves as one of the earliest clinical signs of lumbar spine degeneration [19]. The pain is largely attributed to the degeneration of intervertebral discs and facet joints, which are essential to the spine's mechanical support. Over time, the intervertebral discs undergo degenerative alterations, losing hydration, elasticity, and their inherent biomechanical function. This results in a diminished ability of the spine to distribute mechanical loads evenly, which increases pressure on surrounding structures. This stress is particularly concentrated on adjacent vertebrae, facet joints, and ligaments, often intensifying the pain. The facet joints themselves may also degenerate, with changes such as cartilage wear and osteophyte formation, leading to inflammation, stiffness, and localized discomfort.

In addition to the degeneration of discs and joints, muscle spasms frequently develop as a compensatory response to the instability caused by these degenerative changes. The paraspinal muscles, which support the spine, can become overworked in their efforts to stabilize the affected area, leading to painful spasms. Ligamentous strain, particularly in the ligaments surrounding the spine that provide support and limit excessive movement, can contribute to pain when these structures are overstretched or injured as a result of the degenerative process. Mechanical back pain may also result from spinal instability that develops with degenerative conditions such as disc collapse, facet subluxations, facet effusions, and dynamic translation of degenerative spondylolisthesis.

Although axial low back pain may worsen with activity, many patients report relief through rest or when adopting positions that reduce mechanical stress on the lumbar spine. However, the pain may become chronic and persistent as degeneration progresses. Addressing this pain requires a thorough understanding of its multifactorial causes, which include not only disc and facet joint pathology but also the involvement of muscular and ligamentous factors [1, 7, 51].

12.4.2 Lumbar Radiculopathy

Radicular pain or radiculopathy is typically a result of compression or irritation of the spinal nerve roots, often arising from degenerative changes such as disc herniation, foraminal narrowing, or osteophyte formation. Disc herniation can be triggered by an acute injury or the gradual degeneration of the disc, while spondylosis narrows the spinal canal through degenerative changes, including osteophyte formation. Prolonged nerve compression can lead to ischemia, inflammation, and edema, further contributing to nerve root damage. The L4-L5 and L5-S1 levels are the most commonly affected, with approximately 90% of compressive lumbosacral radiculopathies occurring at these levels [4].

When the lumbar spine is involved, the pain—commonly referred to as sciatica—radiates along the affected nerve root. The patient may present with a typical sciatic list due to the nerve root compression (Fig. 12.3). Each lumbar nerve root from L2 to S1 presents with distinct clinical signs, which include myotomal weakness or dermatomal sensory loss are crucial for accurate diagnosis and treatment (Fig. 12.4) [45].

L2 Nerve Root Compression Symptoms manifest as pain that radiates to the anterior thigh and groin, often accompanied by sensory disturbances such as numbness or tingling in these regions. Patients may also experience weakness in hip flexion due to the involvement of the iliopsoas muscle. Under normal conditions, the L2 nerve root plays a pivotal role in hip flexion, which is necessary for movements like lifting the thigh while walking or climbing stairs. Compression of this nerve root impairs these activities, resulting in notable functional limitations [49].

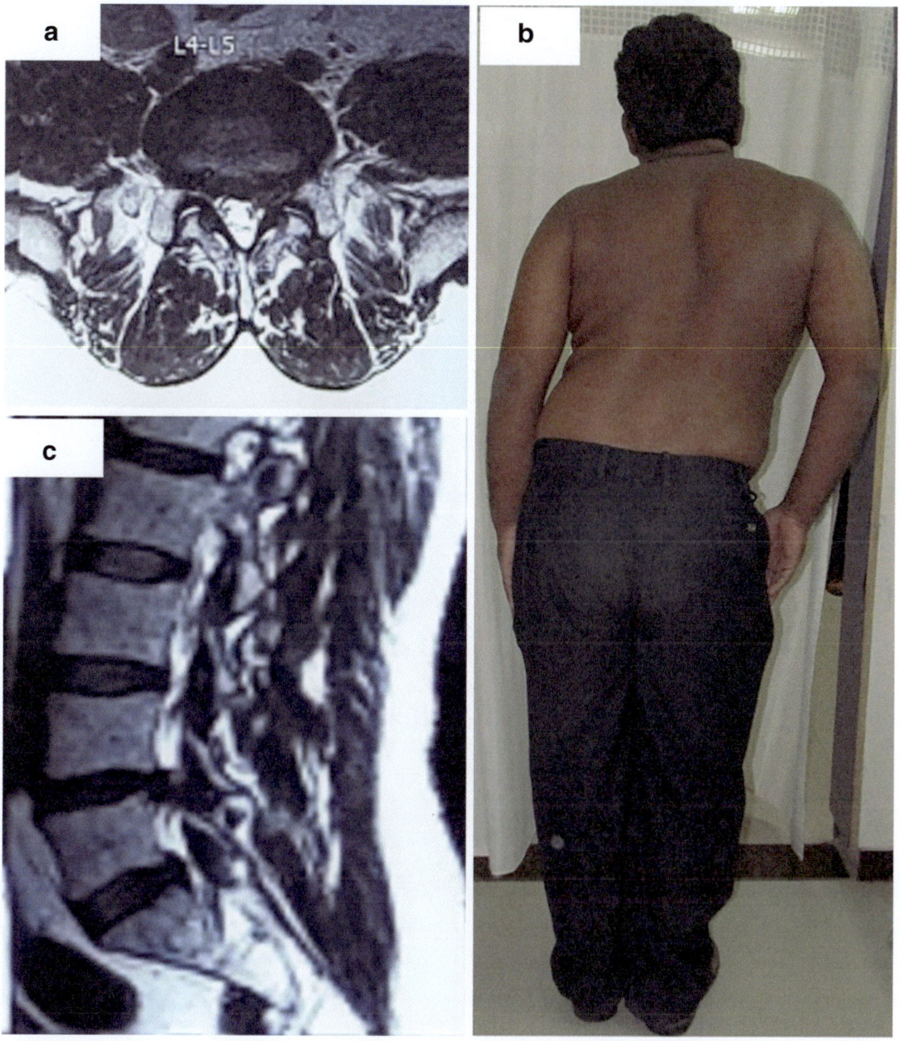

Fig. 12.3 (**a**) Axial T2 weighted MRI showing a left paracentral disc extrusion with compression in the left L5 traversing root. (**b**) Sagittal T2 weighted MRI image showing the disc extrusion. (**c**) The clinical image of the patient showing a classical sciatic list on examination

L3 Nerve Root Compression Symptoms manifest as pain that radiates from the lower back to the anterior and medial thigh, often extending to the knee. Sensory disturbances such as numbness may occur along the same path. The quadriceps muscle, responsible for knee extension, may weaken due to the involvement of the L3 nerve root. Normally, L3 plays a key role in knee extension, enabling smooth

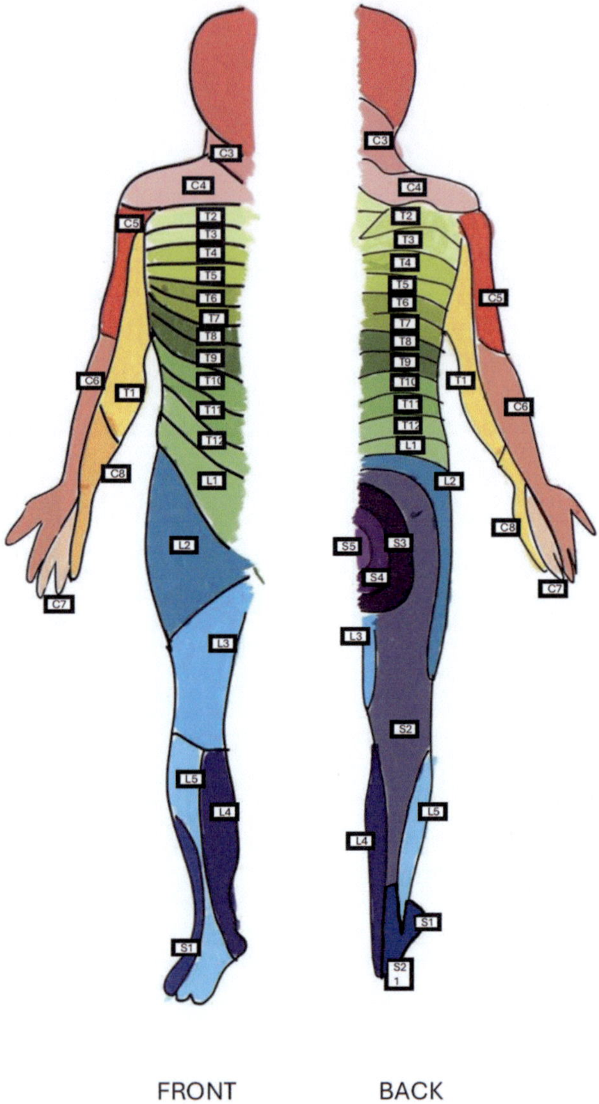

Fig. 12.4 Sensory dermatomal distribution of spinal nerve roots

walking and the ability to stand from a seated position. A reduced patellar reflex is often seen with L3 compression, impacting the patient's ability to maintain balance and strength in the lower extremities [5].

L4 Nerve Root Compression Symptoms manifest as pain that radiates along the anterior thigh, knee, and medial leg. Sensory disturbances such as numbness or tingling are commonly reported in these areas. The quadriceps muscle and the tibialis anterior are innervated by the L4 nerve root and are essential for knee extension and foot dorsiflexion. Weakness in the Tibialis anterior can lead to a foot drop which can make activities such as standing up from a seated position or walking difficult. A decrease in the patellar reflex is another common indicator of L4 nerve root compression [49, 50].

L5 Nerve Root Compression Compression of the L5 nerve root is one of the most common clinical presentations in lumbar degenerative spine disease. Patients typically report pain radiating down the lateral aspect of the thigh, leg, and into the dorsum of the foot. Sensory disturbances, such as numbness or tingling, may also be noted, particularly over the top of the foot and great toe. The L5 nerve root plays a crucial role in controlling dorsiflexion of the foot and toes, an essential movement for walking. When this nerve root is compressed, it often results in foot dorsiflexion and toe extension. Individuals with L5 weakness may show hip abduction weakness resulting in a modified gait with abductor lurch. In healthy individuals, the L5 nerve root facilitates smooth foot dorsiflexion, which is critical for proper foot clearance during the swing phase of walking [38].

S1 Nerve Root Compression Compression of the S1 nerve root produces pain that typically radiates along the posterior thigh, calf, and lateral part of the foot, often extending to the heel. Commonly associated sensory disturbances include numbness and tingling in these regions. The gastrocnemius and soleus muscles, which are essential for plantarflexion of the foot, are innervated by the S1 nerve root. Under normal circumstances, the S1 nerve root facilitates plantarflexion, allowing individuals to push off their toes while walking and to stand on their tiptoes. Compression of this nerve root leads to weakness in these muscles, impairing the patient's ability to perform these movements. A diminished or absent Achilles reflex is a key diagnostic sign often observed in patients with S1 nerve root compression [18, 24, 45, 50].

12.4.3 Cauda Equina Syndrome

Cauda equina syndrome (CES) is a critical neurological condition arising from compression of the cauda equina nerve roots within the lower spinal canal. Key clinical features include bladder and bowel dysfunction, saddle anesthesia, and sexual dysfunction, often accompanied by lower limb motor and sensory deficits. Early identification and intervention are essential to mitigate irreversible neurological deficits.

Bladder disturbances are among the hallmark symptoms, typically beginning with altered sensation in urination, including poor stream, hesitancy, or a need to strain. Advanced cases may progress to painless urinary retention, a sign of significant neurogenic dysfunction. Bowel symptoms include incontinence or constipation due to compromised anal sphincter control, representing late-stage CES manifestations.

Saddle anesthesia, or loss of sensation in the perineal region, is a distinctive feature that aids in diagnosis. This sensory deficit often encompasses the inner thighs, buttocks, and perianal region, indicating sacral nerve root involvement. Sensory impairments may extend to the lower extremities, presenting as numbness or tingling.

Sexual dysfunction, though less commonly discussed, is a vital component of CES symptomatology. Patients may report reduced genital sensation or erectile dysfunction, significantly impacting quality of life [17, 27].

12.4.4 Special Diagnostic Tests for Nerve Root Compression

Several specialized tests are employed to diagnose lumbar nerve root compression by reproducing pain using provocative limb positioning [36].

Femoral Nerve Stretch Test This test is primarily used to diagnose compression of the L2, L3, and L4 nerve roots. The patient lies prone while the examiner extends the hip with the knee flexed. Reproduction of pain in the anterior thigh suggests irritation or compression of these nerve roots, aiding in the localization of upper lumbar nerve root involvement.

Straight Leg Raise (SLR) Test The SLR test is commonly used to assess irritation of the lower lumbar nerve roots, particularly L4, L5, and S1. The patient lies supine while the examiner lifts the leg with the knee extended. Pain or paresthesia radiating down the posterior leg, calf, or foot during this maneuver indicates nerve root irritation. This test is particularly effective in detecting nerve compression caused by conditions such as a herniated disc [35].

Manual Muscle Testing for Nerve Root Weakness Manual muscle testing is a valuable tool for evaluating motor deficits associated with nerve root compression, as shown Table 12.1 [18, 50].

Table 12.1 Key muscle group testing for motor power and sensory dermatomal distribution

Level	Motor muscle group	Action	Sensory dermatome distribution	Reflexes
L2	Iliopsoas	Hip flexion	Anterior thigh	None
L3	Quadriceps	Knee extension	Medial thigh	Patellar (partial)
L4	Tibialis anterior	Ankle dorsiflexion	Medial lower leg, medial malleolus	Patellar (primary)
L5	Extensor hallucis longus, gluteus medius	Great toe extension, hip abduction	Lateral lower leg, dorsum of foot	None
S1	Gastrocnemius, soleus	Ankle plantarflexion	Lateral foot, sole of foot	Achilles (primary)

12.4.5 Neurogenic Claudication in Lumbar Degenerative Spine Disorders

Neurogenic claudication is a hallmark clinical feature of lumbar spinal stenosis, characterized by cramping and pain in the lower limbs triggered by ambulation and exercise. It may be associated with sensory symptoms of tingling, numbness, or paresthesia in the lower limbs. It is defined as "a condition in which there is reduced space available for neural elements in the lumbar spine due to degenerative changes in the spinal canal" [54]. The degenerative processes leading to spinal stenosis include hypertrophy of the ligamentum flavum, disc herniation, and osteophyte formation (Fig. 12.5). *Lumbar canal stenosis* is indeed a condition characterized by a constellation of symptoms [45].

Spinal stenosis is predominantly observed in individuals over 60 years of age, with lumbar spinal stenosis being the most common pre-operative diagnosis for adults over 65 who are undergoing spinal surgery. Despite many individuals showing radiographic evidence of stenosis, a significant number remain asymptomatic, making the true incidence of the condition difficult to estimate [33].

Neurogenic claudication is apparent particularly when the lumbar spine is extended during activities like standing or walking, patients experience leg pain, numbness, and weakness. Unlike axial low back pain, neurogenic claudication causes symptoms that radiate into the lower limbs and is typically relieved by sitting or adopting a lumbar flexion posture. Flexion of the lumbar spine increases the canal's diameter, temporarily alleviating the compression of the neural structures. This mechanism explains why patients often find relief in positions such as sitting or leaning forward, which reduces nerve root compression. A key feature of neurogenic claudication is its positional dependence. This positional relief distinguishes neurogenic claudication from vascular claudication, where the pain is due to insufficient blood flow to the lower limb muscles. In vascular claudication, pain is typically relieved by simply ceasing activity, without the need for specific postural adjustments.

Patients with neurogenic claudication, often suffering from advanced degenerative spine disease, may experience significant limitations in mobility. They may find

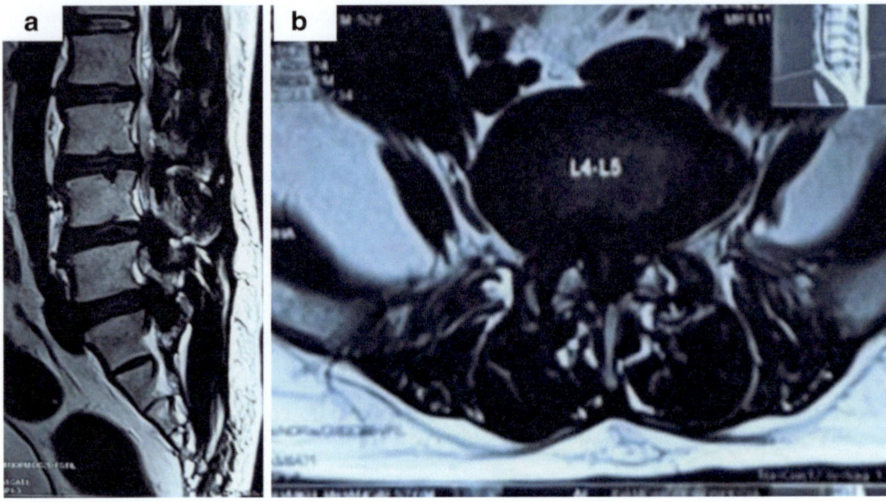

Fig. 12.5 T2 weighted MRI showing (**a**) sagittal and (**b**) axial section with lumbar canal stenosis with multiple factors contributing to the reduction of the canal dimensions including disc protrusion, flavum hypertrophy, facet hypertrophy, synovial facet effusion and facetal osteophytes

it difficult to walk long distances or remain standing for prolonged periods. Accurate diagnosis is achieved through clinical assessment combined with imaging techniques such as MRI or CT, which confirm the extent of spinal stenosis and the associated neural compression [52].

12.4.6 Difference Between Vascular and Neurogenic Claudication (Table 12.2)

Radiculopathy and claudication, although both seen in lumbar degenerative spine disease, stem from different pathological mechanisms and present distinct clinical features.

Radiculopathy occurs due to irritation or compression of a spinal nerve root, most commonly caused by a herniated disc or narrowing of the neural foramen. This condition manifests as sharp, radiating pain that follows the dermatomal distribution of the affected nerve. Patients often experience additional symptoms such as numbness, tingling, or burning sensations, along with motor deficits including muscle weakness or reduced reflexes. For example, in cases of radiculopathy involving the L5 or S1 nerve roots, patients may experience sciatica, with pain radiating down the leg along the affected nerve. The pain is typically sharp and electric, and activities that increase intraspinal pressure, such as coughing or sneezing, tend to aggravate the symptoms.

Neurogenic claudication, in contrast, is caused by a narrowing of the spinal canal (spinal stenosis), which compresses the cauda equina or multiple nerve roots instead of a single nerve. Unlike the sharp, radiating pain associated with radiculopathy, neurogenic claudication presents as a more diffuse aching or cramping sensation, typically affecting the buttocks, thighs, and calves. It is often triggered by activities such as walking or standing, with relief commonly achieved by sitting or leaning forward. The key distinction between these conditions lies in the fact that neurogenic claudication symptoms are alleviated through postural changes, whereas radiculopathy symptoms are generally constant and tend to worsen with direct pressure on the affected nerve root [16].

12.5 Functional Impairment in Lumbar Degenerative Spine Disease

Functional impairment is a major concern for patients with lumbar degenerative spine disease, as pain, neurological deficits, and mechanical instability can significantly reduce their ability to perform everyday tasks. Both LBP and radicular pain often limit mobility, making activities such as walking, bending, or lifting difficult. Neurogenic claudication, which is commonly observed in more advanced stages, further compromises a patient's ability to walk, reducing endurance and forcing frequent breaks or changes in posture, such as leaning forward, to relieve symptoms. These limitations severely affect a patient's capacity to carry out basic tasks such as climbing stairs, completing household chores, or standing for extended periods [15].

Neurological deficits, including muscle weakness and sensory disturbances, compound these impairments. For instance, foot drop can result in gait disturbances,

Table 12.2 Differentiation of symptoms of vascular claudication from symptoms of neurogenic claudication

Evaluation	Vascular	Neurogenic
Walking distance	Fixed	Variable
Provocative factors	Walking	Walking/standing
Walking uphill	Painful	Painless
Palliative factors	Standing	Sitting/bending
Bicycle test	Positive (painful)	Negative
Pain character	Cramping—Distal to proximal	Numbness, aching—Proximal to distal
Pulses	Absent	Present
Skin	Loss of hair; shiny	Normal
Weakness	Rarely	Occasionally
Back pain	Occasionally	Commonly
Back motion	Normal	Limited
Atrophy	Uncommon	Occasional

increasing the risk of falls and further limiting physical activity. Patients may also experience balance and coordination issues. This often leads to a reliance on external support for basic activities, contributing to a diminished quality of life. Reduced activity levels over time can result in physical deconditioning, which exacerbates both pain and functional limitations, creating a cycle of disability that is difficult to break without targeted intervention.

As the disease progresses, patients often experience increasing difficulties with mobility, posture, and gait, leading to a more sedentary lifestyle. This, in turn, contributes to further deconditioning and symptom exacerbation. Chronic pain and reduced mobility can also lead to psychological effects, perpetuating a cycle of pain, disability, and emotional distress [40].This functional disability can be assessed with various patient-reported outcome measures and tools such as The Oswestry Disability Index (ODI), Short Form 36 (SF-36), and Short Form 12 (SF 12) [11, 29].

12.6 Restricted Mobility and Flexibility of the Lumbar Spine

One of the most prominent functional impairments in patients with lumbar degenerative spine disease is restricted mobility and flexibility of the lumbar spine. Morning stiffness is a common complaint among these patients, and it may persist throughout the day, especially after periods of inactivity. As lumbar degeneration advances, spinal stiffness, and reduced flexibility become more permanent, limiting the range of motion and diminishing functional capacity [28].

12.7 Postural Changes and Deformity in Lumbar Degenerative Spine Disorders

Postural changes are a hallmark of functional impairment in individuals with lumbar degenerative spine disease. As the condition progresses, patients often adopt compensatory postures to alleviate pain, particularly in cases involving lumbar canal stenosis. A *forward-flexed posture* is frequently adopted by patients to relieve the symptoms of neurogenic claudication, as this position increases the available space for compressed neural structures, offering temporary symptom relief. However, prolonged use of this forward-leaning posture can lead to musculoskeletal imbalances over time. Tightness in the hip flexors, combined with weakness in the spinal extensor and core muscles, are common consequences of this compensatory posture. These imbalances increase the strain on other parts of the musculoskeletal system, leading to further discomfort and dysfunction. Additionally, patients may develop degenerative kyphotic or scoliotic deformity, characterized by a sagittal or coronal plane deformity and derangement of spinopelvic parameters such as lumbar lordosis, pelvic tilt, sacral slope, and sagittal vertical axis.

In advanced cases, the development of a degenerative deformity disrupts normal spinal biomechanics, increasing mechanical stress on the intervertebral discs and facet joints. As a result, degenerative changes accelerate, intensifying the pain and dysfunction experienced by patients and further limiting their mobility and quality of life [10].

12.8 Gait Disturbance

Gait disturbance is a frequent complication in patients with advanced lumbar degenerative spine disease, particularly in those experiencing neurogenic claudication, radiculopathy, or significant motor weakness. The leg pain which is often triggered by walking, forces patients to adopt an altered gait to reduce discomfort resulting in antalgic gait patterns. In patients with significant motor weakness, a high-stepping gait may develop as a way to compensate for foot drop.

In more severe cases, patients may develop a slow, shuffling gait, which further restricts their mobility and increases the risk of falls. These gait abnormalities severely impact a patient's independence. Over time, some patients may require assistive devices like canes or walkers to maintain mobility and balance [34].

12.9 Chronic Pain and Psychological Impact

Chronic pain is a common consequence in patients with lumbar degenerative spine disease, particularly when the condition is not effectively managed. Over time, acute pain can transition into chronic pain through a process known as central sensitization, where the nervous system becomes increasingly responsive to pain signals. This heightened sensitivity can cause even mild pain stimuli to feel severe, complicating the treatment process and contributing to long-term disability. Chronic pain often has a profound psychological impact on patients [37].

Depression, anxiety, and fear-avoidance behaviors are common psychological responses to chronic pain. Many patients may avoid physical activity out of fear that it will worsen their symptoms, which can lead to further declines in physical fitness and mobility. The psychological toll of chronic pain extends beyond the physical symptoms, affecting a patient's social life, relationships, and mental well-being [53].

References

1. Andersson GB. Epidemiological features of chronic low-back pain. Lancet. 1999;354(9178):581–5.
2. Ando K, Imagama S, Kobayashi K, Ito K, Tsushima M, Morozumi M, Tanaka S, Machino M, Ota K, Nakashima H, Nishida Y, Ishiguro N. Clinical features of thoracic myelopathy: a single-center study. JAAOS Glob Res Rev. 2019;3(11):e18.00090.
3. Bajwa NS, Toy JO, Young EY, Ahn NU. Establishment of parameters for congenital stenosis of the cervical spine: an anatomic descriptive analysis of 1066 cadaveric specimens. Eur Spine J. 2012;21(12):2467–74.

4. Berry JA, Elia C, Saini HS, Miulli DE. A review of lumbar radiculopathy, diagnosis, and treatment. Cureus. 2019;11:e5934. Available from: https://www.cureus.com/articles/19778-a-review-of-lumbar-radiculopathy-diagnosis-and-treatment Accessed 16 Oct 2024
5. Breivik H, Nicholas M, Campbell W, Newton-John T. Clinical pain management: practice and procedures. 2nd ed. CRC Press; 2008. Available from: https://www.taylorfrancis.com/books/9781444109825 Accessed 17 Oct 2024
6. Briggs AM, Van Dieën JH, Wrigley TV, Greig AM, Phillips B, Lo SK, Bennell KL. Thoracic kyphosis affects spinal loads and trunk muscle force. Phys Ther. 2007;87(5):595–607.
7. Casiano VE, Sarwan G, Dydyk AM, et al.. Back pain. [Updated 2023 Dec 11]. In: StatPearls [internet]. Treasure Island: StatPearls Publishing; 2024. Available from: https://www.ncbi.nlm.nih.gov/books/NBK538173/
8. Chikuda H, Seichi A, Takeshita K, Shoda N, Ono T, Matsudaira K, Kawaguchi H, Nakamura K. Correlation between pyramidal signs and the severity of cervical myelopathy. Eur Spine J. 2010;19(10):1684–9.
9. Chung NL, Espinoza Orías AA, He J, Inoue N, An HS. Facet joints. In: Spine phenotypes. Elsevier; 2022. p. 319–38. Available from: https://linkinghub.elsevier.com/retrieve/pii/B9780128227787000158 Accessed 20 Oct 2024.
10. Deane JA, Lim AKP, Phillips ATM, McGregor AH. Symptomatic individuals with lumbar disc degeneration use different anticipatory and compensatory kinematic strategies to asymptomatic controls in response to postural perturbation. Gait Posture. 2022;94:222–9.
11. El-Hady AO, El Molla SS, Elwan SI, Ibrahim RA. Evaluation of health related quality of life with the use of Oswestry disability index in degenerative discogenic low back pain. Egypt Rheumatol Rehabil. 2023;50(1):4.
12. Fogwe DT, Petrone B, Munakomi S, et al. Thoracic Discogenic syndrome. [updated 2024 mar 20]. In: StatPearls [internet]. Treasure Island: StatPearls Publishing; 2024. Available from: https://www.ncbi.nlm.nih.gov/books/NBK470388/.
13. Fotakopoulos G, Georgakopoulou VE, Lempesis IG, Papalexis P, Sklapani P, Trakas N, Spandidos DA, Faropoulos K. Pathophysiology of cervical myelopathy (review). Biomed Rep. 2023;19(5):84.
14. Galbusera F, Wilke H-J. Biomechanics of the spine: basic concepts, spinal disorders and treatments. London: Academic press; 2018.
15. Gautschi O, Smoll N, Corniola M, Joswig H, Chau I, Hildebrandt G, Schaller K, Stienen M. Validity and reliability of an objective measurement of functional impairment in lumbar degenerative spine disease: the timed-up-and-go (TUG) Test. J Neurol Surg A: Central Eur Neurosurg. 2015;76(S 01):s-0035-1564542.
16. Genevay S, Atlas SJ, Katz JN. Variation in eligibility criteria from studies of radiculopathy due to a herniated disc and of neurogenic claudication due to lumbar spinal stenosis: a structured literature review. Spine. 2010;35(7):803–11.
17. Hawa A, Denasty A, Elmobdy K, Mesfin A. The most impactful articles on Cauda Equina Syndrome. Cureus. 2023;15(4):e38069.
18. Hoppenfeld J-D, Hoppenfeld S. Orthopaedic neurology: a diagnostic guide to neurologic levels. 2nd ed. Philadelphia: Wolters Kluwer; 2018.
19. Huygen F, Kallewaard JW, Van Tulder M, Van Boxem K, Vissers K, Van Kleef M, Van Zundert J. "Evidence-based interventional pain medicine according to clinical diagnoses": update 2018. Pain Pract. 2019;19(6):664–75.
20. Inoue T, Soshi S, Kubota M, Marumo K. New method for the quantitative assessment of sensory disturbances in cervical myelopathy: application for neurological level diagnosis. Spine Surg Relat Res. 2020;4(3):216–22.
21. Jaumard NV, Welch WC, Winkelstein BA. Spinal facet joint biomechanics and mechanotransduction in normal, injury and degenerative conditions. J Biomech Eng. 2011;133(7):071010.
22. Kang K-C, Lee HS, Lee J-H. Cervical radiculopathy focus on characteristics and differential diagnosis. Asian Spine J. 2020;14(6):921–30.
23. Katzman WB, Wanek L, Shepherd JA, Sellmeyer DE. Age-related Hyperkyphosis: its causes, consequences, and management. J Orthop Sports Phys Ther. 2010;40(6):352–60.

24. Konno T, Aota Y, Kuniya H, Saito T, Qu N, Hayashi S, Kawata S, Itoh M. Anatomical etiology of "pseudo-sciatica" from superior cluneal nerve entrapment: a laboratory investigation. J Pain Res. 2017;10:2539–45.
25. Lacy J, Bajaj J, Gillis CC. Atlantoaxial instability. In: StatPearls [online]. Treasure Island: StatPearls Publishing; 2024. Available from: http://www.ncbi.nlm.nih.gov/books/NBK519563/ Accessed 21 Oct 2024.
26. Lannon M, Kachur E. Degenerative cervical myelopathy: clinical presentation, assessment, and natural history. J Clin Med. 2021;10(16):3626.
27. Lavy C, Marks P, Dangas K, Todd N. Cauda equina syndrome–a practical guide to definition and classification. Int Orthop. 2022;46(2):165–9.
28. Lee BH, Moon S-H, Suk K-S, Kim H-S, Yang J-H, Lee H-M. Lumbar spinal stenosis: pathophysiology and treatment principle: a narrative review. Asian Spine J. 2020;14(5):682–93.
29. Lee C-P, Fu T-S, Liu C-Y, Hung C-I. Psychometric evaluation of the Oswestry disability index in patients with chronic low back pain: factor and Mokken analyses. Health Qual Life Outcomes. 2017;15(1):192.
30. Lukasiewicz AM, Basques BA, Bohl DD, Webb ML, Samuel AM, Grauer JN. Myelopathy is associated with increased all-cause morbidity and mortality following anterior cervical discectomy and fusion: a study of 5256 patients in American College of Surgeons National Surgical Quality Improvement Program (ACS-NSQIP). Spine. 2015;40(7):443–9.
31. Maezawa Y, Uchida K, Baba H. Gait analysis of spastic walking in patients with cervical compressive myelopathy. J Orthop Sci. 2001;6(5):378–84.
32. Misawa T, Kamimura M, Kinoshita T, Itoh H, Yuzawa Y, Kitahara J. Neurogenic bladder in patients with cervical compressive myelopathy. J Spinal Disord Tech. 2005;18(4):315–20.
33. Munakomi S, Foris LA, Varacallo M. Spinal stenosis and neurogenic claudication. In: StatPearls [Internet]. Treasure Island: StatPearls Publishing; 2024. Available from: https://www.ncbi.nlm.nih.gov/books/NBK430872/.
34. Natarajan P, Fonseka RD, Kim S, Betteridge C, Maharaj M, Mobbs RJ. Analysing gait patterns in degenerative lumbar spine diseases: a literature review. J Spine Surg. 2022;8(1):139–48.
35. Nee RJ, Coppieters MW, Boyd BS. Reliability of the straight leg raise test for suspected lumbar radicular pain: a systematic review with meta-analysis. Musculoskelet Sci Pract. 2022;59:102529.
36. Nygaard OP, Kloster R, Mellgren SI. Recovery of sensory nerve fibres after surgical decompression in lumbar radiculopathy: use of quantitative sensory testing in the exploration of different populations of nerve fibres. J Neurol Neurosurg Psychiatry. 1998;64(1):120–3.
37. Ozgur B, Benzel E, Garfin S, editors. Minimally invasive spine surgery: a practical guide to anatomy and techniques [online]. New York, NY: Springer; 2009. Available from: https://link.springer.com/10.1007/978-0-387-89831-5. Accessed 17 Oct 2024
38. Pećina MM, Krmpotić-Nemanić J, Markiewitz AD. Tunnel syndromes. Boca Raton: CRC Press; 1991.
39. Pollintine P, Przybyla AS, Dolan P, Adams MA. Neural arch load-bearing in old and degenerated spines. J Biomech. 2004;37(2):197–204.
40. Ravindra VM, Senglaub SS, Rattani A, Dewan MC, Härtl R, Bisson E, Park KB, Shrime MG. Degenerative lumbar spine disease: estimating global incidence and worldwide volume. Global Spine J. 2018;8(8):784–94.
41. Robblee J, Katzberg H. Distinguishing radiculopathies from Mononeuropathies. Front Neurol. 2016;7:111.
42. Rong X, Liu Z, Wang B, Chen H, Liu H. The facet orientation of the subaxial cervical spine and the implications for cervical movements and clinical conditions. Spine. 2017;42(6):E320–5.
43. Rujeedawa T, Mowforth OD, Davies BM, Yang C, Nouri A, Francis JJ, Aarabi B, Kwon BK, Harrop J, Wilson JR, Martin AR, Rahimi-Movaghar V, Guest JD, Fehlings MG, Kotter MR. Degenerative thoracic myelopathy: a scoping review of epidemiology, genetics, and pathogenesis. Global Spine J. 2024;14(5):1664–77.
44. Seidenwurm DJ, Expert Panel on Neurologic Imaging. Myelopathy. AJNR Am J Neuroradiol. 2008;29(5):1032–4.

45. Solomon L, Warwick D, Nayagam S. Apley and Solomon's concise system of orthopaedics and trauma [online]. 0th ed. CRC Press; 2014. Available from: https://www.taylorfrancis.com/books/9781444174328. Accessed 17 Oct 2024
46. Swanson BT. Tandem spinal stenosis: a case of stenotic cauda equina syndrome following cervical decompression and fusion for spondylotic cervical myelopathy. J Man Manip Ther. 2012;20(1):50–6.
47. Van Kleef M, Stolker RJ, Lataster A, Geurts J, Benzon HT, Mekhail N. 10. Thoracic pain. Pain Pract. 2010;10(4):327–38.
48. Vitzthum H-E, Dalitz K. Analysis of five specific scores for cervical spondylogenic myelopathy. European Spine J. 2007;16(12):2096–103.
49. Vucetic N, Astrand P, Guntner P, Svensson O. Diagnosis and prognosis in lumbar disc herniation. Clin Orthop Relat Res. 1999;361:116–22.
50. Wang H, Wang Y, Li Y, Wang C, Qie S. A diagnostic model of nerve root compression localization in lower lumbar disc herniation based on random forest algorithm and surface electromyography. Front Hum Neurosci. 2023;17:1176001.
51. Will JS, Bury DC, Miller JA. Mechanical low back pain. Am Fam Physician. 2018;98(7):421–8.
52. Wu L, Munakomi S, Cruz R. Lumbar spinal stenosis. In: StatPearls [Internet]. Treasure Island: StatPearls Publishing; 2024. Available from: https://www.ncbi.nlm.nih.gov/books/NBK531493/.
53. Yücetaş ŞC, Yenilmez Y, Yıldırım CH, Hüseyinoğlu N, Ehi Y, Tunç S, Yıldırım K, Üçler N. Psychiatric disorders in lumbar stenosis with chronic pain and their effects on lumbar stenosis surgery. Kafkas J Med Sci. 2016;6(3):155–61.
54. Zileli M, Crostelli M, Grimaldi M, Mazza O, Anania C, Fornari M, Costa F. Natural course and diagnosis of lumbar spinal stenosis: WFNS spine committee recommendations. World Neurosurg X. 2020;7:100073.

Treatment Modalities: Non-surgical Management Options 13

Vishal Kumar and Aditya Gupta

13.1 Introduction

It is essential to comprehend the pathophysiology of DDD to understand the mechanism of action of nontreatment modalities. The intervertebral discs are made up of an outer fibrous ring (Annulus Fibrosus) and an inner gel-like core (Nucleus Pulposus). The disc loses its hydration and elasticity with aging leading to decreased disc height and integrity. Pain is produced due to the stimulation of receptors through direct nerve compression or inflammation due to chemical mediators released from the damaged disc. Aging, Nutrition, Genetic and Environmental factors all play a pivotal role in disc degeneration.

13.2 Non-surgical Treatment Modalities

Non-surgical options for DDD include watchful waiting, physical therapy, medications, spinal injections, and surgical referrals. They are generally useful in the majority of patients and the pain gradually subsides. The patient's symptoms and level of disability dictate the treatment modality. Longevity and progression of the symptoms as well as the response to any past interventions, including physical therapy, medications, or injections, help in determining the further course of action [1].

More than 90% of patients with symptomatic chronic back pain do not require surgical intervention. Watchful waiting is indicated in patients with mild or primarily axial symptoms. Medications used commonly to treat pain and inflammation include opiates, steroids, or Non-Steroidal Anti-inflammatory Drugs (NSAIDs) which are usually combined with other conservative measures such as physical therapy and corticosteroid injections [2]. These do not treat the underlying cause of

V. Kumar · A. Gupta (✉)
Department of Orthopaedics, PGIMER, Chandigarh, India

V. Kumar, P. Mishra (eds.), *A Comprehensive Guide to Degenerative Spine Disorders*, https://doi.org/10.1007/978-981-96-9091-6_13

the degeneration and the natural progression of the disease. Surgery is usually reserved for refractory cases usually. Nowadays, the focus is shifting towards biologic-based therapies. Biomolecular therapies (e.g., genes and proteins) and cell-based therapies (e.g., stem cells and chondrocytes) are the new broader horizons of research in biologics for DDD.

13.3 Physical Therapy

Physical therapy, equipment, and modalities are recommended as the first line of management to treat DDD. The aim is to strengthen the spinal muscles and enhance spinal function which can reduce the load on the degenerated discs and alleviate pain.

Physical therapy includes Back and Core strengthening exercises (Fig. 13.1) to help in correcting the posture and address radicular symptoms. Lumbosacral corsets help in reducing lumbar lordosis and increase walking capacity. Techniques such as spinal manipulation and mobilization may improve spinal alignment and reduce pain.

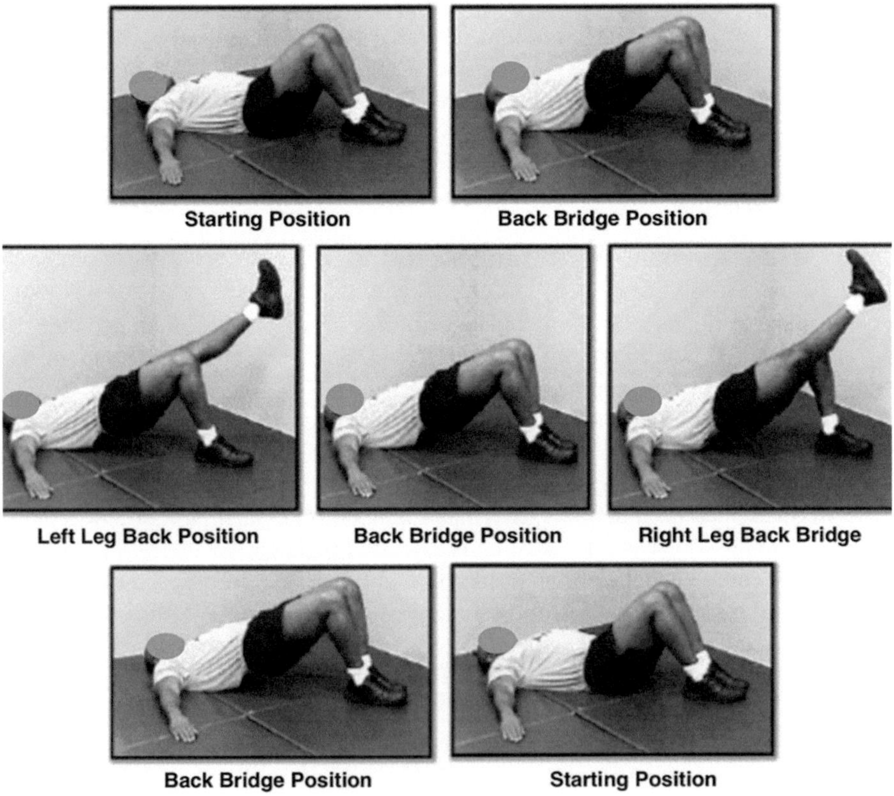

Fig. 13.1 Back and core strengthening exercises

Physiotherapy includes transcutaneous electrical nerve stimulation, ultrasound, heat or cold therapy, and traction. The success of therapy often depends on the patient's adherence to the prescribed exercises. Other miscellaneous modalities include chiropractic care, acupuncture, massage therapy, and Cognitive Behavioral Therapy (CBT).

13.4 Lifestyle Modifications

Lifestyle changes improve overall health and are recommended as part of a comprehensive treatment plan to manage the symptoms of DDD. These include the following:

- Reducing body weight decreases the load on the spine.
- Better posture reduces strain on the back.
- Quitting smoking slows the progression of DDD.
- Ensuring adequate intake of balanced diet and nutrients including calcium and vitamin D supports bone and disc quality.

13.5 Pharmacological Treatment

Pharmacological treatment offers symptomatic relief and improves the quality of life of the patients. A variety of drugs with distinct mechanisms of action are available including NSAIDs, analgesics, muscle relaxants, corticosteroids, and antidepressants.

13.6 Guidelines for Pharmacological Management

Stepwise Approach Acetaminophen or NSAIDs are used in the beginning for pain relief. Topical NSAIDs or combination therapy are used in patients with contraindications to systemic NSAIDs. Muscle relaxants or short courses of corticosteroids are used for acute exacerbations or if the pain does not subside. For chronic pain, antidepressants can be tried. Epidural steroid injections are reserved for refractory severe cases.

Patient-Centered Considerations Pharmacological treatments are tailored based on individual Risk Factors like comorbidities, age, and overall health status. This includes combining pharmacologic agents with physical therapy and psychological support followed by regular monitoring and follow-up to assess pain levels, function, and quality of life and alter treatment.

13.7 Non-steroidal Anti-inflammatory Drugs (NSAIDs)

NSAIDs are the most commonly used medications for DDD. Various studies have established the efficacy of NSAIDs in reducing pain and inflammation associated with DDD. The mechanism of action involves inhibition of the Cyclooxygenase(COX) enzymes. Both COX-1 and COX-2 inhibitors are effective, but selective COX-2 inhibitors, such as celecoxib are preferred especially in younger patients without cardiovascular risk due to their lower gastrointestinal side effect profile.

Side effects include gastrointestinal toxicity, renal impairment, and cardiovascular events and are contraindicated in patients with peptic ulcers, kidney disease, or cardiovascular risk factors.

13.8 Analgesics

Analgesics are widely used for mild to moderate pain in DDD. Centrally acting drugs like acetaminophen act by reducing prostaglandin synthesis, although its exact mechanism remains unclear. It has a favorable safety profile compared to NSAIDs, but high doses can lead to hepatotoxicity, particularly in patients with existing liver disease.

13.9 Muscle Relaxants

Muscle relaxants are indicated in the short-term management of acute exacerbations of DDD-related pain (Table 13.1). They are often prescribed to relieve muscle spasms associated with DDD. These medications act on the central nervous system to reduce muscle tone and alleviate spasm-related pain.

Long-term use is avoided due to the risk of sedation and dizziness. These drugs are to be used moderately with caution in patients whose job requires them to stay attentive like drivers and machinery operators.

Table 13.1 Classification of muscle relaxants

Peripherally acting (neuromuscular blockers)			Centrally acting skeletal muscle relaxants		Direct acting
Non-depolarizing neuromuscular blockers		Depolarizing neuromuscular blockers	Mephenesin congeners	Benzodiazepines	Dantrolene
Isoquinoline derivatives	Steroid derivatives	Suxamethonium (succinylcholine)	Mephenesin	Diazepam	
D-Tubocurarine	Pancuronium	Decamethonium	Carisoprodol	*GABA mimetic*	
Gallamine	Vecuronium		Chlorzoxazone	Baclofen	
Atracurium	Rapacuronium		Chlormezanone	Thiocolchicoside	
Doxacurium	Pipecuronium		Methocarbamol	*Central α2 agonist*	
Mivacurium	Rocuronium			Tizanidine	

13.10 Corticosteroids

Corticosteroids, e.g., prednisone are indicated in acute flare-ups for a short duration. They can also be used as epidural steroid injections for targeted pain relief. These agents reduce inflammation and nerve root irritation. Their immunosuppressant and anti-inflammatory action reduces the production of inflammatory mediators. Although they are effective but used in moderation for the short term due to potential side effects including weight gain, osteoporosis, hyperglycemia, and decreased immunity.

13.11 Antidepressants

Antidepressants have been proven effective in managing chronic pain. They modulate the neurotransmitters in the Central Nervous System, which alters pain perception. Tricyclic Antidepressants (TCAs) and Serotonin-Norepinephrine Reuptake Inhibitors (SNRIs) are an adjunct therapy in the treatment of DDD in patients with symptoms of depression or anxiety. They reduce chronic pain and improve sleep quality in anxious patients, thus relieving symptoms [3].

Safety and adverse effects include dry mouth, constipation, and sedation. SNRIs are better tolerated but cause nausea, dizziness, and insomnia so start at lower doses and are titrated slowly.

13.12 Spinal Injections

Spinal injections deliver medication directly to the source of pain, providing targeted relief. Intralaminar epidural injections are used to treat symptoms related to neurogenic claudication. Patients with radiculopathy often experience better relief with transforaminal epidural injections. Effectiveness and longevity can vary depending on the cause and severity of the DDD [4].

The different types of injections include epidural steroid injections, facet joint injections, and selected nerve root blocks. Spinal injections provide significant short-term pain relief but, their long-term efficacy is variable requiring repeated injections. In an article published in Pain Practice in 2020, 54 patients were treated with transforaminal epidural steroid injections for lumbar radicular pain from spinal stenosis, only about 15% of the patients reported complete resolution of the initial pain, while about 50% of the patients had significant pain and required additional injections every 2–6 months or oral medications.

13.13 Pain Management Programs

Pain management programs offer a holistic approach to improving pain, function, and quality of life for patients with DDD. They combine multiple treatment modalities to address the physical, psychological, and social aspects of pain. A multidisciplinary approach involves a team of doctors, physical therapists, psychologists, and pain specialists to create individualized treatment plans tailored to the patient's specific needs and conditions [5].

13.14 Regenerative Medicine

The aim of regenerative medicine is to repair or replace damaged tissues. Stem Cell and Platelet-Rich Plasma (PRP) therapy can be effective in treating DDD. Platelet-rich-plasma (PRP) contains factors such as TGF-b, platelet-derived growth factor (PDGF), epidermal growth factor (EGF), vascular endothelial growth factor, and insulin-like growth factor-1 (IGF-1) which increase collagen content, accelerate epithelial regeneration, promote angiogenesis, improve wound healing and stimulate IVD metabolism. They enhance cell viability, stimulate ECM metabolism, and stimulate the proliferation of IVD cells. This can be used as an intradiscal therapy to stimulate regeneration or at least slow the progression of degeneration within a diseased IVD [6].

13.15 Key Emerging Treatments for DDD

1. *Biologic Therapies*:
   - *Growth Factors and Cytokine Modulators*: These treatments target the inflammatory processes within the disc and promote regeneration. Researchers are exploring recombinant proteins that can reduce disc aging by minimizing catabolic processes at the genetic level, leading to the production of molecules that encourage tissue repair.
2. *Regenerative Medicine*:
   - *Stem Cell Therapy*: Mesenchymal stem cells (MSCs), particularly from bone marrow, are used to address chronic low back pain associated with DDD. These cells can enhance disc regeneration by boosting cell viability and stimulating extracellular matrix (ECM) activity. However, harvesting MSCs can be invasive and costly.
   - *Platelet-Rich Plasma (PRP) Therapy*: PRP contains several growth factors (e.g., TGF-β, PDGF, EGF, VEGF, IGF-1) that contribute to tissue repair, accelerate healing, stimulate disc metabolism, and promote the proliferation of disc cells. It is being explored as a treatment to slow disc degeneration when injected directly into the disc.

   - *Bone Marrow Concentrate (BMC) Therapy*: BMCs, which include a mixture of stem and progenitor cells such as MSCs, can be auto-transplanted during surgery. Studies suggest that higher concentrations of colony-forming unit fibroblasts (CFU-F) from bone marrow aspirates lead to significant pain relief.
3. *Specific Targeted Therapies*:
   - *TNF and IL Inhibitors*: These therapies aim to control the inflammation within degenerating discs, potentially slowing the progression of degeneration.
   - *Growth Factor Therapy (Bone Morphogenetic Proteins—BMPs)*: BMPs, including Recombinant Human Growth/Differentiation Factor-5 (GDF-5), part of the TGF-β superfamily, are being studied for their role in promoting disc repair.
   - *Autologous Disc Chondrocyte Transplantation (ADCT)*: This approach involves transplanting a patient's own disc chondrocytes to repair damaged or inflamed disc tissue. Although this method is available in some countries like Germany, it is not yet approved in the USA by the FDA.

13.16 Challenges and Considerations

These innovative treatments are still undergoing research, and their full safety profiles are not yet established. Potential risks include the following:

- *Immune Suppression*: Particularly with therapies targeting inflammatory cytokines like TNF and IL.
- *Infection Risk*: Due to the introduction of autologous or biological materials into the body.
- *Systemic Side Effects*: Resulting from growth factor or cytokine modulation, which could have broader physiological effects.

While these therapies are still in experimental stages, they offer significant potential to slow or reverse the progression of disc degeneration, providing new hope for individuals with chronic low back pain associated with DDD [7].

13.17 Gene Therapy for DDD

Gene therapy has shown promising results in biological treatment strategies for DDD. The injection of biological molecules into the disc allows for direct delivery of protein products to address the causes of degenerative disc disease at the source. It has emerged as a potential solution to the shortcomings of biological molecules like short half-life. The recombinant genes are delivered and incorporated with the DNA of the host cell allowing for long-term expression of a protein to facilitate healing of the degenerated disc space. Since viral carriers are often used for transfection, serious concerns involving unexpected mutations create challenges for Food and Drug Administration (FDA) approval and patient inclusion [8].

13.18 Conclusions

Non-surgical treatment modalities for degenerative disc disease offer a wide variety of options for managing symptoms and improving quality of life. Physical therapy, pharmacological treatments, lifestyle modifications, cognitive behavioral therapy, spinal injections, and regenerative medicine each have different mechanisms and varying degrees of efficacy. A multidisciplinary approach, tailored to the individual patient's needs, is often the most effective strategy. Future research is needed to continue improving these treatments and exploring new options to provide better outcomes for patients with DDD. Surgical referral should be considered when patients have persistent or progressive weakness or numbness, changes in bowel or bladder function, or when significant symptoms persist despite the above medical management interventions.

References

1. Sahu R. Non-drug non-invasive treatment in the Management of low back pain. Ann Med Health Sci Res. 2014;4(5):780–5. https://doi.org/10.4103/2141-9248.14156.
2. Chen C, Liu L, Li Y, Fu W. Efficacy of platelet-rich plasma in the treatment of degenerative disc disease: a systematic review and meta-analysis. Eur Spine J. 2022;31(9):2351–61. https://doi.org/10.1007/s00586-022-07111-2.
3. Dahal S, Bhandari S. Impact of psychological therapies on chronic pain management in patients with degenerative disc disease: a review. J Spine Surg. 2021;7(4):387–98. https://doi.org/10.21037/jss-21-40.
4. Jensen RK, Leboeuf-Yde C, Wedderkopp N. Conservative treatment of lumbar disc herniation with radiculopathy: a narrative review of recent evidence. J Clin Med. 2023;12(2):460. https://doi.org/10.3390/jcm12020460.
5. Park CH, Lee SH, Lee DC. The effects of manual therapy on pain and disability in patients with lumbar degenerative disc disease: a systematic review and meta-analysis. J Manip Physiol Ther. 2023;46(1):31–40. https://doi.org/10.1016/j.jmpt.2022.09.001.
6. Pereira H, Soares D, Correia FD, Ferreira A. Digital therapeutics in the management of chronic pain in degenerative disc disease: a comprehensive review. Pain Res Manag. 2022;2022:1294517. https://doi.org/10.1155/2022/1294517.
7. Sigmundsson FG, Kang HS, Jonsson B. Long-term outcomes of non-surgical management in patients with lumbar degenerative disc disease: a 10-year follow-up study. Spine J. 2021;21(12):2069–79. https://doi.org/10.1016/j.spinee.2021.05.014.
8. Vadalà G, Russo F, Papalia R. Biologic treatment of degenerative disc disease: a narrative review. Int J Spine Surg. 2020;14(S1):S91–9. https://doi.org/10.14444/7061.

14 Surgical Intervention for Degenerative Spine Disorders

Sanjay Yadav, Ankith Kesagodu Virupaksha, and Surabhi Das

14.1 Introduction

Symptoms emanating from degenerative lumbar spine disease are managed conservatively to begin with. In cases where conservative treatment proves ineffective, prior research has demonstrated that surgical intervention can effectively reduce both the duration of symptoms and the time required to resume employment [1, 2]. Nevertheless, the achievement of favorable results is contingent upon the careful selection of patients and the implementation of appropriate surgical techniques.

14.1.1 Indications of Surgical Intervention

Surgery for degenerative spine disease should be considered in the following scenarios [3]:

1. Failed conservative treatment given for 6–12 weeks.
2. Severe pain refractory to conservative management.
3. Severe acute or rapidly progressive neurological deficit.
4. Cauda equina syndrome. It is a true surgical emergency and requires immediate decompression surgery.
5. "Red-flag" signs present [4].

S. Yadav (✉) · A. K. Virupaksha · S. Das
Department of Orthopaedics, Institute of Medical Sciences, BHU, Varanasi, India

V. Kumar, P. Mishra (eds.), *A Comprehensive Guide to Degenerative Spine Disorders*, https://doi.org/10.1007/978-981-96-9091-6_14

14.1.2 Surgical Options

Surgical options available for the treatment of lumbar degenerative spine disease can be broadly divided into fusion and non-fusion procedures. The indication for each varies with symptoms and radiological signs in the patient. Some hybrid procedures have also been introduced in recent times [5].

Various approaches have been designed to access the spine to perform these procedures.

14.1.3 Approaches to Lumbar Spine

14.1.3.1 Posterior Approach to Lumbar Spine

The posterior approach (Fig. 14.1) is the most common approach to the lumbar spine. It provides exposure, to the intervertebral discs, the spinal cord, and most importantly the posterior elements, namely, the spinous processes, laminae, facet joints, and pedicles.

Indications of posterior approach [6]:

1. Excision of a prolapsed disc.
2. Nerve root exploration.
3. Decompression of the spinal cord.
4. Fusion procedures of the spine.

Patient Positioning The patient is positioned in a prone position on a radiolucent table, using bolsters to avoid chest and abdominal compression (Letting the abdomen

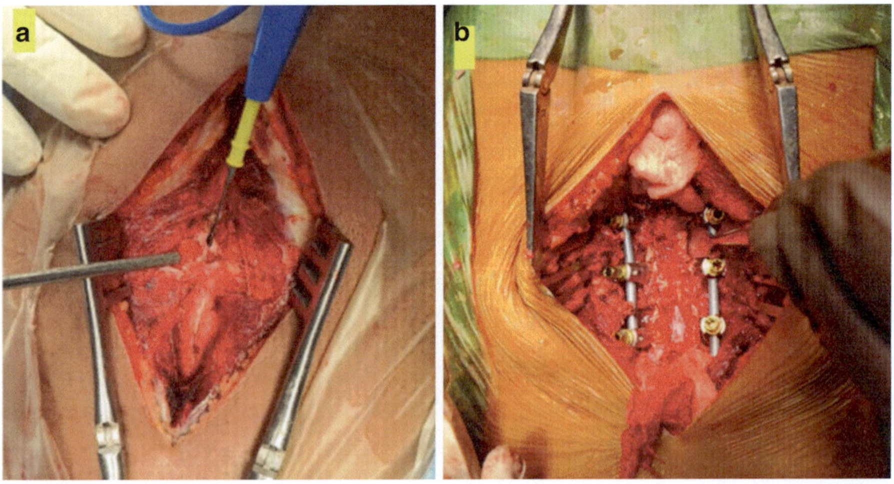

Fig. 14.1 (**a**) Posterior approach to lumbar spine. (**b**) Posterior instrumentation of lumbar spine showing pedicle screws and rods

free decreases the intravenous pressure and blood loss due to collapse of the epidural venous plexus. It also prevents superior mesenteric artery syndrome) [7].

Incision Make a longitudinal midline incision over the spinous processes, centered over the pathological vertebral level. This level may be identified by palpation keeping L4–L5 disc space as reference (line joining the highest points of both iliac crests passes through L4–5 disc space), or under image intensification [8]. Extend the incision depending on the number of vertebral levels involved.

Superficial Dissection Perform blunt dissection through subcutaneous fat to reach the facia. Incise the facia in line with the incision.

Deep Dissection Detach the paraspinal muscles subperiosteally, using a Cobb elevator or cautery. Dissect down the spinous process and along the lamina to the facet joint, using electro-cautery. Care should be taken not to dissect the muscle, which will result in necrosis and may cause infection. If required, dissect laterally and strip the facet joint capsule from the facets below and above, and expose the mammillary and transverse processes. Do not dissect anterior to the transverse processes as it may injure the exiting spinal nerves lying just in front of the transverse processes. Use bipolar cautery to establish hemostasis. The spinal cord can be exposed via the removal of the lamina, and the disc space can be exposed by cutting through the ligamentum flavum.

Complications of long-duration prone positioning are as follows [7]:

- Facial swelling.
- Airway swelling.
- Muscle injury (myositis).
- Wilke Syndrome.

Closure A drain should be placed beneath the fascia. Watertight closure of the fascial layer is key and should be done in an interlocking continuous fashion using absorbable sutures. This allows for the reduction of dead space. The skin should be closed in layers.

14.1.3.2 Posterior Paraspinal Approach (Wiltse and Spencer)

The posterior paraspinal approach (Fig. 14.2) follows the principles of minimally invasive procedure. It provides exposure, to the intervertebral discs, the spinal cord, and most importantly the posterior elements, namely, the spinous processes, laminae, facet joints, and pedicles, but is not as invasive as the posterior approach.

Indications of the posterior paraspinal approach are the same as the posterior approach.

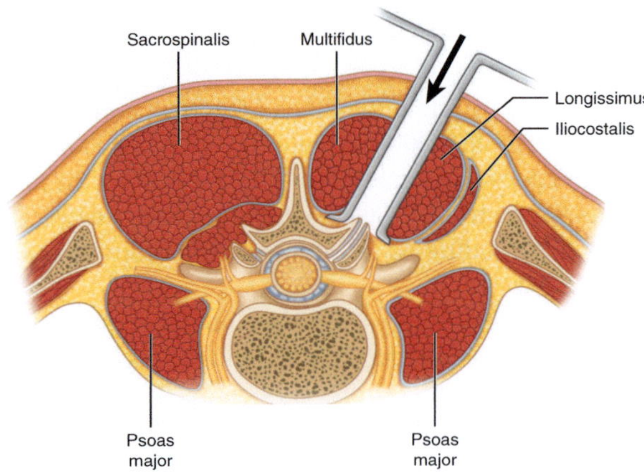

Fig. 14.2 Wiltse and Spencer's paraspinal approach. [Cross-sectional anatomical diagram at lower lumbar vertebral level, Arrow indicates the plane of approach.]

Patient Positioning The patient is positioned in a prone position on a radiolucent table, using bolsters to avoid chest and abdominal compression.

Incision Make a longitudinal midline incision over the spinous processes, centered over the pathological vertebral level. Extend the incision depending on how many levels of vertebrae are involved. (Infiltrate with 1:500,000 epinephrine. before incision, to help with hemostasis).

Superficial Dissection Perform blunt dissection through subcutaneous fat to reach the facia. Incise the facia 2 cm lateral to the incision.

Deep Dissection Enter using blunt finger dissection between the multifidus and longissimus muscles and apply a self-retaining retractor between them. Palpate the facet joints at L4–5. Use electrocautery or an elevator to separate the multifidus fibers from their fascial attachments, and expose the transverse processes, facet joints, and laminae subperiosteally. Dissection anterior to the transverse processes should not be done as it may cause injury to the exiting spinal nerves lying just in front of transverse processes. Use bipolar cautery to establish hemostasis.

Closure A drain should be placed beneath the fascia. Watertight closure of the fascial layer is key and should be done in an interlocking continuous fashion using Absorbable sutures. This allows for the reduction of dead space. The skin should be closed in layers.

14.1.3.3 Anterior (Retroperitoneal) Approach to the Lumbar Spine

Indications:

- Fusion of L5 to S1.
- Fusion of L4 to L5 (involves mobilization of the great vessels).

Patient Positioning Supine on a radiolucent operating table.

Incision It is imperative to ensure that the skin incision is precisely aligned with the level of approach, often positioned to the left of the midline. The recommended incision should be of minimal size, horizontal in orientation, often measuring 6–7 cm in length, and positioned slightly to the left, resembling the Pfannenstiel incision configuration. The consideration of alternative incisions should be based on factors such as the patient's body size or other technical parameters. It is imperative to consider the sacral slope when making the incision.

Superficial Dissection Dissect through the fat in line with the incision to reach the anterior fibrous rectus sheath. Incise the rectus sheath longitudinally at midline.

Deep Dissection The medial border of the intrafascial rectus muscle is mobilized cranio-caudally by approximately 10 cm. Subsequently, mobilize the muscle laterally to expose the underlying arcuate line. Identify the arcuate ligament. It serves as the caudal boundary of the incomplete posterior rectus sheath. By inserting the fingers and subsequently the entire hand into the retroperitoneal space, sweep the intraperitoneal contents superiorly, inferiorly, and medially to expose the spinal column in the midline (Fig. 14.3). To locate and palpate the left great vessels, it is necessary to identify the psoas muscles. Additionally, precautions must be taken to prevent tears in the peritoneal membrane. To prevent inadvertent injuries, it is necessary to identify the ureter. A sufficient corridor to the disc space can now be maintained by placing deep, self-retaining abdominal retractors. The disc is typically situated below the bifurcation of the major vessels at the L5–S1 level. Ligate the middle sacral artery and vein using a bipolar electrocautery. The superior hypogastric parasympathetic plexus lies over the sacral promontory and aorta. Mobilize and retract the great vessels (aorta and vena cava) as required for exposure to the desired level (L4–L5). Expose the disc spaces subperiosteally.

> Superior hypogastric parasympathetic plexus injury causes retrograde ejaculation in males [9].

Closure Closure should be done in layers. The rectus sheath should be carefully repaired to prevent diastasis and incisional hernias.

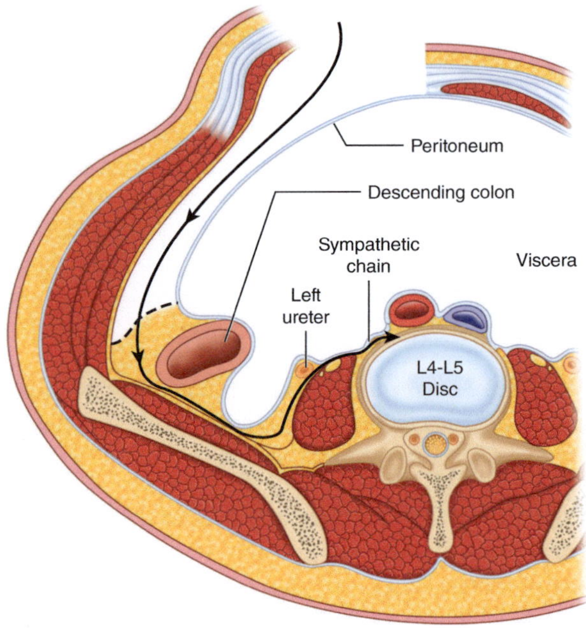

Fig. 14.3 Anterior (retroperitoneal) approach to the lumbar spine. [Cross-sectional anatomical diagram at the level of L4-L5 intervertebral disc. Arrow depicts the plane of access.]

14.1.3.4 Anterolateral (Retroperitoneal) Approach to the Lumbar Spine

Advantages of the Anterolateral (Retroperitoneal) Approach over the trans-peritoneal approach are as follows [10]:

- It allows access to all vertebrae from L1 to sacrum, whereas the trans-peritoneal approach is difficult to use above L4.
- It allows drainage of psoas abscess, without risking contamination of the peritoneal cavity, preventing peritonitis.

However, it is difficult to access L5–S1 disc space using this approach.

Patient Positioning Partial-lateral position on a radiolucent table, with either of the sides up depending on the preference of the surgeon.

Incision Make an oblique incision from the posterior half of rib-12, to the lateral border of the rectus abdominis muscle, staying between the umbilicus and the pubic symphysis.

Superficial Dissection Bluntly dissect through the subcutaneous fat to reach the external oblique aponeurosis, and divide it in the line of its fibers, which is in line with the skin incision. Split the internal oblique muscle in the same line, perpendicular to the muscular fibers. Follow it with the division of the transversus abdominis muscle, in line with the incision. This exposes the retroperitoneal space.

Deep Dissection Bluntly dissect and develop a plane between the retroperitoneal fat and the psoas fascia, using your finger. Carefully mobilize the peritoneal cavity contents. Depending on the side that requires exposure, dissect starting from either the right upper quadrant or the left lower quadrant. Retract the peritoneal contents along with the ureter, to the right upper quadrant using a Deaver-type retractor. Follow the surface of the psoas muscle medially to reach the anterolateral surface of the vertebral bodies. The lumbar arteries and veins tie the aorta and vena cava to the waist of the vertebral bodies. The ones on the involved vertebra should be located and ligated to mobilize the aorta and vena cava and access the anterior part of the vertebral body. Location can be determined under image intensification, by tagging a disc space with a k wire/needle.

Closure Closure should be done in layers. The external oblique aponeurosis should be well repaired.

14.2 Surgical Interventions for Lumbar Degenerative Spine

14.2.1 Laminectomy

The most accepted treatment of lumbar canal stenosis (LCS) is decompressive laminectomy.

Indications for laminectomy include the following [11]:

1. Central or lateral spinal canal stenosis not responding to at least 12 weeks of conservative therapy.
2. New onset or progressive neurological deficits.
3. Cauda equina syndrome.
4. Debilitating refractory pain not responding to at least 6 to 8 weeks of conservative management.

Contraindications of laminectomy [11]:

- Spondylolisthesis/ instability.
- Scoliosis.
- Lateral listhesis.

Approach: Posterior approach with midline incision.

Procedure After reflecting the muscles subperiosteally, resect spinous processes with dorsal laminae with bone cutting rongeur or a burr, to expose ligamentum flavum. Using a Woodson elevator and spatula, cut and remove the ligamentum flavum off its attachments to the superior, or leading edge of the inferior lamina. Perform laminectomy using a nibbler to start with, then switch to a Kerrison punch forceps to remove the lamina meticulously. Right below are the epidural fat and the dura. Bluntly dissect with caution, keeping lateral to the dura, down to the floor of the spinal canal, while you retract the spinal cord and nerve roots medially. This causes decompression of the spinal cord at that level. Decompression is said to be satisfactory when there is no bulging or kinking of the spinal cord, and the nerve roots are circumferentially free with some amount of excursion possible.

Laminectomy can also be performed with a minimally invasive technique using a smaller incision, and less traumatic dissection.

Did You Know?

Laminotomy is the removal of a small section of lamina at the pathological level of the spine.

Laminoplasty is the splitting of lamina on one side of the midline, and swinging it open like a door. It increases the sagittal diameter of the spinal canal. It is done in the cervical spine.

Complications of laminectomy [11]:

Instability: Due to damage to more than 50% of facets on both sides or pars interarticularis.

Dural tear: Causes persistent cerebrospinal fluid leak.

Bony re-growth.

Spinal epidural hematoma: maximum risk at the L2–L3 level.

Kyphosis: Due to disruption of posterior tension banding function of the posterior Osseo-ligamentous complex.

14.2.2 Discectomy

Indications [12]:

1. Cauda equina syndrome.
2. Debilitating refractory pain not responding to at least 6–8 weeks of conservative management.
3. New onset or progressive neurological deficits.

Contraindications [12]:

1. Bony spinal canal stenosis.
2. Neurological or vascular pathologies mimicking disc herniations.
3. Concurrent segmental instability.
4. Malignant tumors with dural involvement.
5. Requirement of fusion or instrumentation in vertebral fracture.
6. Local or systemic infection.

The Approach Used Posterior approach with midline incision.

Procedure After reaching the lamina, insert an angled Woodson elevator anterior to the ligamentum flavum, and direct it caudally, to protect the dura beneath it. This should be done cautiously. Using a curette, release the ligamentum flavum from its superior vertebral attachment on its anterior surface. Sharply incise the ligamentum flavum and retract it using a Penfield elevator. Exiting nerve root and associated epidural fat can be visualized now. Resect the medial aspect of the inferior facet of the superior vertebra if necessary to get adequate exposure. Insert a Penfield or blunt probe into the neuroforamen to mobilize the root, and retract it medially. After clearly visualizing the intervertebral disc space, remove the herniated disc using pituitary rongeurs. Meticulous hemostasis should be maintained using bipolar electrocautery.

Technical Tip

In instances where a segment of the ruptured disc persists behind the posterior longitudinal ligament, the surgeon may be required to employ a scalpel to make an incision in the annulus in order to get access. To ensure the complete removal of any excess disc or ligamentous tissue, it is imperative to methodically probe the epidural space in all directions with a Woodson elevator. Furthermore, it is advisable to irrigate the disc space with saline using a bulb syringe in order to remove any loose disc pieces that may have escaped visualization.

Evidentially, the above technique is associated with a higher rate of recurrent disc herniation, however, a more aggressive discectomy may lead to accelerated symptomatic disc degeneration and back pain.

14.2.2.1 Microdiscectomy

Microdiscectomy is a discectomy aided by a microscope. It allows for a smaller incision, less traumatic dissection, and better visualization of the operative field than a standard open discectomy. It is considered the gold-standard surgical procedure for the removal of herniated discs [13].

Minimally invasive discectomy and endoscopic discectomy are recent advances in the technique and are discussed later in this chapter.

Complications of discectomy [14]:

- Persistent symptoms.
- Residual or recurrent stenosis or disc herniation.
- Cerebrospinal fluid leak due to dural tear.
- Infection.
- Spinal instability due to more than required laminectomy or facet distortion.

14.2.3 Fusion Procedures

Degenerative spine disease can cause spinal instability, as discussed earlier. Fusion of a selected lumbar spinal segment is required to reduce the pain-producing stimuli produced by disrupted disc material and the motion between unstable segments. Fusion procedures are considered the "gold standard" for lumbar degenerative disorders [15].

Following are the three main fusion techniques currently employed:

1. *Posterolateral fusion (PLF)*:
   Posterolateral fusion (PLF) involves the fusion of only the posterior elements.

Approach Posterior or Wiltse approach through a midline incision.

Procedure After sub-periosteal elevation of muscles to reach facet joints and transverse processes bilaterally, they are decorticated. Local grafts from spinous processes or autologous bone grafts from the iliac crest are packed into the posterolateral gutters to facilitate fusion. Posterolateral fusion used to be performed without instrumentation. However, due to the comparatively high non-fusion rate in the absence of instrumentation [16, 17], instrumentation with pedicle screws is considered standard now. Some clinical studies have shown that patients with instrumented fusion have better clinical functional outcomes and a higher rate of fusion than patients without instrumented fusion [18, 19].

Studies have mentioned the persistence of lower back pain even after posterolateral fusion in some patients, which was ultimately ascribed to the presence of remnant nociceptive disc [20]. Such patients were found to experience relief after subtotal disc clearance and anterior interbody fusion, thus emphasizing the importance of disc clearance and interbody fusion.

2. *Interbody Fusion*:
   The advantages of interbody fusion over posterolateral fusion are as follows:

- In patients with discogenic pain, interbody fusion eliminates the nociceptive foci by subtotal removal of the disc.
- 80% of the body's weight is supported by the anterior column of the spine [5], which is majorly made up of the vertebral bodies. Interbody fusion devices placed between two such vertebral bodies provide a large surface area for the compressive load they bear, and thus biomechanically facilitate fusion.
- Interbody devices help restore the intervertebral height and sagittal balance, and correct lumbar lordosis depending on their design and final positioning on the endplates. They may even indirectly decompress the neural elements.

The interbody device consists of either a cage (typically manufactured from Peek and carbon fiber) or a bone graft spacer.

Approach Posterior or Anterior approach to lumbar spine.

Interbody fusion can be done by various approaches to the disc space (Fig. 14.4), namely:

A. *Posterior Lumbar Interbody Fusion (PLIF)*:

This technique provides access to both anterior and posterior columns through a single posterior approach. It entails a wide laminectomy, partial or complete facetectomy, a subtotal discectomy, endplate preparation, and finally insertion of the interbody device between the end plates, with or without posterior instrumentation. The disc is approached through the angle formed by the dural sac and exiting the upper nerve root.

Advantages [21] include the access to do an excellent spinal canal decompression to treat a concurrent central spinal canal stenosis. Wider resection allows for lesser neural retraction to access the diseased disc.

Disadvantage [22] of this technique is the resultant instability it may cause, and thus the need to restore stability with posterior pedicle screw instrumentation, especially above L5–S1 and when multiple levels are involved.

PLIF can be combined with posterolateral fusion to facilitate fusion rates.

B. *Transforaminal Lumbar Interbody Fusion (TLIF)*:

TLIF is a modification of the PLIF wherein the intervertebral disc is exposed on one side using a transforaminal approach paired with subtotal facetectomy and pedicle screw instrumentation. The nerve root needs to be retracted to expose the disc and thus increases the risk of nerve injury and radiculitis. A bilateral posterior pedicle screw instrumentation is advocated to restore stability.

In a manner akin to PLIF, the inclusion of contralateral posterolateral fusion has the potential to enhance fusion rates.

A wide spectrum of pathologies can be addressed through this approach, including degenerative spondylolisthesis.

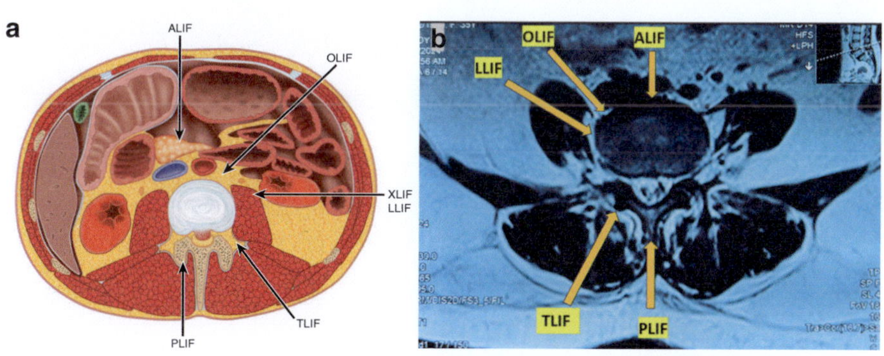

Fig. 14.4 Various surgical approaches for lumbar interbody fusion. (**a**) Cross-section at the level of L5–S1. (**b**) Axial MRI at the level of L5–S1. [Anterior lumbar interbody fusion (ALIF), lateral or extreme lateral interbody fusion (LLIF or XLIF), oblique lumbar interbody fusion/anterior to psoas (OLIF/ATP), transforaminal (TLIF or MI-TLIF), and posterior (PLIF)]

TLIF however, is a more demanding technique for insertion of the interbody device, which can potentially hinder adequate achievement of lumbar lordosis and subtotal disc clearance [23].

Figure 14.5a–g shows a case of degenerative L5–S1 spondylolisthesis managed with TLIF

C. *Anterior Approach for Lumbar Interbody Fusion (ALIF)*:

Approach used: Anterior transperitoneal or retroperitoneal approach.

ALIF allows access to the lumbar discs from L2 to S1. Proximal access is limited by the presence of renal vessels and the diaphragm. Distal access may be hindered by pubic symphysis, blocking L5–S1 disc space exposure, in patients with deep-seated L5–S1 levels relative to the pelvis. Hence, preoperative planning must include lateral radiographs of the lumbosacral spine including the pubis. The preparation of end plates and insertion of graft or implant are similar to PLIF and TLIF.

The advantage of ALIF lies in direct front-on visualization of disc space, also allowing for the accommodation of larger-sized implants with greater capacity to increase disc height and lordosis [24].

D. *Lateral Lumbar Interbody Fusion (LLIF/DLIF/XLIF)*:

A minimally invasive lateral approach (Fig. 14.6), where access is gained through the retroperitoneal space, to reach the surface of the iliopsoas muscle, and then the disc space through the muscle, is used. Next, dilatation of this path is done using serial tubular dilators. This allows access up to the L4–L5 disc space and proximal.

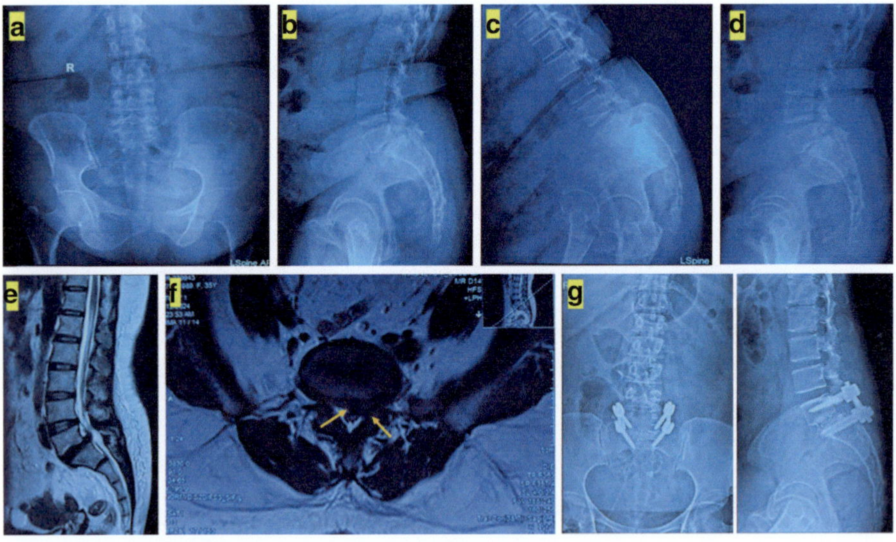

Fig. 14.5 A 35-year-old female with grade II isthmic spondylolisthesis of L5–S1 with bilateral lower limb radiculopathy. (**a–d**) Preoperative radiographs of LS spine (anteroposterior view, lateral view, lateral flexion view, and lateral extension view, respectively). (**e, f**) Preoperative sagittal and axial MR images, respectively. (**g**) Post L5/S1 TLIF with PEEK cage AP and Lateral radiographs

Intraoperative neuromonitoring is employed to avoid injury to the lumbar plexus that is present in this region.

Advantages of this technique include the following [25]:

- Better restoration of disc space height.
- Indirect decompression of the neural elements.

Complications are rare with LLIF, including visceral and vascular injury in the retroperitoneal space.

Both the ALIF and the DLIF procedures may be performed as stand-alone techniques or may require a posterior instrumented stabilization depending on the presence of instability.

E. *Oblique Lumbar Interbody Fusion (OLIF)/ Anterior to Psoas (ATP) Approach*:

It is a variant of LLIF and is also a minimally invasive technique. The interval used to access the intervertebral disc space lies between the peritoneum and psoas muscle (Fig. 14.7). This eliminates the need for splitting of the psoas muscle.

Did You Know?

360-degree or circumferential fusion is interbody fusion combined with posterolateral fusion.

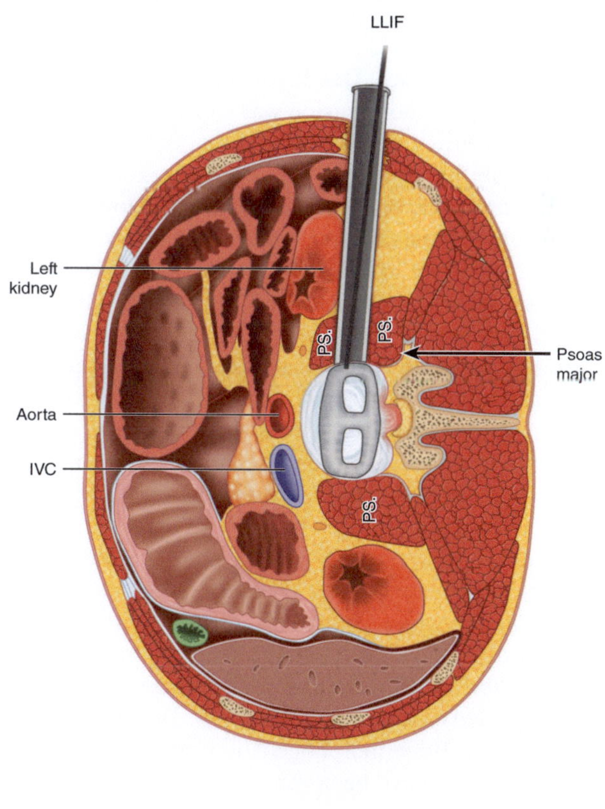

Fig. 14.6 Lateral lumbar interbody fusion (LLIF). It is a psoas splitting approach

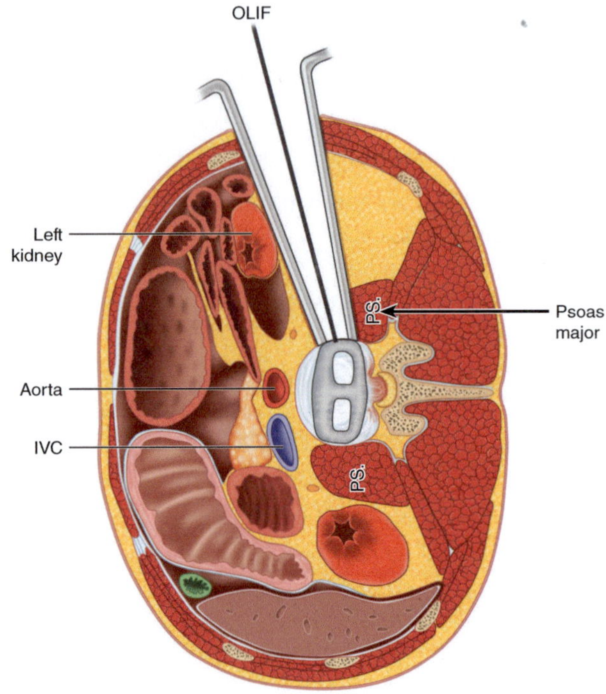

Fig. 14.7 Oblique lumbar interbody fusion/anterior to psoas (OLIF/ATP). (PS-Psoas Major; IVC-Inferior vena cava)

14.2.3.1 Interbody Devices and Graft Options

Historically, interbody fusion was carried out using tricortical iliac crest grafts. The associated difficulties included donor site morbidity, correct sizing of the graft blocks, stability of the graft after impaction in disc space, and the problems of subsidence and collapse of the graft. The development of interbody devices and their instrumentation has made the procedure easier with its design. Currently, interbody fusion devices are available in a wide range of materials, in conjunction with various graft options to enhance fusion. It started with the use of titanium cages, which gained popularity over the years, and have been associated with subsidence. Currently, interbody cages made of carbon fiber and non-absorbable, biocompatible material like polyetheretherketone (PEEK) are available. These are radiolucent and have Young's modulus closer to bone. Despite the controversial incorporation of bone into PEEK cages, as opposed to titanium ones, these cages have been found to have lower subsidence rates in addition to being visible on radiographs, allowing easier assessment of fusion rates. PEEK cages are thought to stimulate fibrous, nonmineralized tissue, instead of bony incorporation.

These interbody devices also have design characteristics that may help in restoring sagittal balance, lumbar lordosis, sagittal balance, indirect neuroforaminal decompression, and physiological load through the anterior spinal column.

Bone graft substitutes like demineralized bone matrix and tricalcium phosphate can be used in case of unavailability of iliac crest graft, to provide a scaffold for new bone growth. Bone morphogenetic proteins (BMPs) are osteoinductive bone graft substitutes that have been reported to be at least as effective as autologous bone graft substitutes or extenders [26]; however, extensive osteolysis resulting in graft subsidence and cage migration has also been reported with their use [27].

14.2.3.2 Non-fusion Procedures

Lumbar Disc Arthroplasty (Dynamic Stabilization and Motion Preservation)
Fusion procedures cause a rigid construct and take away the physiological movements present at the disc spaces which allow for mobility of the spine with posture to provide sagittal and coronal balance. Moreover, according to Wolff's law, bone grows when exposed to loading. Micromotion also allows for bone formation. Rigid fusions have also been postulated to produce increased loading on adjacent segments above and below, causing accelerated degeneration in adjacent discs, known as Adjacent Segment Disease (ASD). Hence, an alternative to a rigid fixation and fusion, flexible instrumentation to the lumbar spine, in the form of lumbar disc replacement has been introduced. Charite artificial disc is one such lumbar disc prosthesis in use (Fig. 14.8).
Indications of LDA are as follows [28]:

1. Symptomatic degenerative disc disease refractory to at least 6 months of conservative treatment.
2. 18 and 60 years of age.
3. Post-laminectomy syndrome or prior failed lumbar microdiscectomy.
4. Back pain without radiculopathy.
5. Only 1- or 2-level degenerative disc disease.

Considerations while choosing Lumbar Disc Arthroplasty over Lumbar Interbody Fusion are as follows:

1. Disc height was not significantly reduced.
2. Sufficient motion is still present at the disc level.

Contraindications of LDA are as follows [28]:

1. Ossified posterior longitudinal ligament.
2. Significantly reduced disc height.
3. No movement at that disc level.
4. Any spinal deformity/scoliosis.
5. Spinal instability or spondylolysis.
6. Spondylolisthesis.
7. Radiculopathy below knee.
8. Allergy or sensitivity to implant materials.
9. Objective evidence of nerve root compression.
10. Facet arthrosis.
11. Spinal stenosis.
12. Osteoporosis/osteopenia.
13. Previous lumbar fusion or fracture.
14. 3- or higher-level degenerative disc disease
15. Local infection, pregnancy, diabetes, autoimmune disorders, obesity.
16. Spinal tumor.

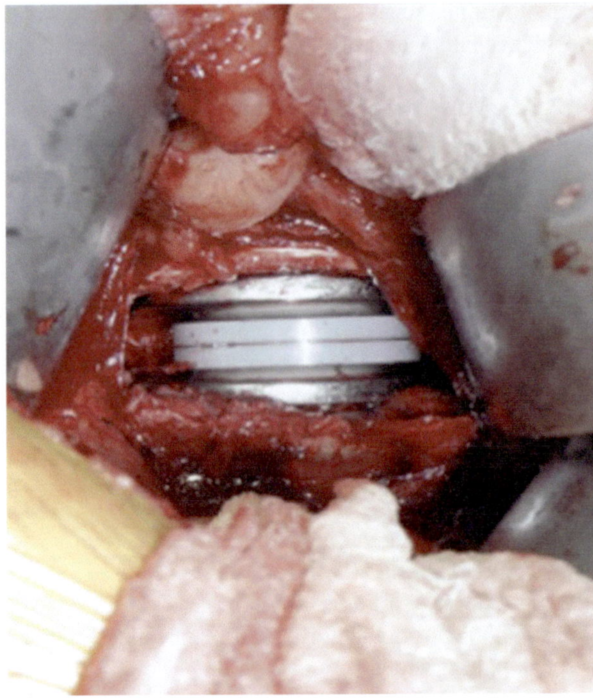

Fig. 14.8 Intraoperative image of Charite artificial disc between intervening vertebrae [3] (Eliyas JK, 2011,p.592–606)

Approach Used Anterior at lower lumbar levels (L4/5 and L5/S1).

Though there is no long-term evidence of its outcomes, mid-term evidence suggests satisfactory clinical results, implant survival, and comparable complication profiles to fusion.

The proposed advantages of LDA are as follows [29]:

- Decreases incidence of ASD seen with fusion procedures.
- Eliminates the need for grafting or screw fixation.
- Lower reoperation rate due to ASD.
- Clinical outcomes and rates of return-to-work are equivalent to fusion.
- Lower rates of secondary sacroiliac joint dysfunction.
- Faster patient recovery and higher patient satisfaction in the short term compared to the fusion techniques, with higher rates of return to work.

Disadvantages of LDA are as follows [28]:

- It is technically taxing and has a steep learning curve.
- No long-term outcomes are known yet.
- Lower versatility in indications compared to fusion.

Complications associated with LDA [28]:

- Implant extrusion.
- Vascular injury linked to inadequate training.
- Improper sizing of the implant.

- Lack of confirmation of satisfactory placement on imaging.
- Metal ion and polyethylene wear particle release from the articulation interface can cause systemic reactions.

> Whether to perform a multiple-level disc replacement or a hybrid disc replacement and fusion surgery in case of multiple lumbar levels requiring surgical intervention, depends on the surgeon's discretion. There is no literature that holds one higher than the other.

14.2.3.3 Recent Advances

1. *Minimally Invasive Surgery Interbody Fusion*: Due to increasing patient demands of faster recovery, and lower morbidity, minimally invasive surgery (MIS) techniques have been developed to allow access to the intervertebral discs while limiting soft tissue dissection and muscle damage. They provide the same clinical outcomes as an open interbody fusion, but with reduced intraoperative blood loss and muscle damage, faster return to work, and decreased opioid dependence for the patient.

MIS adaptation of TLIF utilizes the Wiltse paraspinal approach. This technique reduces muscle stripping, preserves blood supply and muscular attachment, and thereby reduces erector muscle dysfunction and fibrosis.

Minimally invasive LLIF and anterior-to-psoas approaches allow us to access the intervertebral disc space anterior to the psoas muscle, rather than through the muscle.

MIS-ATP interbody fusion: Here, the patient is positioned in the lateral decubitus position. Access is gained through the retroperitoneal space via a small lateral incision. Neural monitoring probes are then placed in the psoas to identify the lumbosacral plexus and help steer clear of it. The safe zone to access the lumbar spine is within the anterior one-third to one-half of the psoas.

Disadvantages of MIS are that the learning curve is very steep, and the reported neurologic side-effects overall are as common as in 18–40% of patients [30].

2. *Endoscopic Spine Surgery*:

With improvements in the optics, high resolution camera, light source, high-speed burr, and irrigation pump, minimally invasive spine surgeries can be performed with various endoscopic techniques for lumbar, cervical, and thoracic regions.

Advantages of endoscopic spine surgeries include the following [31]:

- Reduced tissue dissection and muscle trauma.
- Low blood loss.
- Reduced damage to the epidural blood supply and consequent epidural fibrosis and scarring.
- Reduced hospital stay.
- Early functional recovery and improvement in the quality of life.
- Better cosmesis.

With a precise indication, proper diagnosis, and good training, endoscopic spine surgery can give equally good results as open spine surgery. Use of endoscopic technique is wide, applicable for all spinal levels, and all severities of disc herniations. In the lumbar region, endoscopic technique can also be used for decompression of spinal canal stenosis, apart from treated disc herniations. Endoscopy-assisted fusion surgeries have also been developed. Appropriate indications, clear imaging prior to surgery, and preplanning are keys to successful outcomes.

14.3 Conclusion

The degeneration of the lumbar spine is a prevalent clinical presentation. Fortunately, the majority of the associated disorders resulting from this process can be effectively managed with nonsurgical interventions. Lumbar interbody fusion is considered the gold standard in these cases. However, recent advancements in technology have made it possible to employ more efficient and minimally invasive procedures for many of the cases that do not respond to conservative therapy or require surgical intervention.

References

1. Fritzell P, Hägg O, Jonsson D, Nordwall A, Swedish Lumbar Spine Study Group. Cost-effectiveness of lumbar fusion and nonsurgical treatment for chronic low back pain in the Swedish Lumbar Spine Study: a multicenter, randomized, controlled trial from the Swedish Lumbar Spine Study Group. Spine. 2004;29(4):421–34. discussion Z3
2. Fritzell P, Hägg O, Wessberg P, Nordwall A. Swedish Lumbar Spine Study Group. 2001 Volvo award winner in clinical studies: lumbar fusion versus nonsurgical treatment for chronic low back pain: a multicenter randomized controlled trial from the Swedish Lumbar Spine Study Group. Spine. 2001;26(23):2521–32. discussion 2532–4
3. Eliyas JK, Karahalios D. Surgery for degenerative lumbar spine disease. Dis Mon DM. 2011;57(10):592–606.
4. DePalma MG. Red flags of low back pain. JAAPA Off J Am Acad Physician Assist. 2020;33(8):8–11.
5. Lee YC, Zotti MGT, Osti OL. Operative management of lumbar degenerative disc disease. Asian Spine J. 2016;10(4):801–19.
6. Kwon BK, Vaccaro AR, Grauer JN, Beiner J. Indications, techniques, and outcomes of posterior surgery for chronic low back pain. Orthop Clin North Am. 2003;34(2):297–308.
7. Cunha PD, Barbosa TP, Correia G, Silva R, Cruz Oliveira N, Varanda P, et al. The ideal patient positioning in spine surgery: a preventive strategy. EFORT Open Rev. 2023;8(2):63–72.
8. Chakraverty R, Pynsent P, Isaacs K. Which spinal levels are identified by palpation of the iliac crests and the posterior superior iliac spines? J Anat. 2007;210(2):232–6.
9. Kanemura T, Satake K, Nakashima H, Segi N, Ouchida J, Yamaguchi H, et al. Understanding retroperitoneal anatomy for lateral approach spine surgery. Spine Surg Relat Res. 2017;1(3):107–20.
10. Mehren C, Mayer HM, Zandanell C, Siepe CJ, Korge A. The oblique anterolateral approach to the lumbar spine provides access to the lumbar spine with few early complications. Clin Orthop. 2016;474(9):2020–7.
11. Estefan M, Munakomi S, Camino Willhuber GO. Laminectomy. In: StatPearls [Internet]. Treasure Island (FL): StatPearls Publishing; 2024 [cited 2024 Aug 24]. Available from: http://www.ncbi.nlm.nih.gov/books/NBK542274/

12. Butler AJ, Munakomi S, Iii CJD. Diskectomy. In: StatPearls [Internet] [Internet]. StatPearls Publishing; 2024 [cited 2024 Aug 24]. Available from: https://www.ncbi.nlm.nih.gov/books/NBK544281/
13. Dowling TJ, Munakomi S, Dowling TJ. Microdiscectomy. In: StatPearls [Internet]. Treasure Island (FL): StatPearls Publishing; 2024 [cited 2024 Aug 24]. Available from: http://www.ncbi.nlm.nih.gov/books/NBK555984/
14. Bombieri FF, Shafafy R, Elsayed S. Complications associated with lumbar discectomy surgical techniques: a systematic review. J Spine Surg. 2022;8(3):377–89.
15. Donnally III CJ, Hanna A, Varacallo M. Lumbar Degenerative Disk Disease. In: StatPearls [Internet]. Treasure Island (FL): StatPearls Publishing; 2024 [cited 2024 Sep 1]. Available from: http://www.ncbi.nlm.nih.gov/books/NBK448134/
16. Bono CM, Lee CK. Critical analysis of trends in fusion for degenerative disc disease over the past 20 years: influence of technique on fusion rate and clinical outcome. Spine. 2004;29(4):455–63; discussion Z5.
17. Bono CM, Lee CK. The influence of subdiagnosis on radiographic and clinical outcomes after lumbar fusion for degenerative disc disorders: an analysis of the literature from two decades. Spine. 2005;30(2):227–34.
18. Bjarke Christensen F, Stender Hansen E, Laursen M, Thomsen K, Bünger CE. Long-term functional outcome of pedicle screw instrumentation as a support for posterolateral spinal fusion: randomized clinical study with a 5-year follow-up. Spine. 2002;27(12):1269–77.
19. Lorenz M, Zindrick M, Schwaegler P, Vrbos L, Collatz MA, Behal R, et al. A comparison of single-level fusions with and without hardware. Spine. 1991;16(8 Suppl):S455–8.
20. Weatherley CR, Prickett CF, O'Brien JP. Discogenic pain persisting despite solid posterior fusion. J Bone Joint Surg Br. 1986;68(1):142–3.
21. Lestini WF, Fulghum JS, Whitehurst LA. Lumbar spinal fusion: advantages of posterior lumbar interbody fusion. Surg Technol Int. 1994;3:577–90.
22. Cole CD, McCall TD, Schmidt MH, Dailey AT. Comparison of low back fusion techniques: transforaminal lumbar interbody fusion (TLIF) or posterior lumbar interbody fusion (PLIF) approaches. Curr Rev Musculoskelet Med. 2009;2(2):118–26.
23. Sakeb N, Ahsan K. Comparison of the early results of transforaminal lumbar interbody fusion and posterior lumbar interbody fusion in symptomatic lumbar instability. Indian J Orthop. 2013;47(3):255–63.
24. Hsieh PC, Koski TR, O'Shaughnessy BA, Sugrue P, Salehi S, Ondra S, et al. Anterior lumbar interbody fusion in comparison with transforaminal lumbar interbody fusion: implications for the restoration of foraminal height, local disc angle, lumbar lordosis, and sagittal balance. J Neurosurg Spine. 2007;7(4):379–86.
25. Arnold PM, Anderson KK, McGuire RA. The lateral transpsoas approach to the lumbar and thoracic spine: a review. Surg Neurol Int. 2012;3(Suppl 3):S198–215.
26. Burkus JK, Gornet MF, Dickman CA, Zdeblick TA. Anterior lumbar interbody fusion using rhBMP-2 with tapered interbody cages. J Spinal Disord Tech. 2002;15(5):337–49.
27. Burkus JK, Gornet MF, Schuler TC, Kleeman TJ, Zdeblick TA. Six-year outcomes of anterior lumbar interbody arthrodesis with use of interbody fusion cages and recombinant human bone morphogenetic protein-2. J Bone Joint Surg Am. 2009;91(5):1181–9.
28. Othman YA, Verma R, Qureshi SA. Artificial disc replacement in spine surgery. Ann Transl Med. 2019;7(Suppl 5):S170.
29. Guyer RD, McAfee PC, Banco RJ, Bitan FD, Cappuccino A, Geisler FH, et al. Prospective, randomized, multicenter Food and Drug Administration investigational device exemption study of lumbar total disc replacement with the CHARITE artificial disc versus lumbar fusion: five-year follow-up. Spine J Off J North Am Spine Soc. 2009;9(5):374–86.
30. Park J, Ham DW, Kwon BT, Park SM, Kim HJ, Yeom JS. Minimally invasive spine surgery: techniques, technologies, and indications. Asian Spine J. 2020;14(5):694–701.
31. Chen KT, Kim JS, Huang APH, Lin MHC, Chen CM. Current indications for spinal endoscopic surgery and potential for future expansion. Neurospine. 2023;20(1):33–42.

Future Trends and Innovations in the Management of Degenerative Spine Disorders

15

Syed Ifthekar and Deepankar Satapathy

15.1 Introduction

As the ageing population increases across the world, the incidence of degenerative spine disorders is on the rise [1]. Degenerated intervertebral discs, changes in facet joints and ligamentum flavum are common radiologic findings in population more than 50 years [1].

The common clinical presentation of individuals with degenerative spine are axial back/neck pain, radiating pain to upper and/or lower limbs and less commonly symptoms of myelopathy or claudication [2, 3]. The treatment of degenerative spine disorders has a wide-spectrum approach ranging from targeted physiotherapy/strengthening exercises to decompression and fusion/replacement surgeries [3]. The operative treatment though relieves the symptoms of the patient, it does not address the underlying disease process. It is needless to say that the decompression and fusion procedures come with their own set of procedure-related complications. This chapter deals with the future possibilities or advanced treatment methods of targeting the underlying disease process or advanced minimally invasive techniques to treat such disease process.

The degenerative process in the spine starts from the disc which is pivotal in absorbing the day-to-day forces. If the disc degeneration is addressed in a biological way which cures the degeneration and maintains the native spine anatomy, the complications of complex surgeries can be avoided. The protection of intervertebral disc at earlier stages and restoration of intervertebral disc in later stages have been tried in the literature [4]. Both in vitro and in vivo models have tried these methods. In the younger disc which is prone for earlier degeneration, the administration of growth factors is thought to decrease the rate of degeneration [5].

S. Ifthekar (✉) · D. Satapathy
Department of Orthopaedics, AIIMS Bibinagar, HMR Region, Hyderabad, India

V. Kumar, P. Mishra (eds.), *A Comprehensive Guide to Degenerative Spine Disorders*, https://doi.org/10.1007/978-981-96-9091-6_15

The direct administration of growth factors into the intervertebral disc space stimulates the cell-matrix production [6]. The TGF-β family of the growth factors have reproducible results on the anabolic effect of intervertebral discs [7–9]. Few in vivo studies conducted showed increased disc height and increased matrix production after administration of growth factors [10–12]. Klein et al. in his study used few matrix components and aiding component in the treatment of degenerated discs and the results were promising at 13 months of follow-up. There was significant reduction of pain and disability [13]. Slow release formulations may be sought for continuous benefits of growth factors in the disc [5].

Using the viral vectors to transfer the growth factors into the intervertebral discs using gene transfection showed sustained improvement in TGF-β levels for 6 weeks [14]. The transfection process can also be used to reduce the rate of disc degeneration by reducing the protease expression and matrix degradation by transferring IL-1RA and IL-1 inhibitors [15].

These techniques of stimulating the intervertebral disc to produce more matrix is possible only if sufficient viable cells are present. In advanced degeneration, where the reserve of healthy disc is very meagre, transplantation of healthy and functional cell is required [16, 17]. The practical application of this technique is difficult due to unavailability of the donor grafts to implant in the disc space. The tissue engineering of these cells followed by transplantation can be a future prospect in the advanced degenerated discs. The restoration of the intervertebral disc mainly focuses on nucleus pulposus restoration with scaffolds and cell containing biomatrices [5]. These scaffolds can be derived from synthetic sources and biological sources. The biological sources such as fibrin, collagen, alginate or chitosan-based matrices replicate the native disc environment and reduce the chances of hypersensitivity [18–20]. Synthetic scaffolds like polyglycolic acid have the advantage of easily modifiable properties [21]. After selecting a suitable scaffold, an environment is created to encourage the attachment, proliferation and differentiation of cells into intervertebral disc-like material [21]. In a study by Alini et al., bovine coccygeal Nucleus Pulposus were seeded on a collagen-hyaluronic scaffold [22]. The study group noted proteoglycan production in 2 months period though the levels were considerably lower. In a similar study by Seguin et al., the study group used Calcium Polyphosphate bone substitute material as a scaffold [23]. After 6 weeks of culture, Proteoglycans levels were comparable to native intervertebral disc. The other scaffolding materials used for intervertebral cell culture are Poly(D,L-Lactide), Poly-L-Lactic acid, Collagen and gelatin [24, 25].

Though scaffolding materials showed some initial promise, the ability to implant in a human intervertebral tissue was a challenge. This led to the development of crosslinked hydrophilic polymer chains which have the property of swelling up when contacted with water. They also had a property not to dissolve upon contact with water. Such substances were known as hydrogels [26, 27]. A polysaccharide hydrogel in the form of chitosan had similar loading properties as the intervertebral disc tissue [28]. Few synthetic hydrogels were also developed like poly vinyl alcohol, polyvinyl pyrrolidone and polyethylene glycol. These materials were used to develop nucleus pulposus which allowed sufficient nutrient diffusion through them [29, 30].

15.2 Role of PRP in IVD Regeneration

Platelet-rich plasma (PRP) which is used in various degenerative conditions is also tried in the degenerated discs. The growth factors present in Platelet-rich plasma have been proven to increase annulus cell proliferation and increased matrix [31]. Few studies have concluded that PRP injection into the rabbit and rat degenerated disc models is shown to delay the progression of early degenerative disc disease [32, 33]. Interleukin-1 receptor antagonist showed the decrease in cytokines and proteolytic enzymes from the nucleus pulposus [34]. Few other studies demonstrated a similar effect on nucleus pulposus by using anti-TNF drugs [35]. These therapies have a limited effect in the late stage of the degenerative disc disease where the reserve cells are less in number [36].

15.3 MSCs for IVD Regeneration

Mesenchymal stem cells (MSCs) are a good source of reserve cells having regenerative ability. Both the types of MSCs, namely, bone marrow-derived cells and Adipose tissue-derived cells have been proven in multiple studies to differentiate into nucleus pulposus-like material [37–39]. There is one human trial in the literature with a limited number of patients in degenerated disc disorder. The study group showed improved pain and disability scores and the discs showed improved water content after 12 months [40].

Combining Hyaluronic acid (HA) with collagen and fibrin has shown to reduce inflammation and pain in degenerative disc disorders [41, 42]. In a study, adipose-derived MSCs were combined with HA to treat the back pain caused by degenerative disc disease. The results were encouraging with reduced back pain and increased quality of life [43].

Amirdelfan K et al. studied 100 patients with low back pain due to degenerated discs for a period of 36 months. The study participants were divided into two groups with one group given mesenchymal precursor cells (MPCs) and the other group treated with placebo. The study group concluded a significant improvement in clinical and radiological parameters in the group that were treated with MPCs [44].

The only disadvantage or shortcoming for the transplantation of MSCs is their inability to survive under avascular conditions [45]. While the direct load on the disc and the relative hypoxia in the disc are beneficial for cellular differentiation, the high osmolarity and low pH are deleterious for the survival of MSCs.

If the degenerated disc disease is in advanced stage with instability, then the restoration of disc is a futile exercise [46]. When the nucleus pulposus is targeted for restoration, then the annulus fibrosis should be in good shape to resist the pressure from the regenerated nucleus pulposus [46]. If the annulus fibrosis is weak or damaged, then the regeneration process can be supported by screws.

In early degeneration, in which the spontaneous repair of the Nucleus pulposus is not possible, the use of growth factors can be sufficient to induce repair. If injection of the growth factor leads to repair of ECM, then growth factors alone may be sufficient to stimulate the cells [46]. If the cells are not responsive to the growth factors, then it may become necessary to supplement the nucleus pulposus with cell-seeded scaffold or an externally produced nucleus pulposus tissue [46].

Hydrogels are self-fitting shape memory construct owing to their unique properties of high water content, biodegradability, tunability and bio-compatibility [47]. Collagen can be used as an injectable hydrogel for the repair of nucleus pulposus and annulus fibrosis [48]. In a study, type 1 collagen and fibrin were used to prepare injectable hydrogels crosslinked with genipin. This preparation showed significant sealing effect on annular defects in an in vivo rat tail model [49, 50]. The challenges associated with using hydrogels are gel formation, leakage and poor mechanical property [51, 52]. The production of hydrogel with optimum properties like scaffold flexibility and shape memory property has remained a challenge [53, 54].

Intervertebral disc degeneration ensues due to loss of rounded chondrocyte like nucleus pulposus cells and their replacement with fibroblast-like cells [55]. The inflammation is high in the degenerated disc owing to increased levels of pro-inflammatory cytokines like Interleukin-β and Tumour necrosis factor-α. Intervertebral disc degenerative disease occurs as a result of high catabolism and less anabolism in the extracellular matrix [56]. The cycle of degeneration starts with reduced oxygen levels and increasing acidic environment in the disc which are harmful to the extracellular matrix of the intervertebral disc [57].

Genetic factors are implicated in disc degeneration. The lack of balance between anabolism and catabolism in the disc space are influenced by the genetic signalling. It is hypothesised that if gene transfers are done to disc space that regulate the extracellular matrix production, the process of disc degeneration can be alleviated. Few animal models have been studied which showed successful outcomes with gene transfers [58].

Gene editing technology by targeting clustered regularly interspaced short palindromic repeats (CRISPR) system and mammalian target of rapamycin (mTOR) signalling can be used to modify specific target genes to obtain desired outcomes. However, immunogenicity and mutations are the potential side effects that arise from vectors. Selecting suitable vectors to target specific genes involved in the degeneration process of disc may yield promising outcomes in future.

Nano drug delivery systems as studied by Liu et al. are found to have many advantages in treating degenerative disc disorders [59]. The advantages of nano drug delivery systems are as follows:

1. They are bio-degradable, have good bio-compatibility and non-toxic.
2. Ability for prolonged drug release which increases efficacy, reduces the cost and improves compliance [60, 61].
3. The natural materials can be used for nano drug delivery and as the composition is similar to the matrix of intervertebral disc and cartilage, it creates a native environment for the healing of intervertebral disc [59].

The most common nano-carriers used are liposomes, polymer micelles, nanohydrogels, polymeric nanoparticles, inorganic nanoparticles, exosomes and nanofibers [59].

If all the efforts to restore the degenerative disc fails, the only option is to treat the symptoms of the patient. As the science and technology is progressing by each passing day, the minimally invasive techniques have gained upper hand in treating degenerative disc diseases [62]. Kambin, in the late 1990s adapted arthroscope to treat the symptomatic patients with lumbar disc herniations [63]. Arthroscope gradually developed into full-fledged spine endoscope. Multiple studies were done to study the efficacy of endoscopy in comparison to conventional techniques. The studies reported equivalent or better outcomes in comparison to conventional techniques [64–66]. Endoscopic techniques have less post-operative pain owing to minimal tissue injury, short hospital duration and faster recovery [62]. The application of endoscopy at present has the capability to deal with a wide spectrum of degenerative disc disorders ranging from simple decompression to single or multi-level fusions.

The various types of decompression which have become popular in the recent decades are.

Transforaminal endoscopic decompression, Interlaminar endoscopic decompression, Biportal endoscopic decompression and endoscopic foraminoplasties. Even, lumbar stenosis is amenable to be treated by endoscopy with the progress in the instrumentation.

The fusion surgeries are no longer the same open wide decompressions and fusions but various routes and techniques are popularised recently. Endoscopic fusions are becoming popular day by day. The fusions with lateral approaches like OLIF and DLIF are also being done according to etiologies. The transkambin fusion is the latest development and serves fusion of the intervertebral disc through the kambin's triangle.

There are multiple studies that compare the various technique of decompression and the outcomes. In a study by Hwang YH et al., all the modes of decompression, namely, conventional decompression, full endoscopic decompression and biportal decompression were studied [67]. The study group evaluated the laboratory markers like creatine phosphokinase (CPK), Lactate dehydrogenase (LDH), ESR, and CRP which were related to the muscle damage [67]. The study group also studied the radiological parameters and clinical parameters. The findings of this extensive multicentric study were that endoscopic surgery has excellent muscle-preserving ability while the clinical outcomes are similar to the standard techniques.

15.4 Advances in Grafts for Fusion

In some degenerative conditions when decompression alone does not suffice and fusion is required to stabilise the segment, bone grafts are used to facilitate fusion. The natural graft which is time tested is the autograft from iliac crest or the bone from the spine which is obtained during decompression. The iliac crest graft has many disadvantages like pain at the donor site, occasional hernias, hematoma formation, etc. [68]. Allografts are devoid of the above complications but allograft displays only osteoconductive property. There is some risk of transmission of HIV or Hep B/C [68]. With these concerns, synthetic grafts were discovered.

Synthetic grafts are mainly of three types.

1. Polymer-based materials.
2. Ceramics.
3. Bio-active glasses.

Ceramics exist in porous and compact forms. These materials can be moldable into shapes and sizes. Porous forms aid the cell adhesion, proliferation and nutrient infiltration [69]. Ceramics are inert and do not elicit immunogenic response. But the ceramics have low mechanical strength and fragility [70]. Calcium sulfate has reduced strength and susceptible to breakage. Due to this limitation, it is used only in small defects [71]. Calcium phosphate has both osteoconductive and osteointegrative property [68]. It has greater strength under loads. The cement formulations of calcium phosphate have long degradation rate [69–71].

Silicon nitride has greater osteoconductivity and osteointegration. It also has high mechanical strength and improved resistance to thermal and heat shock [68]. At present, third-generation ceramics are being used in the market. AttraX and MagnetOs are third-generation calcium phosphate ceramics with improved bio activity [68]. AttraX demonstrated a fusion rate of 55% compared to 52% when autograft was used [72]. MagnetOs granules and putty with autograft had higher fusion rates of 92% and 83%, respectively [73].

15.4.1 Synthetic Polymers

The most common polymers are derived from poly-a-hydroxy acids [68]. Poly-l lactic acid, Poly lactic-co-glycolic acid, polylactide, polyglycolide and polymethyl methacrylate are few examples. These synthetic polymers can be used along with ceramics, with autografts and for growth factor delivery [68].

15.4.2 Synthetic Peptides

The p-15 substitute is a bone matrix biomimetic composed of mineral, synthetic residue and an amino acid sequence similar to type 1 collagen binding domain [68]. This substitute promotes extracellular matrix formation, cell migration and proliferation [74]. It is commercially known as i-factor. This product has excellent fusion rates in lumbar interbody fusion surgeries [75, 76].

15.4.3 Bio-Active Glass

These are composed of inorganic metallic oxides like silicon di oxide and have osteoconductive properties. Some substitutes may contain sodium di oxide and calcium di oxide. These substitutes have better durability and strength [68].

15.5 Summary

The degenerative spine disorders are on the rise throughout the globe as the life expectancy is increasing. Attempts should be made to prevent the degenerative disorders as much as possible. The newer innovations like mesenchymal stem cells and PRP help in restoration of disc matrix. The advancements and incorporation of 3D printing to create custom scaffolds has changed the treatment in today's world. With substitutes like BMP-2 and i-factor, the fusion rates may reach more than 95%. Combination of scaffolds and autografts or allografts can be used with bone marrow to improve the fusion rates and at the same time reduce the ill effects of auto grafting. If symptoms are severe and intervention is required, then minimally invasive spine surgeries like endoscopic spine surgery can be adapted to alleviate the symptoms with minimal damage to the normal tissues structures.

References

1. Goldberg JL, Garton A, Singh S, Kirnaz S, Sommer F, Carnevale JA, et al. Challenges in the development of biological approaches for the treatment of degenerative disc disease. World Neurosurg. 2022;157:274–81.
2. Badhiwala JH, Ahuja CS, Akbar MA, Witiw CD, Nassiri F, Furlan JC, et al. Degenerative cervical myelopathy — update and future directions. Nat Rev Neurol. 2020;16(2):108–24.
3. Kwon J won, Moon SH, Park SY, Park SJ, Park SR, Suk KS, et al. Lumbar spinal stenosis: review update 2022. Asian Spine J 2022;16(5):789–798.
4. Harmon MD, Ramos DM, Nithyadevi D, Bordett R, Rudraiah S, Nukavarapu SP, et al. Growing a backbone – functional biomaterials and structures for intervertebral disc (IVD) repair and regeneration: challenges, innovations, and future directions. Biomater Sci. 2020;8(5):1216–39.
5. Kalson NS, Richardson S, Hoyland JA. Strategies for regeneration of the intervertebral disc. Regen Med. 2008;3(5):717–29.
6. Thompson JP, Oegema TR, Bradford DS. Stimulation of mature canine intervertebral disc by growth factors. Spine (Phila Pa 1976). 1991;16(3):253–60.
7. Li J, Kim KS, Park JS, Elmer WA, Hutton WC, Yoon ST. BMP-2 and CDMP-2: stimulation of chondrocyte production of proteoglycan. J Orthop Sci. 2003;8(6):829–35.
8. Zhang Y, An HS, Song S, Toofanfard M, Masuda K, Andersson GBJ, et al. Growth factor osteogenic protein-1: differing effects on cells from three distinct zones in the bovine intervertebral disc. Am J Phys Med Rehabil. 2004;83(7):515–21.
9. Masuda K, Takegami K, An H, Kumano F, Chiba K, Andersson GBJ, et al. Recombinant osteogenic protein-1 upregulates extracellular matrix metabolism by rabbit annulus fibrosus and nucleus pulposus cells cultured in alginate beads. J Orthop Res. 2003;21(5):922–30.
10. Masuda K, Imai Y, Okuma M, Muehleman C, Nakagawa K, Akeda K, et al. Osteogenic protein-1 injection into a degenerated disc induces the restoration of disc height and structural changes in the rabbit anular puncture model. Spine (Phila Pa 1976). 2006;31(7):742–54.

11. Walsh AJL, Bradford DS, Lotz JC. In vivo growth factor treatment of degenerated intervertebral discs. Spine (Phila Pa 1976). 2004;29(2):156–63.
12. An HS, Takegami K, Kamada H, Nguyen CM, Thonar EJMA, Singh K, et al. Intradiscal Administration of Osteogenic Protein-1 increases intervertebral disc height and proteoglycan content in the nucleus Pulposus in Normal adolescent rabbits. Spine. 2005;30(1):25.
13. Klein RG, Eek BCJ, O'Neill CW, Elin C, Mooney V, Derby RR. Biochemical injection treatment for discogenic low back pain: a pilot study. Spine J. 2003;3(3):220–6.
14. Nishida K, Kang JD, Gilbertson LG, Moon SH, Suh JK, Vogt MT, et al. Modulation of the biologic activity of the rabbit intervertebral disc by gene therapy: an in vivo study of adenovirus-mediated transfer of the human transforming growth factor beta 1 encoding gene. Spine (Phila Pa 1976). 1999;24(23):2419–25.
15. Le Maitre CL, Hoyland JA, Freemont AJ. Interleukin-1 receptor antagonist delivered directly and by gene therapy inhibits matrix degradation in the intact degenerate human intervertebral disc: an in situ zymographic and gene therapy study. Arthritis Res Ther. 2007;9(4):R83.
16. Gruber HE, Johnson TL, Leslie K, Ingram JA, Martin D, Hoelscher G, et al. Autologous intervertebral disc cell implantation: a model using Psammomys obesus, the sand rat. Spine (Phila Pa 1976). 2002;27(15):1626–33.
17. Okuma M, Mochida J, Nishimura K, Sakabe K, Seiki K. Reinsertion of stimulated nucleus pulposus cells retards intervertebral disc degeneration: an in vitro and in vivo experimental study. J Orthop Res. 2000;18(6):988–97.
18. Stock UA, Vacanti JP. Tissue engineering: current state and prospects. Annu Rev Med. 2001;52:443–51.
19. Shao X, Hunter CJ. Developing an alginate/chitosan hybrid fiber scaffold for annulus fibrosus cells. J Biomed Mater Res A. 2007;82(3):701–10.
20. Halloran DO, Grad S, Stoddart M, Dockery P, Alini M, Pandit AS. An injectable cross-linked scaffold for nucleus pulposus regeneration. Biomaterials. 2008;29(4):438–47.
21. Mouw JK, Case ND, Guldberg RE, Plaas AHK, Levenston ME. Variations in matrix composition and GAG fine structure among scaffolds for cartilage tissue engineering. Osteoarthr Cartil. 2005;13(9):828–36.
22. Alini M, Li W, Markovic P, Aebi M, Spiro RC, Roughley PJ. The potential and limitations of a cell-seeded collagen/hyaluronan scaffold to engineer an intervertebral disc-like matrix. Spine [Internet]. 2003 Mar 1 [cited 2024 Sep 4];28(5). Available from: https://pubmed.ncbi.nlm.nih.gov/12616155/
23. Séguin CA, Grynpas MD, Pilliar RM, Waldman SD, Kandel RA. Tissue engineered nucleus pulposus tissue formed on a porous calcium polyphosphate substrate. Spine [Internet]. 2004 Jun 15 [cited 2024 Sep 4];29(12). Available from: https://pubmed.ncbi.nlm.nih.gov/15187628/
24. Helen W, Gough JE. Cell viability, proliferation and extracellular matrix production of human annulus fibrosus cells cultured within PDLLA/Bioglass composite foam scaffolds in vitro. Acta biomaterialia [Internet]. 2008 Mar [cited 2024 Sep 4];4(2). Available from: https://pubmed.ncbi.nlm.nih.gov/18023627/
25. Ma Z, Gao C, Gong Y, Shen J. Cartilage tissue engineering PLLA scaffold with surface immobilized collagen and basic fibroblast growth factor. Biomaterials. 2005;26(11):1253–9.
26. Kopecek J. Polymer chemistry: swell gels. Nature. 2002;417(6887):388–9. 391
27. Jeong B, Kim SW, Bae YH. Thermosensitive sol–gel reversible hydrogels. Adv Drug Deliv Rev. 2012;(64):154–62.
28. Cloyd JM, Malhotra NR, Weng L, Chen W, Mauck RL, Elliott DM. Material properties in unconfined compression of human nucleus pulposus, injectable hyaluronic acid-based hydrogels and tissue engineering scaffolds. Eur Spine J. 2007;16(11):1892–8.
29. Allen MJ, Schoonmaker JE, Bauer TW, Williams PF, Higham PA, Yuan HA. Preclinical evaluation of a poly (vinyl alcohol) hydrogel implant as a replacement for the nucleus pulposus. Spine (Phila Pa 1976). 2004;29(5):515–23.
30. Thomas J, Gomes K, Lowman A, Marcolongo M. The effect of dehydration history on PVA/PVP hydrogels for nucleus pulposus replacement. J Biomed Mater Res B Appl Biomater. 2004;69(2):135–40.

31. Pirvu TN, Schroeder JE, Peroglio M, Verrier S, Kaplan L, Richards RG, et al. Platelet-rich plasma induces annulus fibrosus cell proliferation and matrix production. Eur Spine J. 2014;23(4):745–53.
32. Gullung GB, Woodall JW, Tucci MA, James J, Black DA, McGuire RA. Platelet-rich plasma effects on degenerative disc disease: analysis of histology and imaging in an animal model. Evid Based Spine Care J. 2011;2(4):13–8.
33. Biological repair of the degenerated intervertebral disc by the injection of growth factors [Internet]. [cited 2024 Sep 4]. Available from: http://ouci.dntb.gov.ua/en/works/4k28xz67/
34. Le Maitre CL, Freemont AJ, Hoyland JA. A preliminary in vitro study into the use of IL-1Ra gene therapy for the inhibition of intervertebral disc degeneration. Int J Exp Pathol. 2006;87(1):17–28.
35. Tobinick EL. Perispinal delivery of CNS drugs. CNS Drugs. 2016;30:469–80.
36. Richardson SM, Kalamegam G, Pushparaj PN, Matta C, Memic A, Khademhosseini A, et al. Mesenchymal stem cells in regenerative medicine: focus on articular cartilage and intervertebral disc regeneration. Methods. 2016;99:69–80.
37. Clarke LE, McConnell JC, Sherratt MJ, Derby B, Richardson SM, Hoyland JA. Growth differentiation factor 6 and transforming growth factor-beta differentially mediate mesenchymal stem cell differentiation, composition, and micromechanical properties of nucleus pulposus constructs. Arthritis Res Ther. 2014;16(2):R67.
38. Peroglio M, Eglin D, Benneker LM, Alini M, Grad S. Thermoreversible hyaluronan-based hydrogel supports in vitro and ex vivo disc-like differentiation of human mesenchymal stem cells. Spine J [Internet]. 2013 Nov [cited 2024 Sep 4];13(11). Available from: https://pubmed.ncbi.nlm.nih.gov/23830827/
39. Buckley CT, Kelly DJ. Expansion in the presence of FGF-2 enhances the functional development of cartilaginous tissues engineered using infrapatellar fat pad derived MSCs. J Mech Behav Biomed Mater. 2012;11:102–11.
40. Orozco L, Soler R, Morera C, Alberca M, Sánchez A, García-Sancho J. Intervertebral disc repair by autologous mesenchymal bone marrow cells: a pilot study. Transplantation [Internet] 2011 [cited 2024 Sep 4];92(7). Available from: https://pubmed.ncbi.nlm.nih.gov/21792091/
41. Omlor GW, Nerlich AG, Lorenz H, Bruckner T, Richter W, Pfeiffer M, et al. Injection of a polymerized hyaluronic acid/collagen hydrogel matrix in an in vivo porcine disc degeneration model. Eur Spine J. 2012;21(9):1700–8.
42. Gansau J, Buckley CT. Incorporation of collagen and hyaluronic acid to enhance the bioactivity of fibrin-based hydrogels for nucleus Pulposus regeneration. J Funct Biomater. 2018;9(3):43.
43. Fuchs S, Erbe T, Fischer HL, Tibesku CO. Intraarticular hyaluronic acid versus glucocorticoid injections for nonradicular pain in the lumbar spine. J Vasc Interv Radiol. 2005;16(11):1493–8.
44. Amirdelfan K, Bae H, McJunkin T, DePalma M, Kim K, Beckworth WJ, et al. Allogeneic mesenchymal precursor cells treatment for chronic low back pain associated with degenerative disc disease: a prospective randomized, placebo-controlled 36-month study of safety and efficacy. Spine J [Internet] 2021 Feb [cited 2024 Sep 2];21(2). Available from: https://pubmed.ncbi.nlm.nih.gov/33045417/
45. Sakai D, Andersson GBJ. Stem cell therapy for intervertebral disc regeneration: obstacles and solutions. Nat Rev Rheumatol. 2015;11(4):243–56.
46. O'Halloran DM, Pandit AS. Tissue-engineering approach to regenerating the intervertebral disc. Tissue engineering [Internet] 2007 Aug [cited 2024 Sep 2];13(8). Available from: https://pubmed.ncbi.nlm.nih.gov/17518718/
47. Koo YW, Lim CS, Darai A, Lee J, Kim W, Han I, Kim GH. Shape-memory collagen scaffold combined with hyaluronic acid for repairing intervertebral disc. Biomaterials research [Internet] 2023 [cited 2024 Sep 2];27(1). Available from: https://pubmed.ncbi.nlm.nih.gov/36991502/
48. Friedmann A, Baertel A, Schmitt C, Ludtka C, Milosevic J, Meisel HJ, et al. Intervertebral disc regeneration injection of a cell-loaded collagen hydrogel in a sheep model. Int J Mol Sci. 2021;22(8):4248.

49. Moriguchi Y, Borde B, Berlin C, Wipplinger C, Sloan SR, Kirnaz S, et al. In vivo annular repair using high-density collagen gel seeded with annulus fibrosus cells. Acta Biomater. 2018;79:230–8.
50. Schek RM, Michalek AJ, Iatridis JC. Genipin-crosslinked fibrin hydrogels as a potential adhesive to augment intervertebral disc annulus repair. Eur Cell Mater. 2011;21:373–83.
51. Tan H, Marra KG. Injectable, biodegradable hydrogels for tissue engineering applications. Materials (Basel). 2010;3(3):1746–67.
52. Liu L, Gao Q, Lu X, Zhou H. In situ forming hydrogels based on chitosan for drug delivery and tissue regeneration. Asian J Pharma Sci. 2016;11(6):673–83.
53. Guillaume O, Daly A, Lennon K, Gansau J, Buckley SF, Buckley CT. Shape-memory porous alginate scaffolds for regeneration of the annulus fibrosus: effect of TGF-β3 supplementation and oxygen culture conditions. Acta Biomater. 2014;10(5):1985–95.
54. Lee J, Kim G. Collagen-based shape-memory biocomposites. App Phys Rev. 2022;9(2):021415.
55. van Uden S, Silva-Correia J, Oliveira JM, Reis RL. Current strategies for treatment of intervertebral disc degeneration: substitution and regeneration possibilities. Biomater Res. 2017;21:22.
56. Roh EJ, Darai A, Kyung JW, Choi H, Kwon SY, Bhujel B, et al. Genetic therapy for intervertebral disc degeneration. Int J Mol Sci. 2021;22(4):1579.
57. Sampara P, Banala RR, Vemuri SK, Av GR, Gpv S. Understanding the molecular biology of intervertebral disc degeneration and potential gene therapy strategies for regeneration: a review. Gene Ther. 2018 Apr;25(2):67–82.
58. Sobajima S, Kim JS, Gilbertson LG, Kang JD. Gene therapy for degenerative disc disease. Gene therapy [Internet]. 2004 Feb [cited 2024 Sep 4];11(4). Available from: https://pubmed.ncbi.nlm.nih.gov/14724681/
59. Liu W, Ma Z, Wang Y, Yang J. Multiple nano-drug delivery systems for intervertebral disc degeneration: current status and future perspectives. Bioact Mater. 2022;23:274–99.
60. Sandhiya S, Dkhar SA, Surendiran A. Emerging trends of nanomedicine–an overview. Fundam Clin Pharmacol. 2009;23(3):263–9.
61. Losi P, Briganti E, Magera A, Spiller D, Ristori C, Battolla B, et al. Tissue response to poly(ether)urethane-polydimethylsiloxane-fibrin composite scaffolds for controlled delivery of pro-angiogenic growth factors. Biomaterials. 2010;31(20):5336–44.
62. Wu B, Yang L, Fu C, Zhuo Y, Feng X, Xiong H. Global trends and hotspots in endoscopic discectomy: a study based on bibliometric analysis. Neurospine. 2022;19(4):1093–107.
63. Kambin P. Arthroscopic microdiscectomy. Arthroscopy. 1992;8(3):287–95.
64. Meyer G, Rocha IDDA, Cristante AF, Marcon RM, Coutinho TP, Torelli AG, et al. Percutaneous endoscopic lumbar discectomy versus microdiscectomy for the treatment of lumbar disc herniation: pain, disability, and complication rate-a randomized clinical trial. Int J Spine Surg [Internet] 2020. Feb 29 [cited 2024 Sep 4];14(1). Available from: https://pubmed.ncbi.nlm.nih.gov/32128306/
65. Jarebi M, Awaf A, Lefranc M, Peltier J. A matched comparison of outcomes between percutaneous endoscopic lumbar discectomy and open lumbar microdiscectomy for the treatment of lumbar disc herniation: a 2-year retrospective cohort study. Spine J. 2021;21(1):114–21.
66. Choi KC, Shim HK, Hwang JS, Shin SH, Lee DC, Jung HH, et al. Comparison of surgical invasiveness between microdiscectomy and 3 different endoscopic discectomy techniques for lumbar disc herniation. World Neurosurg. 2018;116:e750–8.
67. Hwang YH, Kim JS, Chough CK, Cho J, Kim HS, Jang JW, et al. Prospective comparative analysis of three types of decompressive surgery for lumbar central stenosis: conventional, full-endoscopic, and biportal endoscopic laminectomy. Sci Rep. 2024;14(1):19853.
68. Inglis JE, Goodwin AM, Divi SN, Hsu WK. Advances in synthetic grafts in spinal fusion surgery. Int J Spine Surg. 2023;17(S3):S18–27.
69. Ortega B, Gardner C, Roberts S, Chung A, Wang JC, Buser Z. Ceramic biologics for bony fusion-a journey from first to third generations. Curr Rev Musculoskelet Med. 2020;13(4):530–6.
70. Nickoli MS, Hsu WK. Ceramic-based bone grafts as a bone grafts extender for lumbar spine arthrodesis: a systematic review. Global Spine J. 2014;4(3):211–6.

71. Plantz MA, Gerlach EB, Hsu WK. Synthetic bone graft materials in spine fusion: current evidence and future trends. Int J Spine Surg. 2021;15(Suppl 1):104–12.
72. Efficacy of a Standalone Microporous Ceramic Versus Autograft in Instrumented Posterolateral Spinal Fusion: A Multicenter, Randomized, Intrapatient Controlled, Noninferiority Trial – PubMed [Internet]. [cited 2024 Sep 4]. Available from: https://pubmed.ncbi.nlm.nih.gov/32080013/
73. van Dijk LA, Duan R, Luo X, Barbieri D, Pelletier M, Christou C, et al. Biphasic calcium phosphate with submicron surface topography in an ovine model of instrumented posterolateral spinal fusion. JOR Spine. 2018;1(4):e1039.
74. Axelsen MG, Overgaard S, Jespersen SM, Ding M. Comparison of synthetic bone graft ABM/P-15 and allograft on uninstrumented posterior lumbar spine fusion in sheep. J Orthop Surg Res. 2019;14(1):2.
75. Gomar F, Orozco R, Villar JL, Arrizabalaga F. P-15 small peptide bone graft substitute in the treatment of non-unions and delayed union. A pilot clinical trial. Int Orthop. 2007;31(1):93–9.
76. Loenen ACY, Connor J, Johnson S, Davis K, Hannigan N, Barnes T, et al. Peptide enhanced bone graft substitute presents improved short-term increase in bone volume and construct stiffness compared to iliac crest autologous bone in an ovine lumbar Interbody fusion model. Global Spine J. 2022;12(7):1330–7.

Living with Degenerative Spine Disorders: Coping Strategies and Support

16

Nishank Mehta and Khushboo Mehta

16.1 Introduction

Low back pain is ubiquitous—and has been reported to be the number one cause of disability across the world. The Global Burden of Disease Study 2021 has pegged the number of prevalent low back pain cases globally to be a staggering 619 million [1]. This number has an even larger economic and societal impact because it largely affects people in the working-age group—leading to loss of productivity, absenteeism from work and in extreme cases, premature retirement. In fact, low back pain has consistently been the greatest contributor to the world's burden of disability, accounting for 7.7% of all years lost to disability (YLDs) in the year 2020 [1]. While there are some serious causes of low back pain such as vertebral fractures, bone tumors, inflammatory spondyloarthropathies, and spinal infections, they account for a very small fraction of the cases—the overwhelming majority of cases are a result of the natural degenerative process in the various anatomical structures of the spine such as the intervertebral disc, the facet joints, or the vertebral end plates which then become potential nociceptive contributors.

N. Mehta (✉)
Department of Orthopaedics, All India Institute of Medical Sciences, New Delhi, India

K. Mehta
Department of Anaesthesia and Intensive Care, Vardhman Mahavir Medical College & Safdarjung Hospital, New Delhi, India

V. Kumar, P. Mishra (eds.), *A Comprehensive Guide to Degenerative Spine Disorders*, https://doi.org/10.1007/978-981-96-9091-6_16

Over years, it has been recognized and acknowledged that there is more to degenerative spinal disorders than just an anatomical basis for the pain and disability. There is a complex psychological underlay, and the presence of these psychological factors in patients living with degenerative spinal disorders is associated with an increased risk of disability despite the mechanisms not being fully understood. The importance of these psychological factors can be surmised from the fact that these have been designated as 'yellow flags', a term first used by Kendall and colleagues [2]. Studies have consistently proven that the cognitive and behavioral aspects of degenerative spinal disorders and how patients respond to pain and its management is amenable to change, and hence represent an important target for treatment [3]. The purpose of this chapter is to introduce the readers to the importance of various behavioral, cognitive, and psychological factors in the occurrence and persistence of pain in patients living with degenerative spinal disorders, help them identify the coping patterns and what can be done to address these barriers in treatment.

16.2 Coping—What It Means?

Patients living with degenerative spinal disorders suffer from chronic pain and disability—a status that is not amenable to routine pain management methods. Coping refers to a set of behaviors, thoughts, and actions which are a part of the patients' response aimed at diminishing the physical, emotional, and psychological effects of a stressful life event [4]. In the context of degenerative spine disorders, the chronic low back or neck pain is considered to be a typical stressor and hence forces the patients to use myriad coping strategies to deal with the pain and its impact in their daily lives. Coping has been identified as a key to the management of pain and chronic disability in patients with degenerative spine disorders because it determines how patients will function despite their pain and how they will respond to other validated treatments.

Coping responses and strategies have been categorized in many ways—such descriptions are not definitive and have a considerable overlap.

(i) *Active and Passive Coping*

When a patient consciously takes steps to overcome the pain and impairment or makes attempts to live well despite suffering from pain, it is referred to as an active coping strategy. Examples are visiting a physiotherapist and engaging in exercises or performing meditation and other relaxation techniques. On the other hand, passive strategies illicit a defeatist response from the patients wherein they resign or surrender to the pain and fail to take responsibility for their own pain management. Social withdrawal and excessive rest are examples of passive coping strategies. In general, patient who adopt passive coping strategies have inferior long-term outcomes.

(ii) *Problem-Focused and Emotion-Focused Coping*

Problem-focused coping refers to dealing directly with the pain as a symptom or the cause of pain as a source—this involves attempts towards understanding the etiopathogenesis of pain and then making appropriate interventions to reduce it. Examples are taking analgesics for a short term and engaging in physical therapy. Patients who have a negative appraisal of their pain instead focus on the emotional response to the pain and seek to control those emotive responses rather than the pain itself ('distraction', 'over-interpretation', 'catastrophizing')—this is referred to as emotion-focused coping.

(iii) *Adaptive and Maladaptive Coping*

Adaptive coping strategies have a positive connotation wherein patients actively adopt certain processes to manage stressors such as pain arising due to degenerative spinal disorders. In contrast, maladaptive coping strategies are negative where the emotional or behavioral response is not commensurate with the level of pain experienced.

(iv) *Approach and Avoidant Coping*

This dichotomous way of describing coping strategies emphasizes on the patients' engagement with the pain and its source. Approach coping involves efforts directed towards engaging with the pain, while avoidant coping involves efforts made by patients not to engage with pain or ignore it completely.

16.3 Assessment of Coping

Pain is a highly subjective feeling. Some patients may be able to cope extremely well to pain from a severe disease, and others may not be able to tolerate minimal discomfort. It is thus important for the clinician to know how well the patient is able to cope with the disability, so as to help in providing the correct guidance and support for him/her. Without an objective scoring system, it is very difficult to identify the ways of coping adopted by the patient. Hence, there are various available questionnaire available in literature, which may aid in patient assessment. There are two different approaches for this as highlighted by Peres et al. [4]—questionnaires which ask patients to respond to the primary stressor in their life, and questionnaires which allow the patients to tell the ways they use to cope with chronic pain.

The first type allows the clinician to identify whether or not the patient has engaged himself or herself in a strategy for coping with the distressing symptoms. To help with choosing the appropriate strategy for pain management, the pai-specific questionnaires are more advantageous. Table 16.1 enlists the various available questionnaires to understand the coping strategies used commonly.

Table 16.1 Summary of questionnaires to assess coping strategies in patients

Questionnaires for coping	Scoring system	Details
Coping strategies questionnaire—Revised [5]	27-item questionnaires covering six domains	An improvement over the original CSQ proposed in 1983 [6]. Covers domains like distraction, catastrophizing; ignoring pain sensations; distancing from pain; coping self-statements; and praying. The patients report how frequently each method is used as per Likert scale from 0 to 6, with a higher score suggestive of more use.
Pain catastrophizing scale (PCS) [7]	13 items	It is measure of the degree of catastrophizing done either in the presence of actual pain or in anticipation of pain. Each question is rated from 0 (never) to 4 (all the time), based on the frequency of the thoughts/ symptoms. Catastrophizing is broken down into three subscales for better understanding—Rumination (the patient cannot stop thinking about the pain), magnification (anxiety that the symptoms may develop into a more serious condition), helplessness (nothing can be done on the patients' behalf to reduce the pain) [8].
The ways of coping checklist	Original version by Folkman and Lazarus—7 points [9] Revised version—4 points [10]	Measures how frequently the subjects use various methods of coping like wishful thinking, problem-oriented, seeking support, avoidance, blaming. Ranges from 0 (not used at all) to 3 (most used).
Vanderbilt Pain Management Inventory [11]	5 points	Questionnaire to check the usage of active and passive coping strategies and their frequency by patients with a moderate to higher intensity pain. Active and passive coping were two internally reliable scales developed using factor analytic techniques, showing opposite results. Active coping methods showed promising positive results, whereas passive coping resulted depression, flare-up of pain, functional impairment, and reduced efficacy.

16.4 Key Concepts Related to Coping Strategies

A. *Pain, Impairment, and Disability*

While pain is the predominant symptom with which patients with degenerative spine disorders present to physicians, what has greater societal and economic repercussions is the disability brought about by that pain. Physicians must distinguish between pain, disability, and impairment to understand the complex interplay of biomedical and psychosocial factors that affect a patient.

Impairment usually has an anatomical basis and is relatively unaffected by psychosocial factors—examples are prolapsed intervertebral disc and facet joint arthropathy. Pain, however, is subjective and tends to be readily influenced by such factors. Disability refers to how the patient's personal and professional life is affected by the pain—and this is where the coping strategies come into picture. Work loss and reduced productivity are significantly affected by a patient's attitudes, beliefs, behaviors, compensation and litigation matters, emotions, approach of the healthcare providers, and social support.

B. *Bio–Psycho–Social Model*

The fact that findings on magnetic resonance imaging (MRI) often do not correlate with patient symptoms is well recognized—patients having a similar radiological picture and level of degeneration may have completely different symptoms [12]. This suggests that pathoanatomic differences alone cannot explain the pain and disability in patients living with degenerative spine disorders. The basic premise behind the biopsychosocial model in the context of degenerative spinal disorders is that the illness is a complex potpourri of biological, social, emotive, psychological, and cognitive factors—it is wrong to reduce the understanding and treatment of degenerative spinal disorders to a pure biomedical model [13]. This model explains why patients with negative coping strategies such as fear avoidance misinterpretation of symptoms and other psychosocial factors such as familial disputes, involvement in litigation, compensation claims or work-related dissatisfaction have a higher chance of developing chronicity of pain and disability in the presence of underlying disc degeneration than those where these factors are not present or relevant.

C. *Fear-Avoidance Model*

Vlaeyen and Linton described the fear-avoidance model and its consequences in musculoskeletal pain (Fig. 16.1) [14]. The model revolves around the notion

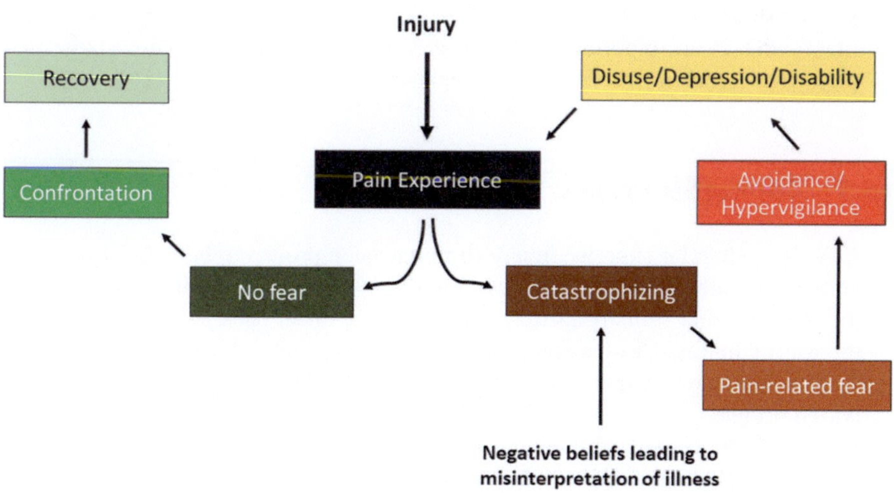

Fig. 16.1 Pictorial representation of the fear-avoidance model

that fear of pain may be more disabling in patients with maladaptive coping strategies than the pain itself. According to this model, the problem begins with a misinterpretation of an acute episode of pain—which may possibly be due to an injury—as threatening (catastrophization). Negative beliefs and attitudes subsequently lead to avoidance and hypervigilance to body sensations. Over a period of time, this develops into a vicious cycle of increasing fear and avoidance and enforces a transition from acute to chronic pain and disability.

D. *Locus of Control Theory*

Locus of control refers to the patients' subjective feeling of agency and conviction of having control over events of their own lives—including the occurrence of pain resulting from degenerative spinal disorders. Locus of control can be categorized as external or internal—patients experiencing the locus of control externally tend to treat their illness or disease as an unhappy situation over which they have no control, and hence feel helpless and respond poorly to pain management techniques. This is usually accompanied by passive coping techniques such as taking time off work, absenteeism, and prolonged rest. Patients with an internal locus of control own their illness, take responsibility for getting better and are more receptive behaviorally to physician-recommended treatments. This increases their pain tolerance and results in active coping strategies such as physical therapy, meditation, and attending back schools.

E. *Self-Efficacy*

Self-efficacy refers to the confidence of an individual to purposefully carry out an activity with the intent of achieving a desired outcome [15]. Self-efficacy has been reported to be the inter-connecting link between pain and disability in chronic musculoskeletal pain syndromes such as degenerative spine disorders. Self-efficacy beliefs, or lack thereof, have been found to be a significant predictor of physical and psychological functioning in the setting of chronic pain. Of note, it has also been suggested that self-efficacy beliefs are not static and can be modifiable in the context of one's experience during the course of treatment—this is an important assumption since it provides a possible target for physician-initiated interventions in degenerative spine disorders [15].

16.5 Coping Strategies

1. *Exercise*—Regular exercise in any form has been proven to be helpful in maintaining a healthy lifestyle. Simple stretching exercises acting on the muscles of the abdomen and hamstrings may help to reduce lower back pain. These involve the use of minimal to no equipment. Examples include knee-to-chest stretch, cat-cow position, trunk rotation, hamstring stretch, pelvic tilt, and supported bridge.

   Yoga includes postures which increase the overall strength and flexibility of the back, reduces muscle tension, and helps to alleviate back pain. However, if performed incorrectly, these postures may do more harm than good. Hence, it is advisable to seek professional help for learning the correct way. Jeng et al. [16] observed significantly less disc degeneration on magnetic resonance imaging among yoga practitioners than a matched control group.

Pilates is also a widely used form of exercise during rehabilitation, aimed at strengthening the deep core muscles, pelvic floor muscles, maintain and improve somatic motor nerve control, increase spinal control, and improve somatic stability. In a meta-analysis by Yu and colleagues [17], it was shown that Pilates has a positive effect in pain relief and improving the functionality of patients with chronic low back pain.

2. *Controlled Use of Analgesics*—Analgesics are often prescribed and taken by patients for acute flare-up of symptoms amidst the chronic complaints of degenerative spinal disorders. While such controlled use of analgesics for overcoming a pain cycle may be considered to be an active form of coping, this must be distinguished from overuse and excessive reliance on medications and pharmacotherapy, especially on a long-term basis. Prolonged intake of any medication hardly has any role in the context of degenerative spinal disorders and if such a tendency is noted in a patient, it may be considered to be a passive coping strategy with the patient refusing to take the responsibility for treatment upon himself or herself and believing that his/her pain can only be dealt with by 'external' agents.
3. *Distraction*—This may be a healthy mechanism of coping in contrast to avoidance, as it may help to temporarily take the patients' mind off the vicious cycle of pain, disability and depression. Ways of distraction may be different for each patient (e.g., change of place, going for a walk, listening to music, etc.) and these short-term strategies may help to reduce the anxiety from the stressor and may help the patient to cope in a more effective manner.
4. *Occupational Therapy and Ergonomics*—One of the most important etiologies/risk factors for back pain, especially, low back pain, is lifestyle or occupation related involving lifting of heavy loads manually, prolonged postures (sedentary lifestyle), and work-related stress. A meta-analysis by Russo et al. [18] showed that certain workplace interventions may result in reduced pain, disability, improved quality of life, and ability to work. These may range from various exercise programs (for strength/stretching/cardiovascular performance), education, use of customized insoles in footwear, stress management, lumbar support, use of mechanical lifting devices for heavy loads.
5. *Spirituality and Religion*—Spirituality is a broad concept, involving the belief in something beyond the self or in a higher power. As mentioned earlier, persistent pain has various components which influence it, ranging from biological, psychological, social, to spiritual. Many patients report using spiritual ways to cope with their pain, and apart from affecting the emotional processes, it may impact the biological mechanisms, thereby directly influencing pain. Positive spiritual coping involves a positive attitude towards problem solving, seeking support, and helping others in need. Whereas, negative forms of this spirituality may involve feelings of punishment/abandonment, blaming, and deferring responsibility to the higher power. Wachholtz and colleagues [19] have classified spiri-

tual beliefs into either positive/negative; public/private; intrinsic/extrinsic; existential/religious. These may result into psycho-social changes (meaning making/attribution/self-efficacy/distraction) which can result in alteration of neurotransmitter levels, changed threshold/pathway for pain conduction, which overall may result in either increased or decreased tolerance to pain.

6. *Praying/Hoping*—People pray when faced with a stressful situation in life and research has shown that there is an inverse relation between religiousness and depression. Such patients, along with a maintaining a positive attitude and self-assurance, show better recovery in terms of pain scores [20]. Reappraisal may help to change ones thoughts/beliefs in response to a stressful situation and may instill self-esteem and confidence to cope with the situation [21]. Hatefi et al. [22] in their research have highlighted that religious, coping in the elderly was significantly correlated with their gender, living condition, marital status, and social support.
7. *Catastrophizing*—It is a cognitive distortion that causes a person to exaggerate the negative consequences of any situation, in this case being pain. The reactions may range from worry, anxiety, repetitive thoughts, helplessness, and an exaggerated response to stress. Originally, this was noticed in patients diagnosed with anxiety or depressive disorders. Such thoughts along with the fear of pain has been proven to be associated with reduced physical activity, poor performance, inability to lift weight, and perceived disability [23].
8. *Rest/Avoidance*—Avoidance involves keeping totally away from activities/tasks/situations with which we are not comfortable. Patients with back pain may resort to avoidance of activities which they think may exacerbate the pain. Passive coping by resting significantly has been shown to be a predictor of disability and depression [24]. In studies done by Samwel et al. [25, 26], it was found that avoidance behavior played an important role in causing reduction in function of patients with chronic pain.

16.6 Summary

Chronic pain due to underlying degenerative spinal disorders can be a subjective, multidimensional experience which is difficult to analyze in isolation. The patients' method of responding to pain has important implications on both the choice and outcome of treatment methods. Patients with negative, maladaptive, and passive coping strategies are known to have a poor prognosis and spend significant time in a state of disability. Developing treatment programs and interventions that address the psychosocial aspect of pain and disability such as involvement of a multidisciplinary team that includes clinical psychologists and counselors, focusing on patient education and emphasizing their role in management of degenerative spinal disorders and creating social support systems can go a long way in improving outcomes in these patients.

References

1. Ferreira ML, de Luca K, Haile LM, Steinmetz JD, Culbreth GT, Cross M, et al. Global, regional, and national burden of low back pain, 1990–2020, its attributable risk factors, and projections to 2050: a systematic analysis of the Global Burden Of Disease Study 2021. Lancet Rheumatol. 2023;5(6):e316–29.
2. Kendall NA. Psychosocial approaches to the prevention of chronic pain: the low back paradigm. Baillieres Best Pract Res Clin Rheumatol. 1999;13(3):545–54.
3. Turk DC. Cognitive-behavioral approach to the treatment of chronic pain patients. Reg Anesth Pain Med. 2003;28(6):573–9.
4. Peres MF, Lucchetti G. Coping strategies in chronic pain. Curr Pain Headache Rep. 2010;14:331–8.
5. Monticone M, Ferrante S, Giorgi I, Galandra C, Rocca B, Foti C. The 27-item coping strategies questionnaire—revised: confirmatory factor analysis, reliability and validity in Italian-speaking subjects with chronic pain. Pain Res Manag J Can Pain Soc. 2014;19(3):153–8.
6. Rosenstiel AK, Keefe FJ. The use of coping strategies in chronic low back pain patients: relationship to patient characteristics and current adjustment. Pain. 1983;17(1):33–44.
7. Sullivan MJL, Bishop SR, Pivik J. The pain catastrophizing scale: development and validation. Psychol Assess. 1995;7(4):524–32.
8. Darnall BD, Sturgeon JA, Cook KF, Taub CJ, Roy A, Burns JW, et al. Development and validation of a daily pain catastrophizing scale. J Pain Off J Am Pain Soc. 2017;18(9):1139–49.
9. Lazarus RS, Folkman S. Stress, appraisal, and coping. Springer Publishing Company; 1984. p. 460.
10. Vitaliano PP, Russo J, Carr JE, Maiuro RD, Becker J. The ways of coping checklist: revision and psychometric properties. Multivar Behav Res. 1985;20(1):3–26.
11. Brown GK, Nicassio PM. Development of a questionnaire for the assessment of active and passive coping strategies in chronic pain patients. Pain. 1987;31(1):53–64.
12. Sigmundsson FG, Kang XP, Jönsson B, Strömqvist B. Correlation between disability and MRI findings in lumbar spinal stenosis: a prospective study of 109 patients operated on by decompression. Acta Orthop. 2011;82(2):204–10.
13. Weiner BK. Spine update: the biopsychosocial model and spine care. Spine. 2008;33(2):219.
14. Vlaeyen JW, Linton SJ. Fear-avoidance and its consequences in chronic musculoskeletal pain: a state of the art. Pain. 2000;85(3):317–32.
15. Bandura A. Self efficacy: toward a unifying theory of behavioral change. Adv Behav Res Ther. 1978;1(4):139–61.
16. Jeng CM, Cheng TC, Kung CH, Hsu HC. Yoga and disc degenerative disease in cervical and lumbar spine: an MR imaging-based case control study. Eur Spine J. 2011;20(3):408–13.
17. Yu Z, Yin Y, Wang J, Zhang X, Cai H, Peng F. Efficacy of Pilates on pain, functional disorders and quality of life in patients with chronic low Back pain: a systematic review and meta-analysis. Int J Environ Res Public Health. 2023;20(4):2850.
18. Russo F, Papalia GF, Vadalà G, Fontana L, Iavicoli S, Papalia R, et al. The effects of workplace interventions on low Back pain in workers: a systematic review and meta-analysis. Int J Environ Res Public Health. 2021;18(23):12614.
19. Rosmarin DH, Wachholtz A, Ai A. Beyond descriptive research: Advancing the study of spirituality and health. J Behav Med. 2011;34(6):409–13.
20. Smith TB, McCullough ME, Poll J. Religiousness and depression: evidence for a main effect and the moderating influence of stressful life events. Psychol Bull. 2003;129(4):614–36.
21. The Role of Positive Affect in Pain and its Treatment – PMC [Internet]. [cited 2024 Aug 29]. Available from: https://www.ncbi.nlm.nih.gov/pmc/articles/PMC4201897/
22. Hatefi M, Tarjoman A, Borji M. Do religious coping and attachment to god affect perceived pain? Study of the elderly with chronic Back pain in Iran. J Relig Health. 2019;58(2):465–75.

23. Swinkels-Meewisse IEJ, Roelofs J, Oostendorp RAB, Verbeek ALM, Vlaeyen JWS. Acute low back pain: pain-related fear and pain catastrophizing influence physical performance and perceived disability. Pain. 2006;120(1–2):36–43.
24. Crombez G, Vlaeyen JWS, Heuts PHTG, Lysens R. Pain-related fear is more disabling than pain itself: evidence on the role of pain-related fear in chronic back pain disability. Pain. 1999;80(1):329.
25. Samwel HJA, Evers AWM, Crul BJP, Kraaimaat FW. The role of helplessness, fear of pain, and passive pain-coping in chronic pain patients. Clin J Pain. 2006;22(3):245–51.
26. Samwel HJA, Kraaimaat FW, Evers AWM, Crul BJP. The role of fear-avoidance and helplessness in explaining functional disability in chronic pain: a prospective study. Int J Behav Med. 2007;14(4):237–41.

Degenerative Spine Disease and Role of Pain Medicine

17

Anurag Agarwal and Shivani Rastogi

17.1 Introduction

The spine comprises a series of vertebrae and intervertebral discs, providing support, stability, and protection for the spinal cord. They act as shock absorbers and help to move, bend, and twist comfortably. Like any other body organ, the spine is subjected to wear and tear during its lifetime. As age increases, the various types of stresses impact the functionality of the spine and its appendages. These degenerative changes may be activity-related (lack of active lifestyle or too much stress), nutritional (Calcium, Vitamin D deficiency), inflammatory origin (common rheumatological diseases like rheumatoid arthritis, ankylosing spondylitis), and degenerative conditions like osteoarthritis [1].

Degenerative changes may affect all parts of the spine, like the vertebral body, intervertebral disc, facet or zygapophyseal joints, ligament flavum, and sacroiliac joints [2]. Many times, these changes in the spine are asymptomatic and only show on some radiological examinations like X-rays, CT scans, and MRIs. However, they warrant active medical intervention only when they are causing signs and symptoms to the patient. Asymptomatic changes do not require active medical management but a strategy to prevent future loss of function through lifestyle modifications, nutritional support, etc.

Pain Medicine is an emerging super-specialty of Anesthesiology, which exclusively deals with the comprehensive management of various chronic pain syndromes, including the spine. The ability and expertise of a Pain Physician is to find the real 'Pain Generator' out of many confounding findings on an X-ray or MRI. The treatment starts conservatively for at least four weeks, but if it does not help, the role of MIPSIs (Minimally invasive Pain and spine Interventions) comes into play. MIPSIs of Pain Medicine are percutaneous and minimally invasive interventions

A. Agarwal (✉) · S. Rastogi
Dr. Ram Manohar Lohia Institute of Medical Sciences, Lucknow, India

V. Kumar, P. Mishra (eds.), *A Comprehensive Guide to Degenerative Spine Disorders*, https://doi.org/10.1007/978-981-96-9091-6_17

that can help not only in treatment but also in the diagnosis of an elusive 'Pain Generator' in a severely degenerative spine.

The common causes of pain in a degenerative spine are usually multifactorial and also depend on the age group [3].

In the Younger age group

- Poor posture (most common).
- Anxiety.
- Depression.
- Strain.
- Sporting or occupational activities.
- Whiplash injury.
- Prolapsed Cervical Disc (Figs. 17.1 and 17.2).

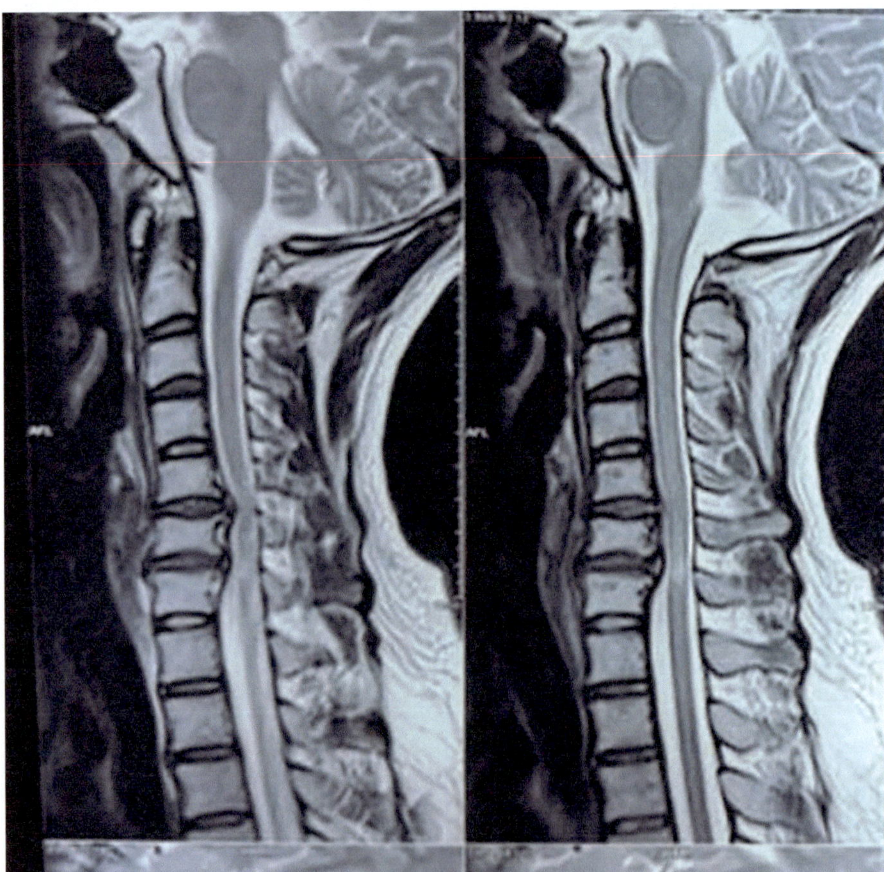

Fig. 17.1 MRI Cervical spine, Mid-sagittal view showing C5-C6 Disc bulge

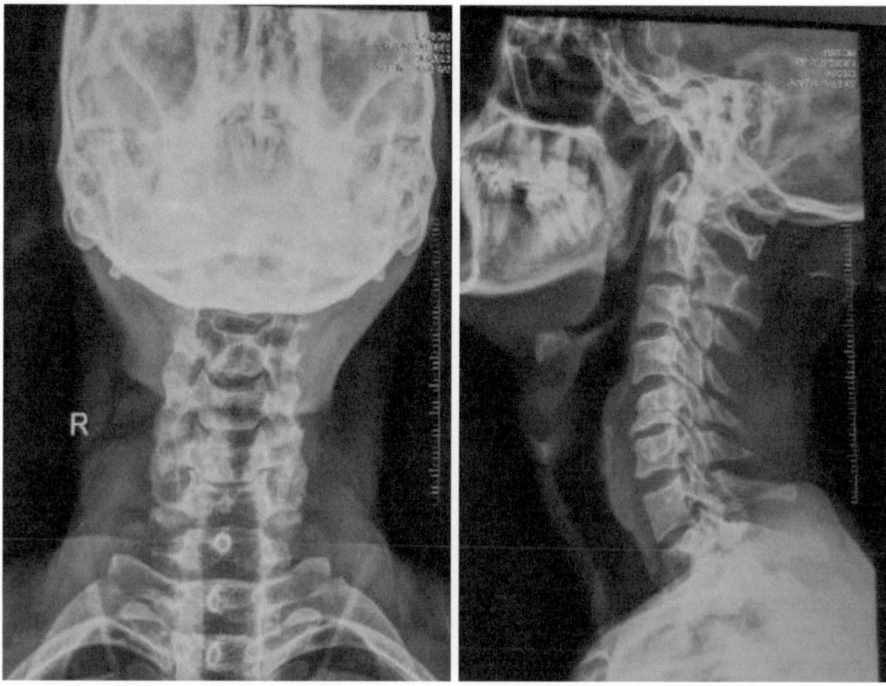

Fig. 17.2 Degenerative changes in cervical spine degenerative changes

In the Elderly age group

- Osteoarthritis of Cervical/ Lumber Facet Joints (Facet Joint Syndrome).
- Osteoporosis.

17.2 Common Red Flags, Which Must Be Ruled Out in Every Patient [4]

Malignancy or infection

- Fever, night sweats.
- Unexpected weight loss.
- History of inflammatory arthritis (rheumatoid arthritis), malignancy, infection, tuberculosis.

- Excruciating pain.
- Intractable night pain.
- Cervical lymphadenopathy.
- Exquisite tenderness over a vertebral body.

Myelopathy

- Gait disturbance or clumsy hands, or both.
- Objective neurological deficit—upper motor neuron signs in the legs and lower motor neuron signs in the arms.
- Sudden onset in a young patient suggests disc prolapse.

Other

- History of severe osteoporosis.
- History of neck surgery.
- Drop attacks, especially when moving the neck, suggest vascular disease.
- Intractable or increasing pain.

17.3 Symptoms and Signs of Cervicalgia (Neck Pain)

Cervicalgia (neck pain) is usually aggravated by movement, which may be referred to occiput, between the shoulder blades and upper limbs. It may also be associated with Cervical stiffness and vague numbness, tingling, or weakness in the upper limbs. In some cases, there may be dizziness, vertigo, or imbalance. This kind of pain is usually due to 'Cervical Facet Joint Syndrome' of cervical disc degeneration.

When neck pain radiates to the upper arm up to the hands and is associated with neuropathic features like tingling, burning, pins and needle sensation, numbness in dermatomal presentation, and motor weakness, it is known as cervical-brachialgia (Fig. 17.3). It is usually due to 'herniated cervical disc and nerve compression.' In these patients, pain is usually aggravated by movement and by weight-bearing positions such as sitting and standing and reduced by lying down posture and by coughing and sneezing (Valsalva maneuver) [5].

Fig. 17.3 Neck pain with Radiation

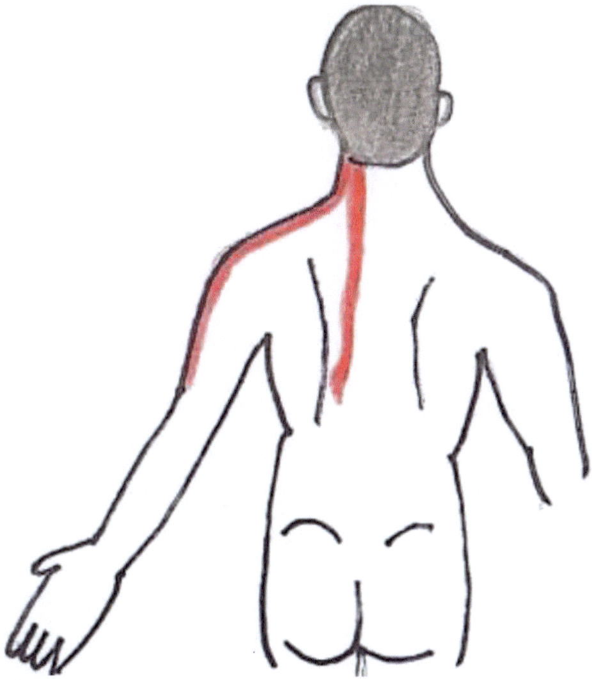

17.4 Signs of Neck Pains

i. Poorly localized tenderness.
ii. Limited range of movement (forward flexion, backward extension, lateral flexion, and rotation to both sides).
iii. Minor neurological changes like inverted supinator jerks (unless complicated by myelopathy or radiculopathy).
iv. Positive Spurling's Test for cervico-brachalgia.

17.5 Common Differential Diagnosis of Neck Pain [6, 7]

- acute neck strain, postural neck ache, or whiplash,
- Fibromyalgia and psychogenic neck pain.
- Mechanical lesions—disc prolapse or diffuse idiopathic skeletal hyperostosis.
- Inflammatory disease—rheumatoid arthritis, ankylosing spondylitis, or polymyalgia rheumatica.
- Metabolic diseases—Paget's disease, osteoporosis, gout, or pseudo-gout.
- Infections—osteomyelitis or tuberculosis.
- Malignancy—primary tumors, secondary deposits, or myeloma.

17.6 Management at Primary Level [5]

- *Use good posture*. When standing and sitting, shoulders should be in a straight line over the hips, and ears should be directly over shoulders. When using cell phones, tablets, and other small screens, keep head up and hold the device straight out rather than bending neck to look down at it.
- *Take frequent breaks*. While traveling long distances or working long hours at the computer, do intermittent stretching exercises for the neck and shoulders.
- *Adjust the desk, chair, and computer* monitor to eye level. Support the arm with the chair's armrests.
- *Quit smoking*. Smoking can increase the risk of developing neck pain.
- *Avoid carrying heavy bags with straps over the shoulder.*
- *Sleep in a healthy position*. Your head and neck should be aligned with your body. Use a small pillow under your neck. Try sleeping on your back with your thighs elevated on pillows, which will flatten your spinal muscles.
- *Stay active*. If you do not move much, increase your activity level.
- Patients should be advised to use only one pillow at night.

17.7 Pharmacological Treatment

- NSAIDs with or without Muscle relaxants.
- Low-dose tricyclic antidepressants, like amitriptyline 10–30 mg per night.
- Topical NSAIDs/Lignocaine patch.
- Hot and cold fomentation.
- TENS.

17.8 MIPSIs for Cervicalgia (Neck Pain) and Cervico-Brachalgia

The most common cause of chronic cervicalgia in younger patients is Myo-fascial pain syndrome; in chronic patients, the most useful MIPSI is *Dry Needling MIPSI* for trigger points.

Facet Joint Syndrome is the most common cause of chronic pain in elderly people; the most useful MIPSI for diagnosis this correctly is Diagnostic Facet Joint MIPSI, a percutaneous minimally invasive intervention where a small amount of local anesthetic agent like injection lignocaine is spilled over the 'cervical medial branches' [8] which supply the cervical facet joints; if patients get relief from the neck pain for the duration of the local anesthetic, the diagnosis of 'Cervical Facet Syndrome' is deemed confirmed.

The long-term treatment of cervical facet joint pain is '*Radiofrequency of Medial Branches for Facet Joint Arthropathy*'; again, a minimally invasive intervention, where a Pain Physician uses specialized Radio-frequency cannulas to ablate the medial branches that supply the facet joints (Figs. 17.4 and 17.5).

In cases of cervico-brachalgia (neck pain radiating to the upper arm) due to nerve compression in the cervical spine, the commonest effective MIPSI is '*Cervical Epidural MIPSI*,' where under a c-arm fluoroscope, a small amount of long-acting steroids are delivered at the site of nerve compression to decrease the nerve edema and pain (Fig. 17.6).

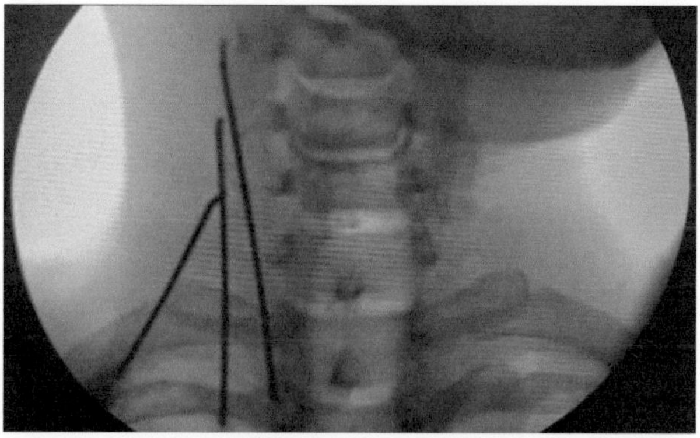

Fig. 17.4 Radio-frequency Treatment of Cervical Facet Syndrome under C-arm fluoroscopic guidance (AP View), using RF Cannulas

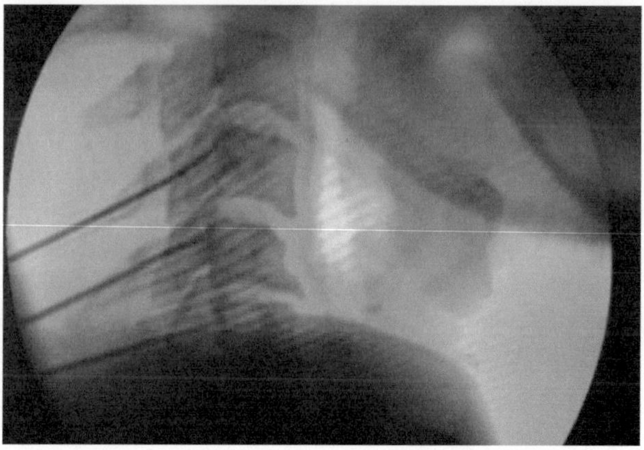

Fig. 17.5 Radio-frequency Treatment of Cervical Facet Syndrome under C-arm fluoroscopic guidance (Lateral View), position of RF cannulas

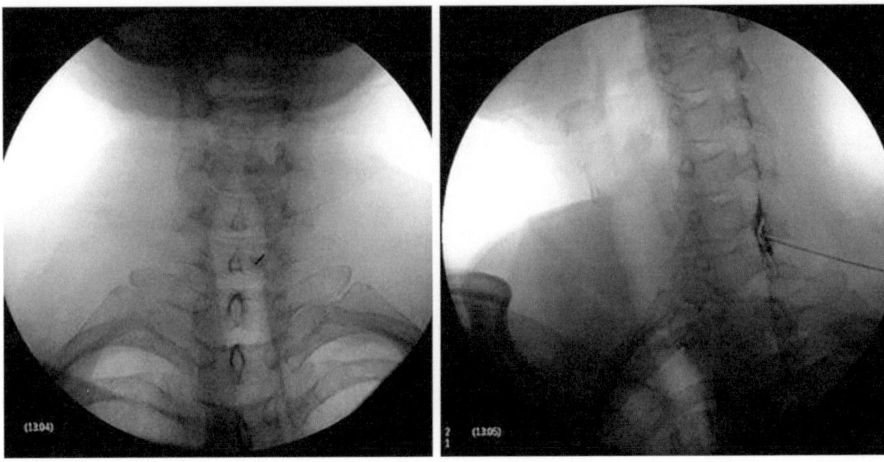

Fig. 17.6 'Cervical Epidural MIPSI' for PIVD; under C-arm fluoroscopic guidance; Left image showing Antero-posterior view showing 'Tuohy's Epidural Needle' in a "Gun-Barrel View' and right image showing the radio-opaque dye contrast in posterior epidural space

17.9 Axial Low Back Pain (Without Radicular Pain)

CLBP can be experienced at any age, and most people experience it at least once in their life. As per the World Health Organization (WHO), in 2020, low back pain (LBP) affected 619 million people globally, and it is estimated that the number of cases will increase to 843 million cases by 2050, mainly driven by population expansion and aging [9]. Prevalence increases with age up to 80 years, while the highest number of CLBP cases occurs at 50–55 years, and it is more prevalent in women [10].

Axial (Non-specific) LBP without radicular symptoms is the most common presentation of LBP (about 90% of cases); it is primarily from the muscles, ligaments, joints (facet joints, sacroiliac joints), or bones in and around the spine [11]. It tends to be localized to the lower back, buttocks, and sometimes the top of the legs, and it usually increases by loading the spine and may feel different based on motion (forward/backward/twisting), activity, standing, sitting, or resting. It may also be associated with morning stiffness when awakening and lessened back pain with activity.

17.10 Red Flags

If back pain does not improve after a few weeks or if any of the following symptoms happen with back pain:

- Numbness and tingling.
- Severe back pain that does not improve with medication.
- Back pain after a fall or injury.
- Back pain along with:

- Trouble urinating.
- Weakness, pain, or numbness in legs.
- Fever.
- Rapid Weight Loss.

17.11 Physical Examination

- Inspection, palpation, range of motion, strength testing, provocative maneuvers, and neurologic (limb strength, sensation, and deep tendon reflex) assessments.
- A straight leg raise (SLR) can be completed by raising the patient's leg to 30 to 70 degrees. Ipsilateral leg pain at less than 60 degrees is a positive test for lumbar disk herniation.
- If the pain reproduction occurs contralaterally, it is a positive test for a lumbar disk herniation.
- One leg hyperextension test/stork test: Have the patient stand on one leg and (supported by the provider) have them hyper-extend their back. Repeat this maneuver on both sides. Pain with hyperextension is positive for a pars interarticularis defect.
- Tests for Facet Joint Syndrome.
  - Extension and twisting of lumbar spine.
  - Presence of para-spinal tenderness.
- Tests for Sacroiliac Joint Syndrome.
  - Patric's/ FABER's test.
  - Yeoman's Test.
  - Sacral and Femoral Thrust Tests.

17.12 Some Common Causes of CLBP and Their Management [12]

17.12.1 Facet Joint Syndrome

Facet joint syndrome occurs when the facet joints in the spine become inflamed or irritated, leading to pain and discomfort. Facet joints are small, paired joints located between the vertebrae of the spine. They provide stability to the spine and allow for various movements, such as bending and twisting. When these joints are affected, facet joint syndrome can result (Fig. 17.7).

Here are some critical points about facet joint syndrome:

1. *Incidence and Prevalence*: facet joints are considered to cause CLBP in 30–45% of patients of the elderly age group.
2. *Causes*:
   - *Degeneration*: Facet joint syndrome is often associated with degenerative changes in the spine, such as osteoarthritis. Over time, the cartilage in the facet joints can wear down, leading to pain and inflammation.

Fig. 17.7 Diagram of Facet Joint Arthritis

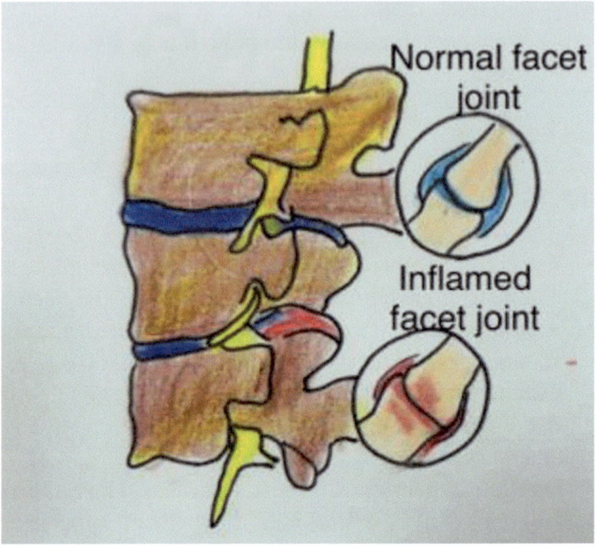

- *Injury or Trauma*: An injury or trauma to the spine, such as a whiplash injury or a fall, can damage the facet joints and trigger facet joint syndrome.
- *Repetitive Stress*: Repetitive movements or activities that place stress on the facet joints, such as heavy lifting or excessive twisting of the spine, can contribute to facet joint pain.
- *Age*: Facet joint syndrome is more common in older adults due to the natural wear and tear of the joints.

3. *Symptoms*:
   - *Localized Pain*: The most common symptom is localized pain in the affected spine. The pain is often described as a dull ache and can be felt in the lower back, neck, or upper back, depending on the location of the affected facet joints.
   - *Pain with Movement*: Pain is typically exacerbated by movements that pressure the facet joints, such as bending backward or to the side.
   - *Stiffness*: Stiffness in the spine, especially in the morning, is a common complaint.
   - *Referred Pain*: In some cases, facet joint pain can radiate to nearby areas, causing referred pain.
4. *Diagnosis*:
   - A thorough physical examination and reviewing the patient's medical history are usually sufficient to suspect Facet Joint Syndrome.
   - Diagnostic tests such as X-rays, MRI scans, or CT scans may be used to visualize the facet joints and rule out other potential causes of back pain.

- Diagnostic MIPSI of the Facet joint, where a local anesthetic is injected into the affected joint or 'Medial Branch Block' to see if it provides pain relief, is the 'Only Validated way' of confirming the diagnosis of Facet Joint Syndrome.

5. *Treatment*:
   - If conservative treatments are not effective, more invasive interventions may be considered, including the following:
     – *Facet Joint MIPSIs*: These injections (Local anesthetic agents with steroids) can relieve temporary pain by delivering medication directly to the affected joint.
     – *Radiofrequency Ablation of Medial Branches*: This procedure uses heat to ablate the dorsal root's medial branches, which transmit pain signals from the facet joints.
     – *Surgery*: In rare cases, surgery may be considered if conservative treatments and other interventions do not provide relief. Surgical options may include facet joint denervation or fusion.

17.12.1.1 Facet Joint Diagnostic and Prognostic MIPSI Technique

Facet joint Diagnostic and prognostic MIPSI is a medical procedure used to diagnose and treat pain originating from the facet joints in the spine. These injections deliver medication directly into the facet joint space to relieve pain and reduce inflammation. Here is an overview of the technique involved in facet joint injections:

Preparation:

1. *Patient Evaluation*: Before the procedure, the patient undergoes a thorough evaluation, including a medical history review and physical examination. Imaging tests such as X-rays, CT scans, or MRI scans may be used to identify the exact location of the affected facet joints.
2. *Informed Consent*: The healthcare provider discusses the procedure, its risks, benefits, and alternatives with the patient and obtains informed consent.

   Procedure: 3. *Patient Positioning*: The patient is typically positioned face down (Prone) on an examination table. The exact positioning may vary depending on the targeted facet joint(s) in the spine. A cushion or pillow may be provided to increase comfort.
4. *Skin Preparation*: The skin over the injection site is cleaned and sterilized to reduce the risk of infection.
5. *Local Anesthesia*: An anesthetic is injected into the skin and tissues, overlying the facet joint(s) to numb the skin and deeper tissues and reducing discomfort during the procedure.
6. *Needle Placement*: Using c-arm fluoroscopy or ultrasound imaging for precise guidance, the Pain Physician inserts a thin needle through the anesthetized area and advances it to the targeted facet joint(s).

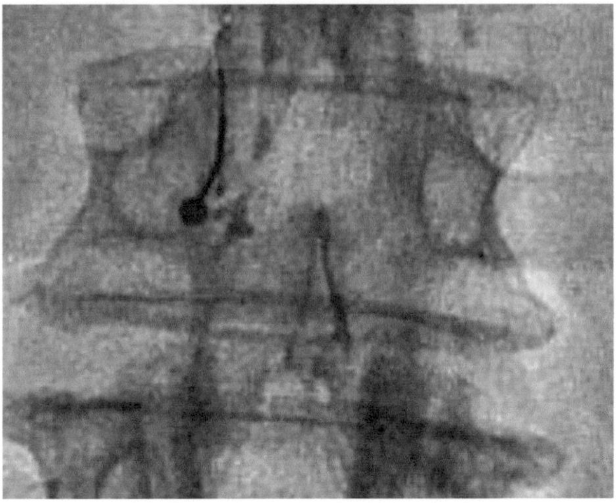

Fig. 17.8 Facet Joint MIPSI, showing a needle in the Facet Joint and radio-opaque dye highlighting the dye spread in the facet joint

7. *Contrast Injection (Optional)*: A contrast dye may be injected into the facet joint(s) through the needle to confirm the correct needle placement by visualizing the dye's spread on fluoroscopy or ultrasound (Fig. 17.8).
8. *Medication Injection*: Once the needle's placement is confirmed, a mixture of medications is injected into the facet joint(s). The medication typically includes a local anesthetic (e.g., lidocaine or bupivacaine) for immediate pain relief and a corticosteroid (e.g., triamcinolone) to reduce inflammation and provide longer-term relief.
9. *Needle Removal*: The needle is carefully withdrawn after the medication is injected.

   Post-Procedure Care: 10. *Observation*: Patients are monitored briefly after the procedure to ensure no immediate adverse reactions or complications.
11. *Activity Restrictions*: Patients may be advised to avoid strenuous activities for a certain period following the injection to allow the medication to take effect.

   Outcome Assessment: 12. *Pain Relief Evaluation*: Over the next several hours or days, patients are typically asked to assess their pain levels and any changes in their symptoms. Pain relief can vary from patient to patient and may last for a variable duration.

   Follow-Up: 13. *Follow-Up Appointments*: The pain Physician may schedule follow-up appointments to evaluate the effectiveness of the facet joint injection and determine the need for additional treatments or interventions.

Facet joint injections can provide diagnostic information (confirming that the facet joint is the source of pain) and therapeutic relief (reducing pain and inflammation). Patients must follow their Pain Physician's instructions and communicate any concerns or changes in symptoms following the procedure. As with any medical procedure, facet joint injections carry some risks, and patients should discuss these with their healthcare provider before undergoing the procedure.

17.12.1.2 Facet Joint Radiofrequency Ablation

Facet joint radiofrequency ablation (RFA), also known as facet rhizotomy, is a minimally invasive procedure used to alleviate chronic back or neck pain that originates from the facet joints in the spine. Facet joints are small, paired joints located between the vertebrae, and they can become a source of pain due to conditions like osteoarthritis or injury. RFA disrupts the nerves that transmit pain signals from these joints, providing long-lasting pain relief. Here is an overview of the facet joint RFA procedure:

Preparation:

1. *Patient Evaluation*: Before the procedure, the patient undergoes a comprehensive evaluation, which includes a medical history review, physical examination, and diagnostic imaging (such as X-rays, CT scans, or MRI scans). These tests help identify the specific facet joints responsible for the pain. Before RFA of Facet Joints, a diagnostic Facet Joint MIPSI must confirm the diagnosis.
2. *Informed Consent*: The healthcare provider discusses the procedure, its risks, benefits, and alternatives with the patient and obtains informed consent.

   Procedure: 3. *Patient Positioning*: The patient is typically positioned face-down on an examination table. The exact positioning may vary depending on the targeted facet joints in the spine.
4. *Skin Preparation*: The skin over the area where the procedure will be performed is cleaned and sterilized to reduce the risk of infection.
5. *Local Anesthesia*: Before RFA, a local anesthetic is administered to numb the skin and deeper tissues, minimizing discomfort during the procedure.
6. *RF Cannula Placement*: Using c-arm fluoroscopy guidance for precision, the Pain Physician inserts a thin, specialized needle (SMK RF cannula) through the anesthetized area and advances it toward the facet joint(s) causing pain.
7. *Radiofrequency Ablation*: Once the needle's placement is confirmed, a radiofrequency electrode is inserted near the targeted facet joint nerve. The electrode emits radiofrequency energy, which heats and cauterizes the nerve, disrupting its ability to transmit pain signals (Fig. 17.9).

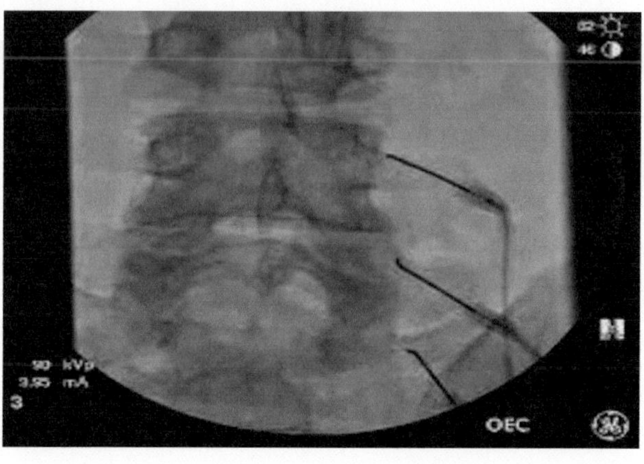

Fig. 17.9 Radiofrequency MIPSI of Lumber Facet Joints; under c-arm fluoroscopic guidance, showing 3 RF cannulas positioned at the junction of transverse process and superior articular process of target vertebrae for medial branch ablation for treatment of Lumber Facet Joint Syndrome

8. *Confirmation*: The patient may be asked to provide feedback during the procedure to help the healthcare provider verify the correct placement of the electrode.
9. *Needle Removal*: After the RFA is completed, the electrode and needle are carefully withdrawn.

   Post-Procedure Care: 10. *Recovery*: Patients are monitored briefly after the procedure to ensure no immediate adverse reactions or complications.

   Outcome Assessment: 11. *Pain Relief Evaluation*: Over the next several weeks, patients are typically asked to assess their pain levels and any changes in their symptoms. Pain relief from facet joint RFA can be significant and may last from several months to a year or more.

   Follow-Up: 12. *Follow-Up Appointments*: Follow-up appointments with the healthcare provider may be scheduled to evaluate the effectiveness of the facet joint RFA and determine the need for additional treatments or interventions.

Facet joint RFA is considered a safe and effective procedure for many individuals with chronic facet joint pain. However, as with any medical procedure, there are potential risks and benefits to consider, and patients should discuss these with their healthcare provider before undergoing the procedure.

17.12.2 Sacroiliac Joint Syndrome

The sacroiliac (SI) joint syndrome, also known as sacroiliitis or sacroiliac joint dysfunction, is an inflammation, irritation, or dysfunction of the sacroiliac joint. This condition can indeed be a cause of chronic low back pain in up to 13–25% of patients with chronic low back pain [13]. The sacroiliac joint is located at the base of the spine and connects the sacrum (the triangular bone at the lower spine) to the ilium (the large pelvic bone). When the SI joint becomes problematic, it can lead to localized pain in the lower back and buttocks. Here are some critical points regarding sacroiliac joint syndrome as a potential cause of chronic low back pain:

1. *Causes of SI Joint Syndrome*:
   - *Inflammation*: Inflammation of the SI joint can occur due to various factors, including trauma, infection, pregnancy-related changes, ankylosing spondylitis, or other inflammatory conditions (Fig. 17.10).
   - *Dysfunction*: Mechanical problems or dysfunction in the SI joint, such as excessive movement (hypermobility) or reduced movement (hypomobility), can lead to pain.
   - *Degeneration*: Similar to other joints, the SI joint can degenerate over time, causing pain.
2. *Symptoms*:
   - *Localized Pain*: Pain is typically felt on one side of the lower back or buttocks and may radiate down the leg. The pain is often described as aching, sharp, or stabbing.
   - *Pain Aggravated by Movement*: Activities like standing, walking, climbing stairs, or transitioning from sitting to standing can exacerbate SI joint pain.

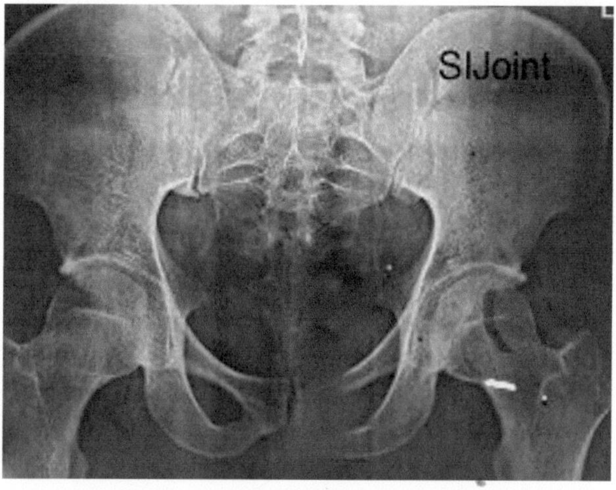

Fig. 17.10 X-ray of Sacroiliac Joint showing 'sclerosis' due to Inflammation

- *Stiffness*: Stiffness in the lower back and hips is a common symptom.
- *Pain with Weight Bearing*: Pain may worsen when the affected side is supported by weight, such as when getting out of a car.

3. *Diagnosis*:
   - *Physical Examination*: A healthcare provider will perform a physical examination to assess the SI joint's mobility and tenderness.
   - *Imaging*: X-rays, MRI scans, or CT scans may be used to visualize the SI joint and assess for structural abnormalities or inflammation.
   - *Diagnostic MIPSI of SI Joint Syndrome*: A diagnostic injection of local anesthetic into the joint may be performed to confirm the SI joint as the pain source. If it provides significant pain relief, it suggests the SI joint is the cause.
4. *Treatment*:
   - *Conservative Approaches*: Initial treatment often involves conservative measures such as physical therapy, exercises to stabilize the SI joint, and medications (e.g., NSAIDs) to manage pain and inflammation.
   - *SI Joint Diagnostic/Therapeutic MIPSI*: Therapeutic injections of corticosteroids or anesthetic into the SI joint can relieve pain and reduce inflammation.
   - *Radiofrequency Ablation*: In cases of chronic SI joint pain that does not respond to other treatments, radiofrequency ablation may disrupt the pain signals from the joint.
   - *Percutaneous SI Joint Fixation Devices*: These are the most advanced MIPSIs for chronic SI Joint syndrome patients who are unresponsive to other conventional treatments.
   - *Surgery*: In rare cases where conservative treatments are ineffective, surgical interventions like SI joint fusion may be considered to stabilize the joint.

Sacroiliac joint syndrome can be a challenging condition to diagnose and treat due to its overlapping symptoms with other causes of lower back pain. A comprehensive evaluation by a Pain Physician is essential to determine the cause of chronic lower back pain and develop an appropriate treatment plan tailored to the individual's needs [14].

17.12.2.1 SI Joint Diagnostic/Therapeutic MIPSI Technique

A sacroiliac (SI) joint Diagnostic/Therapeutic MIPSI is a medical procedure performed to diagnose and treat pain originating from the sacroiliac joint, located at the base of the spine. It connects the sacrum to the ilium in the pelvis. This injection involves the administration of medication, typically a combination of a local anesthetic and a corticosteroid, directly into the SI joint space to alleviate pain and reduce inflammation. Here is an overview of the SI joint injection technique:

Preparation:

1. *Patient Evaluation*: Before the procedure, the patient undergoes a comprehensive evaluation, which includes a medical history review, physical examination, and diagnostic imaging (such as X-rays, CT scans, or MRI scans). These tests help identify the specific SI joint(s) responsible for the pain.
2. *Informed Consent*: The Pain Physician discusses the procedure, its risks, benefits, and alternatives with the patient and obtains informed consent.

    Procedure: 3. *Patient Positioning*: The patient is typically lying face down (prone) on an examination table. The exact positioning may vary depending on the targeted SI joint(s) and the Pain Physician's preferences.
4. *Skin Preparation*: To reduce the risk of infection, the skin over the area where the injection will be performed is cleaned and sterilized.
5. *Local Anesthesia*: A local anesthetic is administered to numb the skin and deeper tissues to minimize discomfort during the procedure.
6. *Needle Placement*: Using c-arm fluoroscopy for precision, the Pain Physician inserts a thin, specialized needle through the anesthetized area and advances it to the targeted SI joint(s).
7. *Contrast Injection*: A contrast dye is injected into the SI joint(s) through the needle to confirm the needle correct position by visualizing the spread of the dye on fluoroscopy (Fig. 17.11).
8. *Medication Injection*: Once the needle's placement is confirmed, a mixture of medications is injected into the SI joint. The medication typically includes the following:
    - *Local Anesthetic*: Provides immediate pain relief by numbing the joint.
    - *Corticosteroid*: Reduces inflammation and provides longer-term relief.
9. *Confirmation*: The patient may be asked to provide feedback during the procedure to help the Pain Physician verify the correct placement of the needle.
10. *Needle Removal*: The needle is carefully withdrawn after the medication is injected.

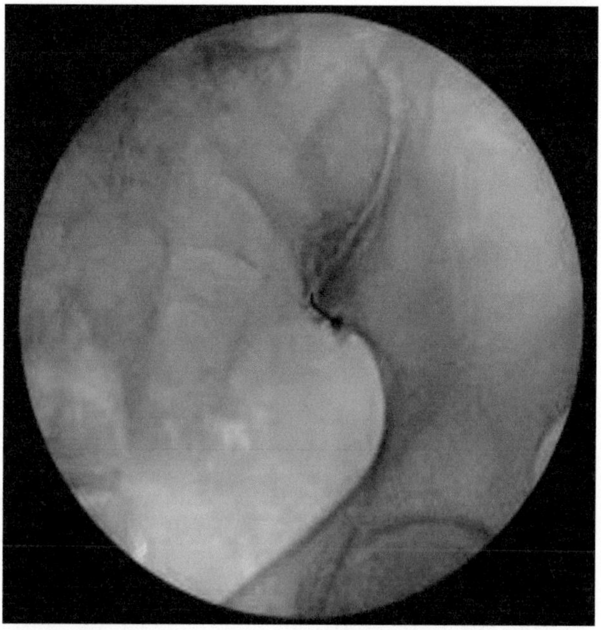

Fig. 17.11 Sacroiliac Joint Intra-articular MIPSI, showing antero-posterior view and a needle placed in right sided SI joint in 'Gun-barrel view' with dye spread inside the joint

Post-Procedure Care: 11. *Recovery*: Patients are monitored for a short period after the procedure to ensure no immediate adverse reactions or complications.

Outcome Assessment: 12. *Pain Relief Evaluation*: Over the next several hours or days, patients are typically asked to assess their pain levels and any changes in their symptoms. Pain relief from SI joint injections can vary from person to person and may last for a variable duration.

Follow-Up: 13. *Follow-Up Appointments*: Follow-up appointments may be scheduled to evaluate the effectiveness of the SI joint injection and determine the need for additional treatments or interventions.

SI joint injections are considered a safe and effective diagnostic tool and treatment for many individuals with SI joint pain. However, as with any medical procedure, there are potential risks and benefits to consider, and patients should discuss these with their healthcare provider before undergoing the procedure.

17.12.2.2 SI Joint Radiofrequency Ablation Technique

Sacroiliac joint (SI joint) radiofrequency ablation (RFA) is a minimally invasive procedure performed to alleviate chronic pain originating from the sacroiliac joint, located at the base of the spine where the sacrum meets the ilium in the pelvis. RFA involves using thermal energy to disrupt the nerves responsible for transmitting pain signals from the SI joint. This procedure is often considered when other conservative treatments have not provided sufficient relief. Here is an overview of the SI joint radiofrequency ablation technique:

Preparation:

1. *Patient Evaluation*: Before the procedure, the patient undergoes a comprehensive evaluation, which includes a medical history review, physical examination, and diagnostic imaging (such as X-rays, CT scans, or MRI scans) to confirm that the SI joint is the source of pain.
2. *Informed Consent*: The Pain Physician discusses the procedure, its risks, benefits, and alternatives with the patient and obtains informed consent.

   Procedure: 3. *Patient Positioning*: The patient is typically lying face down (prone) on an examination table. Proper positioning is crucial to accessing the SI joint and maintaining patient comfort.
4. *Skin Preparation*: The skin over the area where the procedure will be performed is cleaned and sterilized to reduce the risk of infection.
5. *Local Anesthesia*: A local anesthetic is administered to numb the skin and deeper tissues in the area where the RFA is to be done to minimize discomfort during the procedure.
6. *Needle Placement*: Using c-arm fluoroscopy for precision, the Pain Physician inserts a thin, specialized needle/ RF cannula through the anesthetized area and advances it to the vicinity of the SI joint and the nerves responsible for transmitting pain signals from the joint.
7. *Diagnostic Nerve MIPSI*: Before the RFA is performed, a diagnostic MIPSI is conducted to confirm the diagnosis. In this step, a local anesthetic is injected near the targeted nerves to confirm that they are the source of the pain. If the patient experiences temporary pain relief following the nerve block, it indicates that the SI joint nerves are contributing to the pain [15].
8. *Radiofrequency Ablation*: Once the needle's placement is confirmed, a radiofrequency electrode is inserted and positioned near the targeted nerves. The electrode emits radiofrequency energy, which heats and cauterizes the nerves, disrupting their ability to transmit pain signals from the SI joint (Fig. 17.12).
9. *Confirmation*: During the procedure, the patient may be asked to provide feedback to help the Pain Physician verify the correct electrode placement.
10. *Needle Removal*: After the RFA is completed, the electrode and needle are carefully withdrawn.

    Post-Procedure Care: 11. *Recovery*: Patients are monitored for a short period after the procedure to ensure no immediate adverse reactions or complications.

    Outcome Assessment: 12. *Pain Relief Evaluation*: Over the next several weeks, patients are typically asked to assess their pain levels and any changes in their symptoms. Pain relief from SI joint RFA can be significant and may last for a variable duration.

    Follow-Up: 13. *Follow-Up Appointments*: Follow-up appointments may be scheduled to evaluate the effectiveness of the SI joint RFA and determine the need for additional treatments or interventions.

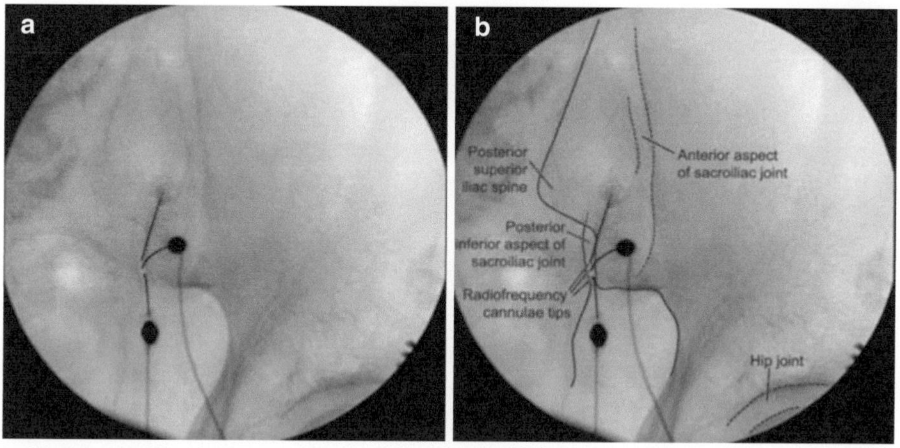

Fig. 17.12 Sacroiliac joint Radiofrequency MIPSI under c-arm fluoroscopic guidance (**a**) showing needle position at SI joint, (**b**) relation with nearby structures with needles

SI joint radiofrequency ablation is a safe and effective procedure for many individuals with chronic SI joint pain. However, as with any medical procedure, there are potential risks and benefits to consider, and patients should discuss these with their healthcare provider before undergoing the procedure.

17.13 Low Back Pain with Sciatica

A prolapsed intervertebral disc, often a herniated or slipped disc, is a common cause of low back pain and sciatica. It occurs when the soft inner core (nucleus pulposus) of an intervertebral disc in the spine protrudes through the rigid outer ring (annulus fibrosus) and compresses nearby nerves. Here is how a prolapsed intervertebral disc can lead to low back pain and sciatica [16].

17.13.1 Low Back Pain

- The protruding disc material can irritate or compress the nerves in the surrounding area, leading to localized low back pain.
- The annular fibers surrounding the disc may also be damaged, contributing to pain.
- Inflammation may occur in response to the disc herniation, causing pain and discomfort in the lower back (Fig. 17.13).

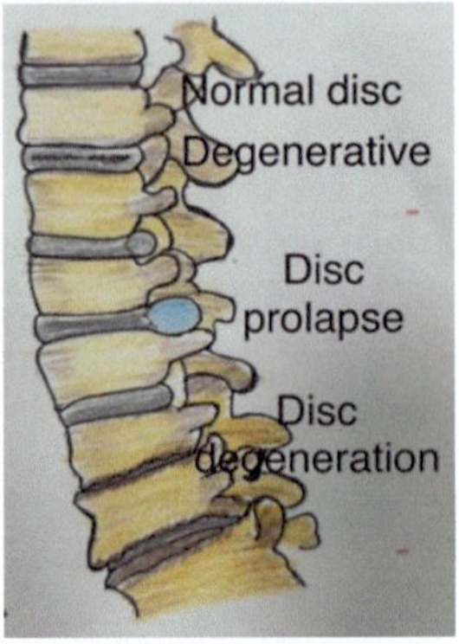

Fig. 17.13 Degenerative disc disease

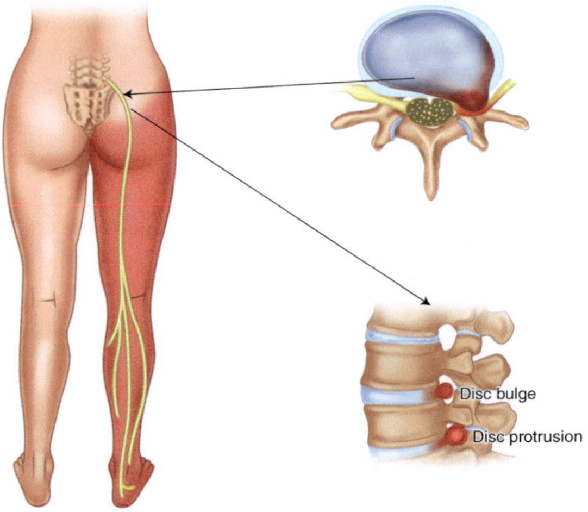

Fig. 17.14 Showing prolapsed disc causing nerve compression

17.13.2 Sciatica

- When the herniated disc material presses on the spinal nerve roots, particularly the sciatic nerve or a bundle of nerves that extends down the back of the leg, it can cause sciatica, a set of symptoms (Fig. 17.14).
- Sciatica typically includes pain, tingling, numbness, or weakness that radiates along the path of the affected nerve. This pain often travels from the lower back down one leg.
- The specific symptoms and their severity can vary depending on the location and size of the disc herniation and which nerve roots are affected.

The characteristic symptoms of sciatica include the following:

1. *Pain*: Sharp, shooting, or burning pain that may be severe and extend from the lower back to the buttocks, thigh, calf, and even into the foot in a 'Dermatomal' pattern (Fig. 17.15).
2. *Tingling and Numbness*: A sensation of tingling or numbness in the leg or foot.
3. *Muscle Weakness*: Weakness in the leg or foot may result in difficulty walking or maintaining balance.

It is important to note that not all disc herniations cause symptoms. Some people may have herniated discs that are asymptomatic or minimally symptomatic and do not require intervention.

Treatment for a prolapsed intervertebral disc that causes low back pain and sciatica may include the following:

- *Conservative Measures*: Many cases of herniated discs can be managed with conservative treatments, including rest, physical therapy, exercises to improve spinal flexibility and strength, and pain relief medications (e.g., NSAIDs).
- *Trans-foraminal Neuroplasty MIPSI*: Doctors may recommend epidural steroid injections for severe pain, where anti-inflammatory medication is injected into

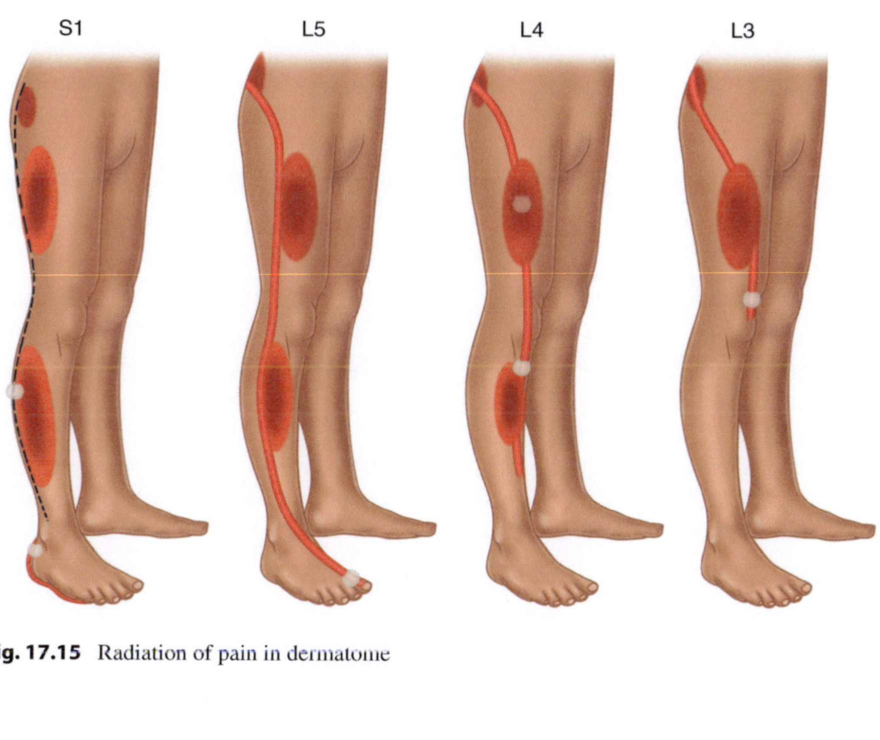

Fig. 17.15 Radiation of pain in dermatome

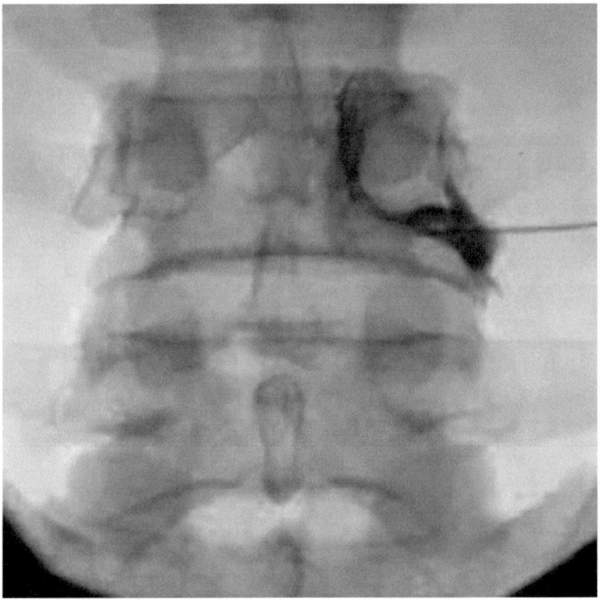

Fig. 17.16 Transforaminal neuroplasty under c-arm fluoroscopy guidance in antero-posterior view, showing a needle in inter-vertebral foramen and dye spread along the nerve root

the anterior epidural space around the spinal nerve roots to reduce inflammation and relieve pain [17] (Fig. 17.16).

Percutaneous and minimally invasive disc interventions are advanced techniques for treating PIVD (Prolapsed Intervertebral Disc), commonly known as a herniated disc or slipped disc. These procedures offer the advantage of smaller incisions, reduced tissue damage, quicker recovery times, and shorter hospital stays compared to traditional open surgery. Here are some of the percutaneous and minimally invasive disc interventions for PIVD [18]:

1. *Percutaneous Discectomy*:
   - *Mechanical Discectomy*: In this procedure, a thin tube or needle is inserted through the skin and into the disc space under fluoroscopic guidance. The Pain Physician then uses specialized instruments to remove or break up the herniated disc material, relieving pressure on the nerve. The procedure can be done with or without laser assistance.
   - *Laser Discectomy*: Laser energy vaporizes or shrinks the herniated disc material, allowing the Pain Physician to remove or decompress the disc with minimal damage to surrounding tissues [20].
2. *Endoscopic Discectomy*:
   - *Transforaminal Endoscopic Discectomy*: In this minimally invasive procedure, an endoscope is inserted through a small incision in the back and guided to the affected disc under fluoroscopic control. The Pain Physician uses the endoscope to visualize and remove the herniated disc material, preserving surrounding structures [19] (Figs. 17.17 and 17.18).

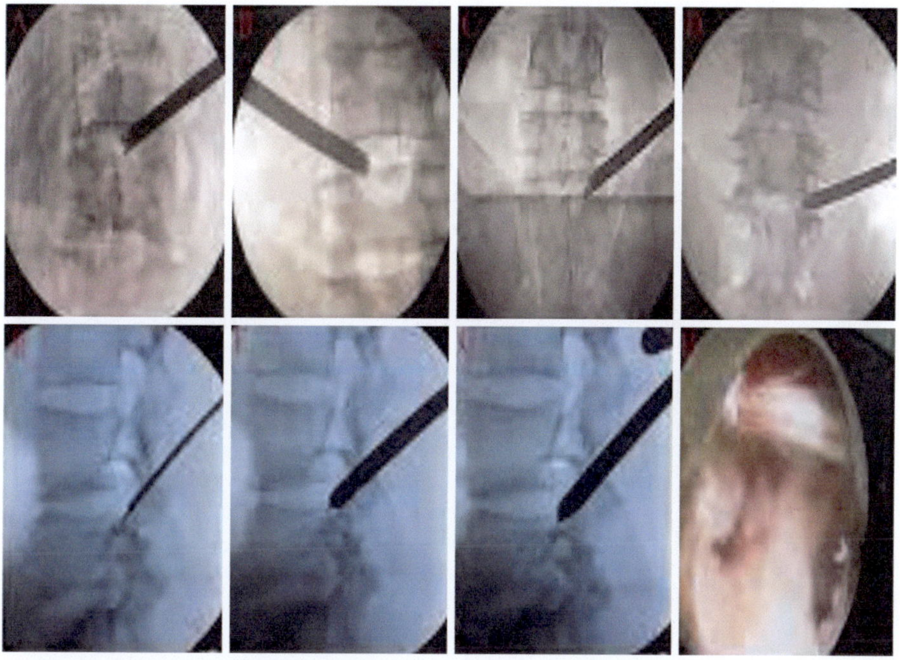

Fig. 17.17 Transforaminal Endoscopic Discectomy

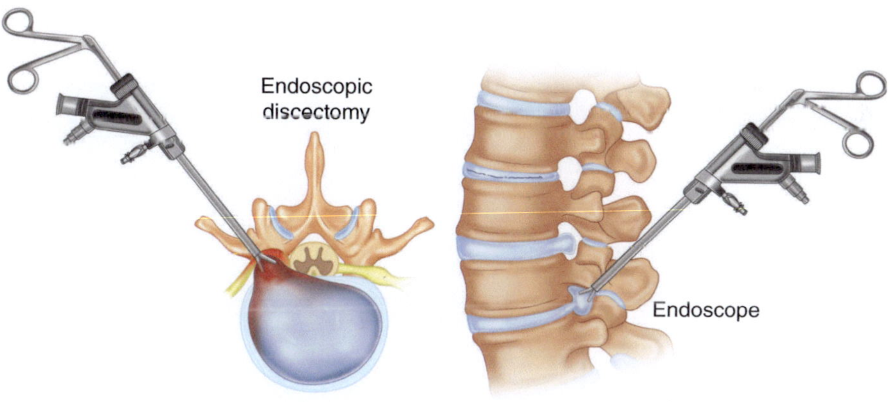

Fig. 17.18 Endoscopic discectomy of prolapsed disc

3. *Nucleoplasty*:
   - Nucleoplasty is a minimally invasive procedure that uses radiofrequency energy to treat PIVD. A needle is inserted into the disc, and the nucleoplasty system delivers energy to reduce the volume of the disc and decompress the nerve.
4. *Intradiscal Electrothermal Therapy (IDET)*:
   - IDET involves inserting a catheter into the disc space under fluoroscopic guidance. The catheter delivers controlled heat to the disc, causing collagen fibers to contract and sealing small disc tears. This procedure aims to reduce pain and improve disc stability [21].(Figs. 17.19 and 17.20).

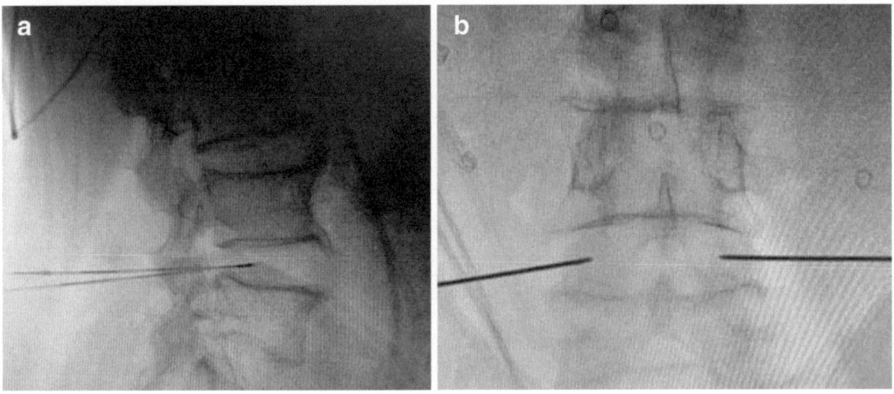

Fig. 17.19 Percutaneous Intra- Discal procedures (**a**) lateral view (**b**) in Anterio-posterior view

Fig. 17.20 Intra Discal Electrothermat (IDET) procedure under c-arm fluoroscopic guidance-lateral view

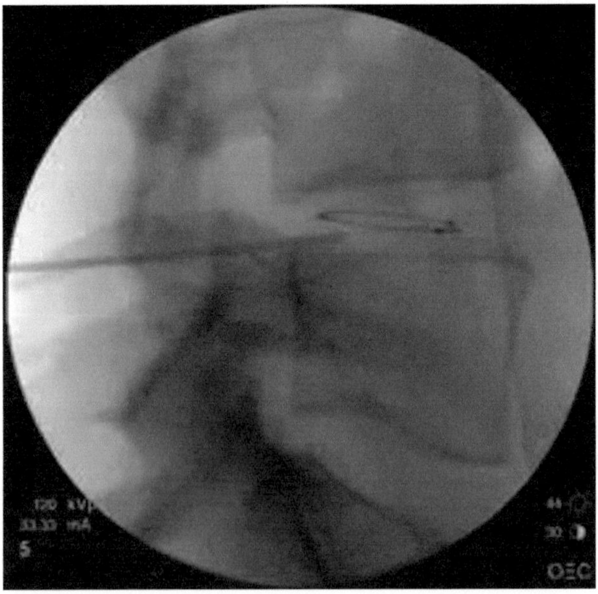

These percutaneous and minimally invasive techniques are typically performed on an outpatient basis or with short hospital stays. They are often preferred when conservative treatments have not provided relief and the herniated disc is causing significant pain or neurological symptoms. The choice of intervention depends on the specific case, including the location and size of the herniation, the patient's overall health, and the surgeon's expertise.

17.14 Percutaneous Spine Endoscopy for Prolapsed Intervertebral Disc

Percutaneous Spine endoscopy is an ultramodern MIPSI (Minimally Invasive Pain and Spine Intervention) technique used to treat various spinal conditions, including prolapsed intervertebral discs (herniated discs). It offers several advantages over traditional open surgery, such as smaller incisions, less tissue damage, reduced blood loss, shorter hospital stays, and faster recovery. Here is an overview of spine endoscopy for the treatment of a prolapsed intervertebral disc [21]:

Procedure:

1. *Preparation*: Before the procedure, a comprehensive evaluation, including medical history, physical examination, and imaging (such as MRI or CT scans) to confirm the diagnosis and assess the specific details of the herniated disc is to be done.
2. *Anesthesia*: Spine endoscopy is typically performed under local or epidural anesthesia where patient remains 'awake & aware' or, in some cases, general anesthesia. The choice of anesthesia depends on the extent and complexity of the procedure.
3. *Incision*: Instead of a large incision, spine endoscopy involves making one or more small incisions (typically less than 1 inch in length) in the skin near the affected disc.
4. *Guidance*: The Pain Physician inserts a thin, flexible endoscope (a tube with a camera and light source) through one of the incisions. The endoscope allows for visualization of the spinal structures, including the herniated disc and surrounding nerves (Fig. 17.21).
5. *Nerve Decompression*: Using specialized endoscopic instruments inserted through additional small incisions, the Pain Physician removes or retracts a portion of the herniated disc material pressing on the spinal nerve or spinal cord.
6. *Closure*: Once decompression and disc removal are completed, the incisions are closed with sutures or adhesive strips. In some cases, a small bandage or dressing may be applied.

Advantages of Percutaneous Spine Endoscopy:

- *Minimally Invasive*: Smaller incisions result in less trauma to surrounding tissues.
- *Reduced Blood Loss*: Compared to traditional open surgery, there is typically less blood loss during spine endoscopy.

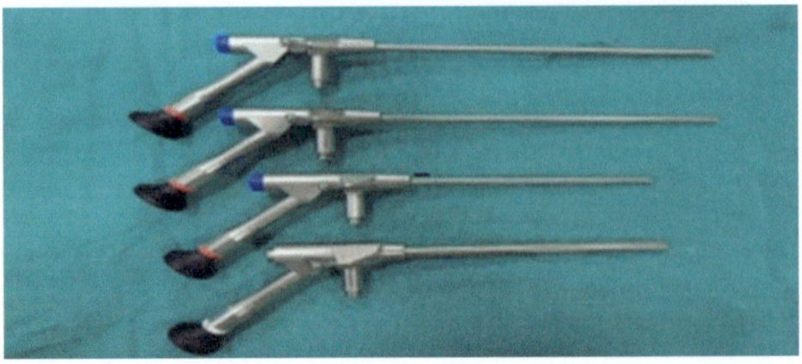

Fig. 17.21 Percutaneous Spine Endoscopes-different sizes for different indications

- *Faster Recovery*: Patients often experience quicker recovery times and shorter hospital stays.
- *Less Scarring*: Small incisions result in minimal scarring.

Candidates for Percutaneous Spine Endoscopy:
Spine endoscopy may be suitable for individuals with a herniated disc if:

- Conservative treatments (such as physical therapy, medications, and epidural injections) have not provided relief.
- There is neurological impairment, such as weakness or numbness in the limbs.
- Imaging studies confirm the location and size of the herniated disc.
- The patient's overall health permits anesthesia and endoscopy.

It is important to note that while percutaneous spine endoscopy is effective for many patients with herniated discs, not all cases are suitable for this approach. The surgical technique and approach may vary depending on the individual's condition and the Pain Physician's expertise. As with any MIPSI procedure, there are potential risks and benefits to consider, and the decision should be made in consultation with a Pain Physician who can assess the patient's unique situation and recommend the most appropriate treatment option.

Most cases of chronic low back pain can be very well managed with MIPSIs (Minimally Invasive Pain and Spine Interventions) of Pain Medicine without major open surgeries, thus obviating the need for major surgeries and general anesthesia.

References

1. Athanassiou L, Kostoglou-Athanassiou I, Koutsilieris M, Shoenfeld Y. Vitamin D and autoimmune rheumatic diseases. Biomolecules. 2023;13(4):709. https://doi.org/10.3390/biom13040709. PMID: 37189455; PMCID: PMC10135889
2. Wilson DJ, de Abreu M. Spine degeneration and inflammation. In: Hodler J, Kubik-Huch RA, von Schulthess GK, editors. Musculoskeletal diseases 2021–2024: diagnostic imaging [Internet]. Cham: Springer. p. 2021. Chapter 14. Available from: https://www.ncbi.nlm.nih.gov/books/NBK570148/; https://doi.org/10.1007/978-3-030-71281-5_14.

3. Saleem S, Aslam HM, Rehmani MA, Raees A, Alvi AA, Ashraf J. Lumbar disc degenerative disease: disc degeneration symptoms and magnetic resonance image findings. Asian Spine J. 2013;7(4):322–34. https://doi.org/10.4184/asj.2013.7.4.322. Epub 2013 Nov 28. PMID: 24353850; PMCID: PMC3863659
4. Enthoven WTM, Geuze J, Scheele J, Bierma-Zeinstra SMA, Bueving HJ, Bohnen AM, Peul WC, van Tulder MW, Berger MY, Koes BW, Luijsterburg PAJ. Prevalence and "red flags" regarding specified causes of back pain in older adults presenting in general practice. Phys Therapy. 2016;96(3):305–12.
5. Binder AI. Cervical spondylosis and neck pain. BMJ. 2007;334(7592):527–31. https://doi.org/10.1136/bmj.39127.608299.80. PMID: 17347239; PMCID: PMC1819511
6. Krasin E, Schermann H, Snir N, Tudor A, Behrbalk E. A quick and comprehensive guide to differential diagnosis of neck and back pain: a narrative review. SN Compr Clin Med. 2022;4(1):232. https://doi.org/10.1007/s42399-022-01321-y. Epub 2022 Oct 27. PMID: 36320816; PMCID: PMC9610337
7. McCormack BM, Weinstein PR. Cervical spondylosis. An update. West J Med. 1996;165(1–2):43–51. PMID: 8855684; PMCID: PMC1307540
8. Le DT, Alem N. Facet Joint Injection. [Updated 2023 Jun 20]. In: StatPearls [Internet]. Treasure Island (FL): StatPearls Publishing; 2024 Jan-. Available from: https://www.ncbi.nlm.nih.gov/books/NBK572125/
9. Wu A, March L, Zheng X, Huang J, Wang X, Zhao J, Blyth FM, Smith E, Buchbinder R, Hoy D. Global low back pain prevalence and years lived with disability from 1990 to 2017: estimates from the Global Burden of Disease Study 2017. Ann Transl Med. 2020;8(6):299. https://doi.org/10.21037/atm.2020.02.175. PMID: 32355743; PMCID: PMC7186678
10. de Souza IMB, Sakaguchi TF, Yuan SLK, Matsutani LA, do Espírito-Santo AS, Pereira CAB, Marques AP. Prevalence of low back pain in the elderly population: a systematic review. Clinics (Sao Paulo). 2019;(74):e789. https://doi.org/10.6061/clinics/2019/e789. PMID: 31664424; PMCID: PMC6807687
11. Hodler J, Kubik-Huch RA, von Schulthess GK, editors. Diseases of the brain, head and neck, spine 2020–2023: diagnostic imaging [Internet]. Cham: Springer; 2020. Chapter 18. https://www.ncbi.nlm.nih.gov/books/NBK554336/. https://doi.org/10.1007/978-3-030-38490-6_18.
12. Casiano VE, Sarwan G, Dydyk AM, et al. Back pain. [Updated 2023 Dec 11]. In: StatPearls [Internet]. Treasure Island (FL):. StatPearls Publishing; 2024.
13. Buchanan BK, Varacallo M. Sacroiliitis. [Updated 2023 Aug 8]. In: Stat-Pearls [Internet]. Treasure Island (FL): Stat-Pearls Publishing; 2024 Jan-. Available from: https://www.ncbi.nlm.nih.gov/books/NBK448141/
14. Barros G, McGrath L, Gelfenbeyn M. Sacroiliac joint dysfunction in patients with low Back pain. Fed Pract. 2019;36(8):370–5. PMID: 31456628; PMCID: PMC6707638
15. Wray JK, Dixon B, Przkora R. Radiofrequency Ablation. [Updated 2023 Jun 12]. In: StatPearls [Internet]. Treasure Island (FL): StatPearls Publishing; 2024 Jan-. Available from: https://www.ncbi.nlm.nih.gov/books/NBK482387/
16. Dydyk AM, Ngnitewe Massa R, Mesfin FB. Disc Herniation. [Updated 2023 Jan 16]. In: StatPearls [Internet]. Treasure Island (FL): StatPearls Publishing; 2024 Jan-. Available from: https://www.ncbi.nlm.nih.gov/books/NBK441822/
17. Patel K, Chopra P, Martinez S, et al. Epidural Steroid Injections. [Updated 2024 Jun 8]. In: StatPearls [Internet]. Treasure Island (FL): StatPearls Publishing; 2024 Jan-. Available from: https://www.ncbi.nlm.nih.gov/books/NBK470189/
18. Agarwal A, Rastogi S, Malviya D, Mahapatra S, Kumar V, Tripathi M, Sindhu K. Functional outcome of percutaneous spine endoscopic intervention in lumbar disc herniation- a retrospective analysis. Indian J Pain. 2021;35(2):150–6. https://doi.org/10.4103/ijpn.ijpn_78_20.
19. Lee SG, Ahn Y. Transforaminal endoscopic lumbar discectomy: basic concepts and technical keys to clinical success. Int J Spine Surg. 2021;15(suppl 3):S38–S46. https://doi.org/10.14444/8162. PMID: 34974419; PMCID: PMC9421271

20. Hosseini B, Allameh F. Laser therapy in lumbar disc surgery – a narrative review. J Lasers Med Sci. 2020;11(4):390–394. https://doi.org/10.34172/jlms.2020.62. Epub 2020 Oct 3. PMID: 33425288; PMCID: PMC7736948
21. Estefan M, Estefan V. IntradiscalElectrothermal Therapy [Updated 2023 Jun 26]. In: StatPearls [Internet]. Treasure Island (FL): StatPearls Publishing; 2024 Jan-. Available from: https://www.ncbi.nlm.nih.gov/books/NBK549805/

Preventive Measures and Spinal Health in Degenerative Spine Diseases

18

Bikram Kar and Punit Gaurav

18.1 Introduction

The five stages of a disease's natural history are susceptible, underlying, subclinical, clinical, and recovery/disability/death. Corresponding preventive health interventions have been categorised into comparable stages to concentrate on the prevention of these stages of a disease. These stages of prevention are called primordial, primary, secondary, and tertiary preventive stages. When combined, these tactics seek to reduce the risk of disease development while also preventing complications that may arise from an illness that has already manifested.

18.2 Primordial Prevention

Primordial prevention is the most recent contribution to preventive tactics, which was first discussed in 1978. It entails reducing risk factors with an emphasis on social and environmental conditions, aimed at a whole population. These kinds of initiatives are usually supported by national policy and legislation. Primordial prevention tries to protect children from as much risk as possible because it is the oldest kind of protection. Primordial prevention aims to address the underlying social factors that facilitate the onset of disease, therefore addressing the underlying stage of natural disease. One example is enhancing the availability of safe pavements in urban neighbourhoods to encourage physical activity; this reduces the risk factors for obesity, cardiovascular disease, type 2 diabetes, etc., and also demonstrates the government's commitment to tobacco and smoking cessation policies.

B. Kar · P. Gaurav (✉)
All India Institute of Medical Sciences (AIIMS), Raipur, India

V. Kumar, P. Mishra (eds.), *A Comprehensive Guide to Degenerative Spine Disorders*, https://doi.org/10.1007/978-981-96-9091-6_18

18.3 Primary Prevention

Primary prevention refers to actions directed at a vulnerable group or person. To stop a disease from ever starting is the goal of primary prevention. Therefore, people in good health are its target demographic. It often involves implementing measures to reduce risk exposure or boost immunity in those who are prone to disease to stop a disease from developing in a person who is vulnerable to subclinical disease. As an instance of primary prevention, vaccinations, adequate healthy and nutritious diet, routine yoga therapy, and exercise programmes are examples.

18.4 Secondary Prevention

The goal of secondary prevention is healthy-looking people who have subclinical versions of the disease; it emphasises early disease detection. Pathologic alterations characterise the subclinical disease; no overt symptoms that can be diagnosed during a visit with a physician are present. Screenings are a common method of secondary prevention. Screening of osteoporosis in the elderly, screening of mental health routine evaluation of eyesight, and hearing checkups are examples.

18.5 Tertiary Prevention

The goal of tertiary prevention is to address a disease's clinical and outcome phases. It is used for patients who exhibit symptoms and seek to lessen the severity of the illness and any related aftereffects. Tertiary prevention tries to lessen the impact of the disease once it has been established in an individual, whereas secondary prevention tries to stop the sickness from ever starting. Rehabilitation initiatives are frequently used as tertiary preventive measures. Examples include preventing contractures, UTIs, and bed sores.

18.6 Quaternary Prevention

Quaternary prevention is defined as "action taken to identify patients at risk of overmedicalisation, to protect him from new medical invasion, and to suggest to him interventions, which are ethically acceptable" by the Wonca International Dictionary for General/Family Practice. When this idea was first put forth by Marc Jamoulle, the majority of the patients he targeted were sick but not sick. Recently, the definition was changed to read, "measure done to shield patients or people from medical procedures that could end up doing more damage than good." Avoiding rigorous treatment of haemangioma in vertebrae, bone infarcts, Schmorl's node are examples [1].

When it comes to spinal diseases, patients requiring preventive treatment frequently need to make more frequent or longer-lasting appointments. A systematic, patient-centred approach to management necessitates the cooperation and coordination of all medical professionals. It is critical to recognise unmet requirements (such as those related to sexual health) and conduct an annual thorough evaluation in a setting that is easily accessible.

Vaccinations are crucial for infection control and preventative health, and they are especially crucial for persons with underlying chronic illnesses, such as cervical spondylotic myelopathy.

Annual influenza vaccination is very strongly advised for adults who have CSM which is associated with chronic medical conditions like diabetes mellitus and chronic kidney disease.

Pneumococcal vaccination is beneficial in adults over 65 years old, especially in those with respiratory impairment resulting in lesions at T8 or above [2].

Mammograms are less common in women with impairments and spinal problems. Lack of health insurance, issues with the qualifications and attitudes of medical professionals, and physical obstacles like inaccessible facilities and equipment are all reasons why getting a mammogram can be difficult.

Papsmear tests for women with spinal problems are frequently hindered. The most evident impediments are those that are physical (e.g. inaccessible examination tables and inaccessible premises). A further possibility is when the practitioner is inexperienced in treating speciality disorders such as bladder problems, autonomic dysreflexia (AD), or spasticity.

In males, prostate cancers and colorectal cancers are often underdiagnosed or diagnosed late due to overlapping symptoms of degenerative spinal disorders and canal stenosis. Judicious colonoscopic examinations and annual prostate-specific antigen (PSA) screening will be of great value.

Given that patients with chronic spinal disorders are more likely to have dyslipidaemia, glycaemic dysregulation, and accelerated atherogenesis, cardiovascular disease has become a major cause of death for these individuals.

Regular screening, cessation of smoking and tobacco consumption, regular exercise, and healthy practices include eating a diet high in fruits, vegetables, low-fat dairy, chicken, fish, legumes, and nuts to establish a neutral energy balance [3].

18.7 Preventive Care for Common Secondary Health Issues in Patients with Degenerative Spinal Disorders

Urinary tract infections and neurogenic urinary tract dysfunction are frequent secondary consequences that can significantly impair the quality of life and cause severe morbidity in people with bladder problems.

These are a few suggestions:

- The patient's bladder care/programme should be regularly reviewed (at least annually).
- Serum creatinine and calculated creatinine clearance to be annually evaluated to assess renal function.

- Annual renal ultrasonography evaluations of the upper tracts are required, or at least every two years.
- At baseline, urodynamic investigations should be carried out to detect any changes in function, such as UTIs, incontinence, difficulties catheterising, autonomic dysreflexia, or urolithiasis, as soon as possible [4].

People who have long-term indwelling catheters require cystoscopy since bladder cancer is more common several years after an injury.

It is best to avoid diagnosing and treating asymptomatic bacteriuria.

The quality of life can be significantly impacted by neurogenic bowel dysfunction (NBD); symptoms might include incontinence, skin breakdown, protracted bowel movements, social isolation, relationship problems, and work-related difficulties.

Regular evaluation of the bowel programme is beneficial, as is keeping an eye on the timing, diet, use of laxatives, problems (such as blood or incontinence), patient satisfaction, and stool consistency (like the Bristol Stool Chart). It is advised to consume a diet rich in fluids and fibre [4].

Autonomic dysreflexia (AD) is a potentially fatal emergency that is more common with a traumatic injury and can arise with cervical spondylotic myelopathy. A 20 mm Hg or greater increase in baseline systolic blood pressure—baseline systolic blood pressure with high degree SCI is frequently 80–100 mm Hg—is the main finding of AD. Significant headache, perspiration beyond SCI threshold, impaired vision, piloerection, and anxiety are further symptoms of AD. It is brought on by unpleasant stimuli below the lesion's level and is frequently brought on by bowel or bladder irritation [5–8].

Here are some suggestions for handling this issue:

- Patients need to be informed about AD, including its symptoms and hazards.
- To be aware of changes, plans of action, severity, and triggers, it should be reviewed frequently.
- Both a home kit and an AD management protocol and kit should be available in the office.
- When referring patients to other medical professionals, AD should be expressly included in their medical records.
- When someone with cervical spondylotic myelopathy stands up straight, they frequently experience orthostatic hypotension (OH).
- Fatigue, light-headedness, dizziness, blurred vision, dyspnoea, and maybe cognitive impairment are among the symptoms [9].

18.8 Respiratory Health

The most common cause of hospitalisation and the main cause of death are still respiratory illnesses, especially pneumonia. Increases in lesion severity and damage levels are associated with increased respiratory problems. It is also an important cause of hospitalisation after surgery in the cervical spine.

Sleep-disordered breathing (SDB) symptoms and indicators should be Spirometry, or monitored pulmonary function testing, could be taken into consideration.

Encouragement of tobacco cessation, regular respiratory muscle training, and weight management are essential.

Patients may be referred to specialists in the worst cases.

18.9 Sexual and Reproductive Health

Sexuality and sexual health are significant subjects that medical professionals frequently fail to appropriately address for people with spinal diseases.

These are the following recommendations:

First, you need to consult, hear, and act upon:

- What state is your sexual health in?
- Have you encountered any challenges concerning your sexual health?
- Have there been any unanswered questions or worries for you or your partner?

Then, one should examine a variety of causes and contributing variables for the above-stated problems.

Also examine pharmacological (such as antispasmodics and painkillers) and psychological (such as depression) variables as possible sources of sexual dysfunction. Then, as directed by a clinician, make referrals.

Sexologists can use both nonpharmacological (like sex gadgets and positive reinforcement) and pharmacological (like phosphodiesterase inhibitors) therapies.

There are six actions one can take to stop or decrease the progression of spinal stenosis.

1. Regular exercise is necessary to maintain the health of one's spine. A training regimen must be customised to the individual for it to become a regular part of that person's life. One must consider his age, present degree of fitness, and any health issues. For someone with spinal stenosis, an exercise programme that will assist him in safely growing his back-supporting core muscles, increasing or maintaining his spinal flexibility, and building endurance is essential. Walking is a fantastic kind of exercise, but if it is too hard for someone, they can try another type of aerobic activity. Swimming, stationary cycling, and aquatic activities with flotation devices are great choices [10].

2. Quit smoking: Smoking is associated with an increased risk of back discomfort in addition to heart disease, respiratory infections, cancer, and other disorders. Smoke inhalation can impede the oxygen and blood flow that support your spine, leading to degenerative changes and an increased sense of pain [11].
3. Achieving and preserving the optimal healthy weight for one's height undoubtedly contributes to the prevention or treatment of spinal stenosis.

   Excess body weight places needless strain on the spine as a whole. Additionally, it may make proper form when exercising difficult. Maintaining proper form when exercising promotes general strength, flexibility, back support, and the capacity to work through the day with little to no muscular soreness [12].
4. Exercises involving relaxation, water exercises, and holistic therapies can also assist in increasing mobility and flexibility while easing pain and other symptoms that are typically connected to spinal stenosis. Try these movements for back release. Alternatively, consult a physical therapist, who could provide customised movement routines and stretching techniques to assist in alleviating any initial problems.
5. Maintaining good posture when sitting or performing daily tasks (such as gardening, heavy lifting, or reaching up to grab objects) can help prevent injuries and wear and tear that can eventually result in spinal stenosis. Maintaining good posture when standing or sitting also involves exercise and postural correction techniques.
6. Wearing the right shoes is important. Biology is unique to a person. Everybody is different, so one should wear proper footwear. Speciality shoe stores exist to fit and test one's feet for the best shoes. High heels are to be avoided and intermittent break is beneficial.

Pressure injuries (PIs) have a significant physical and social impact on people's lives (loss of autonomy, decreased engagement, etc.). Additionally, the expense of treating these illnesses is very high for the healthcare system. Experts and SCI patients alike concur that prevention is often more economical than treatment when it comes to pressure injuries. Preventive measures must be implemented consistently because the prevalence of pressure injuries (PIs) rises sharply with time after injury and is influenced by age and health status. Successful prevention is more likely to occur if people with SCI take an active part, follow advice, and seek expert assistance when necessary.

These are the characteristics of the three prevention styles:

1. Stay Thoughtful.
   - Taking all advised precautions.
   - Capacity to abstain, vast knowledge.
   - Prevention is really important.
   - We must prevent it.
2. Be Selective

3. By using some of the preventive measures that are advised (choice based on experience knowledge). Vast knowledge believes that they are vulnerable to PIs. Prevention is crucial, but it should not get in the way of personal goals. We have to prevent it.
4. Delegator
   - Primarily on "passive" preventative strategies and giving carers responsibility for preventative tasks.
   - Fundamental understanding.
   - Do not believe they are in danger from PIs.
   - There is no great attention to prevention.
   - Everyone must prevent it.
   - Preventing pressure injuries is a lifetime endurance performance that calls for self-efficacy, a sense of personal accountability for one's health, and an understanding of preventive measures and how to implement them [13].

The following are preventive measures:

1. Maintaining good posture.
2. Regular exercise, especially activities that strengthen the core muscles.
3. Ergonomic practices, especially for those who work at desks.
4. Strengthening your core muscles through activities like yoga and Pilates.
5. Applying cold or heat to manage pain or stiffness.

The following are crucial actions to improve the involvement, health, and survival of individuals with spinal disorders:

- Prompt, suitable pre-hospital care: prompt identification of a possible injury, prompt assessment, and start of injury care, which includes spinal immobilisation.
- Acute care (including surgery) should be provided in line with the patient's and their family's wishes and by the kind, severity, degree of instability, and presence of neural compression of the injury.
- Access to continuing medical care, health education, and supplies (such as catheters) to enhance quality of life and lower the chance of developing secondary illnesses.
- To maximise functionality, independence, general well-being, and community inclusion, one should have access to professional rehabilitation and mental health treatments. The control of bowel and bladder function is crucial.
- Access to suitable assistive technology can lessen functional limits and dependency by enabling people to carry out daily tasks they would not otherwise be able to. In low- and middle-income nations, only 5–15% of the population has access to the necessary assistive technologies.

Legislation, policies, and initiatives that support the following are crucial in securing the right to economic participation and education:

Physically accessible residences, employment, medical facilities, schools, and transit.
Outlawing discrimination in the workplace and educational institutions.
Rehabilitation through vocational training to increase job prospects.
Supporting alternate types of economic self-sufficiency through microfinance and other sorts of self-employment advantages.

18.10 Ergonomics

The spine facilitates movement and offers stability as the body's main structural support.

To distribute weight properly and avoid putting unnecessary strain on the vertebrae, discs, and surrounding tissues, proper spinal alignment is essential. However, work-related activities frequently include extended sitting or repetitive motions, which strain the surrounding muscles and spine. Inadequate posture and prolonged sitting can cause spinal misalignment and exacerbate the pressure on the intervertebral discs, which can lead to several health problems like sciatica, herniated discs, and back pain.

Considerations like as posture, workspace, and workstation arrangement can support neutral spine alignment and lower the chance of pain and harm. Posture is a crucial component of workplace ergonomics.

Back pain can result from bad posture. An excessive amount of strain on the spine can result from slouching, hunching forward, and rounding the shoulders. This can cause misalignments and musculoskeletal abnormalities. Maintaining proper posture helps to uniformly distribute body weight, which eases the pressure on joints, muscles, and ligaments. The spine is better able to resist external pressures and gravitational pull when its natural curves are in their correct alignment.

A sitting person's spine should curve into an S when viewed from the side, with the thoracic and cervical areas bending slightly outward and the lumbar and cervical regions slightly inward. Thus, how can you ensure that you maintain this posture of a neutral spine? To have proper posture, follow these four steps:

It is advisable to remember the following points for the workplace.

- Align Your Joints.
- Engage Your Core.
- Relax Your Shoulders.
- Align Your Head and Neck.

The European Journal of Social Psychology discovered that those who were instructed to sit up straight and maintain proper posture were more confident when performing a task than those who were instructed to slouch.

Verify the location of your display. Verify the location of your mouse and keyboard. Make use of the appropriate workplace chair. Make sure your feet are level. Include frequent intervals of rest [14].

18.11 Problems Faced by People with Spinal Disorders

Dr. Lisa Iezzoni, a professor of medicine at Harvard, had been hearing complaints about doctors' attitudes toward caring for people with disabilities for years. Dr. Iezzoni, who has multiple sclerosis and uses a wheelchair herself, decided that the time had come to do a study of what physicians thought when they encountered a patient with a disability in their own office.

The authors conclude, "People with disabilities are frequently not accommodated in health care settings, often receive substandard care and, in some cases, are refused care."

18.12 New Research Study

A research study with the topic "I AM NOT THE DOCTOR FOR YOU" was conducted by Thea Flaum in the journal *Health Affairs*, Northwestern University. The study was conducted to gather information on the prevalence of depression, psychiatric co-occurring illnesses, use of mental health services, and effectiveness of depression therapy in persons with spinal diseases who were either depressed or not. The results of this study show that people with spinal problems and likely serious depression receive little mental health treatment. These discoveries may improve the way that individuals with spinal problems are treated for depression. Depression following a spinal cord injury: comorbidities, utilisation of mental health services, and treatment effectiveness [15].

References

1. Kisling LA, Das JM. Prevention Strategies [Updated 2023 Aug 1]. In: StatPearls [Internet]. Treasure Island (FL): StatPearls Publishing; 2024 Jan-. Available from: https://www.ncbi.nlm.nih.gov/books/NBK537222/
2. Mahoney MC. Adult immunization--influenza vaccine. Am Fam Physician. 2000;61(9):2901–2.
3. McColl MA, Aiken A, McColl A, Sakakibara B, Smith K. Primary care of people with spinal cord injury: a scoping review. Can Fam Physician. 2012;58(11):1207–16. e626–35. PMID: 23152456; PMCID: PMC3498012
4. Faaborg PM, Christensen P, Finnerup N, Laurberg S, Krogh K. The pattern of colorectal dysfunction changes with time since spinal cord injury. Spinal Cord. 2008;46(3):234–8. https://doi.org/10.1038/sj.sc.3102121. Epub 2007 Sep 25. PMID: 17893697
5. Fujioka H. Latent autonomic dysfunction in a chronic cervical spinal injury. Cureus. 2023;15(3):e36785. https://doi.org/10.7759/cureus.36785. PMID: 37123695; PMCID: PMC10134090.Published online 2023 Mar 28

6. Li P, Wei Z, Zhang H, et al. Effects of decompressive operation on cardiac autonomic regulation in patients with cervical spondylotic myelopathy: analysis of blood pressure, heart rate, and heart rate variability. Eur Spine J. 2019;28:1864–71. https://doi.org/10.1007/s00586-019-05972-9.
7. Khashab M, Alem A, Almuatiri A, Rasheed F, Almehmadi M, Felemabn S, Gassass S, Alosaimi M, Sulimani H, Alyami A. Correction: comparison of the effects of regular periods of immobilization and prolonged immobilization on hand function post distal radial fracture. Cureus. 2023;15(8):c134. https://doi.org/10.7759/cureus.c134. Erratum for: Cureus. 2022 Nov 1;14(11):e30986. https://doi.org/10.7759/cureus.30986. PMID: 37664312; PMCID: PMC10472086
8. Ong ET, Yeo LK, Kaliya-Perumal AK, Oh JY. Orthostatic hypotension following cervical spine surgery: prevalence and risk factors. Global Spine J. 2020;10(5):578–82. https://doi.org/10.1177/2192568219863805. Epub 2019 Jul 16. PMID: 32677558; PMCID: PMC7359682
9. Ong ET-E, Yeo LK-P, Kaliya-Perumal A-K, Jacob Yoong-Leong O. Orthostatic hypotension following cervical spine surgery: prevalence and risk factors. Global Spine J. 2019;10(5):578–82.
10. Lee JH, Sung E. The effects of aquatic walking and jogging program on physical function and fall efficacy in patients with degenerative lumbar spinal stenosis. J Exerc Rehabil. 2015;11(5):272–5. https://doi.org/10.12965/jer.150231.
11. Knutsson B, Mukka S, Wahlstrom J, et al. The association between tobacco smoking and surgical intervention for lumbar spinal stenosis: cohort study of 331,941 workers. Spine J. 2017;18(8):1313–7. https://doi.org/10.1016/j.spinee.2017.11.018.
12. Sheng B, Feng C, Zhang D, Spitler H, Shi L. Associations between obesity and spinal diseases: a medical expenditure panel study analysis. Int J Environ Res Public Health. 2017;14(2) https://doi.org/10.3390/ijerph14020183.
13. Zanini C, Brach M, Lustenberger N, Scheel-Sailer A, Koch HG, Stucki G, Rubinelli S. Engaging in the prevention of pressure injuries in spinal cord injury: a qualitative study of community-dwelling individuals' different styles of prevention in Switzerland. J Spinal Cord Med. 202043(2):247–56. https://doi.org/10.1080/10790268.2018.1543094. Epub 2018 Dec 12. PMID: 30540555; PMCID: PMC7054934.
14. Open Article; National Spine health Foundation, VA https://spinehealth.org/
15. Fann JR, Bombardier CH, Richards JS, Tate DG, Wilson CS. Temkin N; PRISMS investigators. Depression after spinal cord injury: comorbidities, mental health service use, and adequacy of treatment. Arch Phys Med Rehabil. 2011;92(3):352–60. https://doi.org/10.1016/j.apmr.2010.05.016. Epub 2011 Jan 20

MIX
Papier aus verantwortungsvollen Quellen
Paper from responsible sources
FSC® C105338

If you have any concerns about our products,
you can contact us on
ProductSafety@springernature.com

In case Publisher is established outside the EU,
the EU authorized representative is:
Springer Nature Customer Service Center GmbH
Europaplatz 3, 69115 Heidelberg, Germany

Printed by Libri Plureos GmbH
in Hamburg, Germany